Coding and Reimbursement for Hospital Inpatient Services

Third Edition

Karen S. Scott, MEd, RHIA, CCS-P, CPC

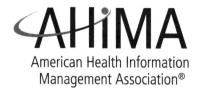

American Health Information
Management Association®

ISBN: 978-1-58426-261-9
AHIMA Product No. AC206210

AHIMA Staff:
Claire Blondeau, MBA, Senior Editor
Cynthia Douglas, Developmental Editor
Katie Greenock, Editorial and Production Coordinator
Ashley Sullivan, Assistant Editor
Ken Zielske, Director of Publications

All information contained within this book, including Web sites and regulatory information, was current and valid as of the date of publication. However, Web page addresses and the information on them may change or disappear at any time and for any number of reasons. The user is encouraged to perform his or her own general Web searches to locate any site addresses listed here that are no longer valid.

All products mentioned in this book are either trademarks of the companies referenced in this book, registered trademarks of the companies of the companies referenced in this book, or neither.

This book is sold, as is, without warranty of any kind, either express or implied. While every precaution has been taken in the preparation of this book, the publisher and author assume no responsibility for errors or omissions. Neither is any liability assumed for damages resulting from the use of the information or instructions contained herein. It is further stated that the publisher and author are not responsible for any damage or loss to your data or your equipment that results directly or indirectly from your use of this book.

American Health Information Management Association
233 North Michigan Avenue, 21st Floor
Chicago, Illinois 60601-5800

ahima.org

Contents

CD-ROM Contents

Exercises

Case Studies

Sample Audit Worksheets, Forms, and Tools

AHIMA Practice Brief: Internet Resources for Accurate
Coding and Reimbursement Practices (Updated)

Detailed Contents

CD-ROM Contents

Exercises

Case Studies

Sample Audit Worksheets, Forms, and Tools

AHIMA Practice Brief: Internet Resources for Accurate
Coding and Reimbursement Practices (Updated)

About the Author

Karen Scott, MEd, RHIA, CCS-P, CPC, is the sole proprietor of Karen Scott Seminars and Consulting. She has been an educator for many years; her experience includes teaching in the HIM programs at the University of Tennessee Health Science Center and Arkansas Tech University. She has worked as an HIM director in an acute care hospital setting, training director for a national transcription company, and reimbursement specialist for a regional physician's group. She is past-president of both the Tennessee and Arkansas Health Information Management Associations, past-chair of the AHIMA Council on Certification, and an elected commissioner for the Commission for Accreditation of Health Informatics and Information Management (CAHIIM).

Ms. Scott is a Certified ICD-10 Trainer. She has won several awards, including the Tennessee Innovator Award and Distinguished Member Award. Karen teaches seminars throughout the country and has written several chapters in HIM and coding textbooks. She is the author of *Medical Coding For Non-Coders: Understanding Coding and Reimbursement in Today's Healthcare Industry.*

Preface

Coding and Reimbursement for Hospital Inpatient Services, Third Edition was written for coding practitioners who have previous knowledge of, and coding experience with, the *International Classification of Diseases, 9th Revision, Clinical Modification* (ICD-9-CM). It includes and expands on the material previously published by AHIMA in the book, *Applying Inpatient Coding Skills under Prospective Payment,* 2004 edition, by Vickie L. Rogers and Ann M. Zeisset.

The reimbursement material in this book is specific to hospital inpatient settings, that is, to hospitals paid under the following Medicare prospective payment systems:

- The inpatient prospective payment system (IPPS)

- The long-term care hospital prospective payment system (LTCH-PPS)

- The inpatient rehabilitation facilities prospective payment system (IRF-PPS)

- The inpatient psychiatric facility prospective payment system (IPF-PPS)

Part I, Reimbursement Systems for Inpatient Services, contains chapters 1 through 4, which provide the reader with a fundamental understanding of reimbursement methodologies under Medicare prospective payment. Chapter 1 provides an introduction to hospital inpatient services and discusses the different types of services provided in various inpatient settings. Chapter 2 presents an in-depth overview of inpatient reimbursement methodologies, focusing on the array of payment systems used to reimburse hospitals for inpatient services and discussing some of the most common payers in the US health system. Chapter 3 contains a detailed discussion of the structure and organization of Medicare prospective payment for inpatient acute care, which centers on the MS-DRG reimbursement system. Chapter 4 explains the structure and organization of other Medicare inpatient prospective payment systems, including the LTCH-PPS, IRF-PPS, and IPF-PPS, with their various patient assignment and payment classifications.

Part II, Coding for Inpatient Services, contains two chapters that deal with the technical and professional aspects of coding practice. Chapter 5 addresses both diagnostic and procedural coding for inpatient services and includes information on the ICD-9-CM Official Guidelines for Coding and Reporting, coding ethics, and billing processes, among other subjects. Chapter 6 discusses coding and DRG assignment, and covers topics such as coding with incomplete information, understanding case mix and case-mix management, understanding paired DRGs and benchmarks, and using physician query forms.

Part III, Processes Related to Coding and Reimbursement for Inpatient Services, contains chapters 7, 8, and 9, which introduce the reader to data quality management, coding compliance, and health record auditing. The chapters are supplemented by exercises, case studies, and appendixes, which include AHIMA's Standards for Ethical Coding and Code of Ethics, an annotated bibliography of coding references, the AHIMA practice brief on developing a coding compliance policy document, and sample audit forms and tools.

Note to Instructors

An answer key for all exercises included in this book is available in online format from the individual book pages in the AHIMA Bookstore and through the Assembly on Education (AOE) Community of Practice (CoP). Instructors who are AHIMA members can sign up for this private community by clicking on the help icon on the CoP home page and requesting additional information on becoming an AOE CoP member. An instructor who is not an AHIMA member or an AHIMA member who is not an instructor may contact the publisher at publications@ahima.org. The instructor materials are not available to students enrolled in college or university programs.

Use of different versions of coding books with this resource will require attention to the code changes after the effective date. Revised answer keys will be created that are consistent with coding changes for the upcoming year soon after the effective date of the new codes. All answer keys are available to instructors in online format from the individual book page in the AHIMA Bookstore and also are posted on the AOE CoP website.

Part I

Reimbursement Systems
for Inpatient Services

Chapter 1

Introduction to Hospital Inpatient Services

An inpatient is defined as "a person who has been admitted at least overnight to a hospital or other health facility for the purpose of receiving diagnostic treatment or other health services" (Southeast Tennessee Legal Services n.d.).

However, there are times when patients are formally admitted to the hospital but, for whatever reason, are either discharged or transferred without actually staying overnight. An inpatient admission begins with the formal acceptance by a hospital of a patient who is to receive healthcare while receiving room and board, continuous nursing, and other related services (CMS 2010). It is the responsibility of the admitting physician to determine the appropriateness of admission to the hospital, but the admission process is monitored by hospital staff to ensure that documentation and clinical information support the need for hospital admission.

The physician typically uses a 24-hour period as a benchmark; that is, he or she orders inpatient admission for patients who are expected to need hospital care for 24 hours or more and treat other patients on an outpatient basis. However, the decision to admit a patient is a complex medical judgment that can be made only after the physician has considered a number of factors, including the patient's medical history and current medical needs, the types of facilities available to inpatients and to outpatients, the hospital's bylaws and admissions policies, and the relative appropriateness of treatment in each setting. Factors to be considered when making the decision to admit include such things as:

- The severity of the signs and symptoms exhibited by the patient

- The medical predictability of something adverse happening to the patient, such as a complication or adverse reaction to medication or other treatment

- The need for diagnostic studies that appropriately are outpatient services (that is, their performance does not ordinarily require the patient to remain at the hospital for 24 hours or more) to assist in assessing whether the patient should be admitted

- The availability of diagnostic procedures at the time when and at the location where the patient presents

This chapter discusses the different services provided in the inpatient setting. The most familiar type of inpatient service is acute care, short-term hospitalization. Most patients in this setting are either medical or surgical patients.

Medical Services

Medical services are those services provided to patients who do not require surgery to correct or enhance body functions. These services may be subdivided according to hospital needs into specific services, such as internal medicine and pediatrics. Common service divisions are as follows:

- *Internal medicine:* Nonsurgical treatment for adults

- *Pediatrics:* Nonsurgical treatment for children

- *Obstetrics/gynecology:* Diagnosis and treatment for female reproductive system conditions including pregnancy-related conditions

- *Cardiology:* Diagnosis and treatment of diseases of the heart and circulatory system

Some services are divided based on body system or organs treated both surgically and medically, such as:

- *Orthopedics:* Treatment of bones and joints

- *Urology:* Treatment of the urinary system

- *Gastroenterology:* Diagnosis and treatment of disorders of the digestive tract

- *Pulmonary medicine:* Diagnosis and treatment of disorders of the respiratory system

- *Neurology:* Treatment of conditions of the nerves

Surgical Services

Surgery is defined as "a procedure to remove or repair a part of the body or to find out whether disease is present" (Webref.org n.d.). General surgery consists of surgeries to correct conditions in various body systems. Traditionally, general surgeons perform surgeries such as cholecystectomies, mastectomies, hernia repairs, and gastric bypass procedures.

Surgical services may be subdivided based on the body system that is treated, such as:

- *Cardiothoracic surgery:* This service refers to the surgical treatment of the heart and other conditions of the vascular system.

- *Bariatric surgery:* This specialty focuses on weight reduction surgery for morbidly obese patients through the use of techniques such as gastric bypass and gastric banding procedures.

- *Plastic surgery:* According to the American Society of Plastic Surgeons, plastic surgery consists of both cosmetic and reconstructive surgery.

  Cosmetic surgery is performed to reshape normal structures of the body in order to improve the patient's appearance and self-esteem. Cosmetic surgery is usually not covered by health insurance because it is elective.

  Reconstructive surgery is performed on abnormal body structures, caused by congenital defects, developmental abnormalities, trauma, infection, tumors, or disease. It is generally performed to improve function, but may also be done to approximate a normal appearance. Reconstructive surgery is generally covered by most health insurance policies, although coverage for specific procedures and levels of coverage may vary greatly (ASPS 2010).

- *Neurosurgery:* This is the surgical treatment of diseases of the nervous system.

- *Oral and maxillofacial surgery:* This comprises surgical treatment of diseases of the mouth and facial region of the body. This type of surgery sometimes includes reconstructive surgery of the face and jaw area.

- *Transplant surgery:* This deals with the transplant of organs such as kidney, liver, heart, and lungs. Transplant surgeons and their staff are involved in preoperative and postoperative treatment of transplant patients, including monitoring for organ rejection.

The Uniform Hospital Data Discharge Set (UHDDS) differentiates between a significant and nonsignificant procedure. A significant procedure is one that:

- Is surgical in nature

- Carries a procedural risk

- Carries an esthetic risk

- Requires specialized training

Rehabilitation Services

Rehabilitation services are provided to patients who have had a previous illness or injury that limits their physical or mental capabilities. These services may be provided as part of the patient's acute care hospitalization or given in an extended care facility. Rehabilitation hospitals or hospital units focus on restoring the patient's functions to the greatest extent possible. Inpatient rehabilitation facilities are known as IRFs.

According to Medicare regulations, inpatient rehabilitation is covered only when the service is considered to be reasonable and medically necessary based on the individual patient's needs.

Preadmission screening is required to help make this determination prior to admission to an IRF. Much of the information that is used in this determination is taken from the documentation in the acute care patient medical record. Examples of the appropriate use of rehabilitation services provided include:

- *After an inpatient hospital stay for rehabilitation care that resulted in little improvement in the patient's condition:* For example, an individual who undergoes surgery for severe contractures as a result of arthritis may require a reassessment of his or her rehabilitation potential in light of the surgery.

- *After an inpatient stay for cerebrovascular accident (CVA) with residual impairments:* The fact that an individual has some degree of mental impairment is not per se a basis for concluding that a multidisciplinary team evaluation is not warranted. Many individuals who have had CVAs have both mental and physical impairments. The mental impairment often results in a limited attention span and reduced comprehension with a resultant problem in communication. With an intensive rehabilitation program, it is sometimes possible to correct or significantly alleviate both the mental and physical problems.

- *After an inpatient admission for an acute traumatic or infectious process, such as a hip fracture, with residual need for rehabilitation:* Absent other complicating medical problems, the type of rehabilitation program normally required by a patient with a fractured hip during or after the period of not bearing weight or a patient with a healed ankle fracture does not require an inpatient hospital stay for rehabilitation care. Accordingly, an inpatient assessment is not warranted in such cases. On the other hand, an individual who has had a CVA that has left him or her unable to perform activities of daily living without assistance (even after physical therapy in a different setting) might be a good candidate for a more extensive inpatient assessment if the patient has the potential for rehabilitation and his or her needs are not primarily of a custodial nature (CMS 2010).

Common criteria used to establish the need for inpatient rehabilitation services include the need for 24-hour medical supervision and nursing care and approximately 3 hours of rehabilitation care per day at least 5 days per week. It must be established that the patient can make significant improvements in recovery through rehabilitation services.

Psychiatric Services

Jonas (1998, 53) defines psychiatric services as "diagnosis and therapy for people of all ages with psychological and emotional problems, using counseling, pharmaceutical, and other interventions." Inpatient psychiatric facilities (IPFs) may be independent or freestanding facilities or may consist of a unit within an acute care facility.

Medicare reimburses facilities for inpatient psychiatric hospital services only for "active treatment" that can reasonably be expected to improve the patient's condition. To ensure that the services provided meet this definition, the physician has to certify that the patient can benefit from inpatient psychiatric treatment. Medicare has established three criteria that must be addressed in the patient's medical documentation:

1. *Individualized treatment or diagnostic plan:* The services must be provided in accordance with an individualized program of treatment or diagnosis developed by a physician in conjunction with staff members of appropriate other disciplines on the basis of a thorough evaluation of the patient's restorative needs and potentialities. Thus, an isolated service such as a single session with a psychiatrist or a routine laboratory test not provided under a planned program of therapy or diagnosis would not constitute active treatment, even though the service was therapeutic or diagnostic in nature.

   The plan of treatment must be recorded in the patient's medical record in accordance with section 405.1037(a)(8) of the regulations on Conditions of Participation for Hospitals.

2. *Services expected to improve the condition or for purpose of diagnosis:* The service must reasonably be expected to improve the patient's condition or must be for the purpose of diagnostic study. It is not necessary that a course of therapy have as its goal the restoration of the patient to a level that would permit discharge from the institution, although the treatment must, at a minimum, be designed to both reduce or control the patient's psychotic or neurotic symptoms that necessitated hospitalization *and* improve the patient's level of function.

   The types of services that meet the above requirements would include not only psychotherapy, drug therapy, and shock therapy, but also such adjunctive therapies as occupational therapy, recreational therapy, and milieu therapy, provided the adjunctive therapeutic services are expected to result in improvement (as defined above) in the patient's condition. If, however, the only activities prescribed for the patient are primarily diversional in nature (that is, to provide some social or recreational outlet for the patient), such services would not be regarded as treatment to improve the patient's condition. In many large hospitals, these adjunctive services are present and part of the life experience of every patient. In a case where milieu therapy (or one of the other adjunctive therapies) is involved, it is particularly important that this therapy be a planned program for the particular patient and not one in which life in the hospital is designated as milieu therapy.

3. *Services supervised and evaluated by a physician:* Physician participation in the services is an essential aspect of active treatment. The services of qualified individuals other than physicians, such as social workers, occupational therapists, group therapists, attendants, and so forth, must be prescribed and directed by a physician to meet the specific psychiatric needs of the individual. In short, the physician must serve as a source of information and guidance for all members of the therapeutic team who work directly with the patient in various roles. It is the responsibility of the physician to periodically evaluate the therapeutic program and determine the extent to which treatment goals are being realized and whether changes in direction or emphasis are needed. Such evaluation should be made on the basis of periodic consultations and conferences with therapists, reviews of the patient's medical record, and regularly scheduled patient interviews, at least once a week (CMS 2010).

Ancillary Services

Ancillary services typically included in an inpatient admission include nursing services, radiology, laboratory, physical and occupational therapy, respiratory therapy, speech therapy, medical social services, and case management services, in addition to other diagnostic and therapeutic services.

Nursing Services

Nursing services are integral to the hospital admission. Nurses are the inpatient's primary caregivers, providing services as diverse as capturing vital signs, giving medications, and ensuring that the patient's needs are met. Nursing documentation assists physicians and other providers in assessing the patient's response to therapy and establishes a plan of action for future care.

Radiology Services

Radiology services in the hospital setting include both diagnostic and therapeutic services. Services such as computed tomography (CT), magnetic resonance imaging (MRI), and ultrasound are commonly used to facilitate diagnosis of medical conditions. Nuclear medicine and interventional cardiology procedures may be used as either diagnostic or therapeutic treatment for diseases such as cancer and heart conditions.

Laboratory Services

According to Medicare, clinical laboratory services "involve the biological, microbiological, serological, chemical, immunohematological, hematological, biophysical, cytological, pathological, or other examination of materials derived from the human body for the diagnosis, prevention, or treatment of a disease or assessment of a medical condition" (CMS 2009b). A hospital medical laboratory is under the direction of a pathologist but is typically managed by medical technologists. Computer technology advances aid medical technologists in performing a variety of laboratory tests designed to help with the diagnosis and evaluation of treatment methodology. Documentation of laboratory test results serves as further clinical proof of the existence of disease or can be used to determine that a patient does not have certain medical conditions.

Physical Therapy Services

Physical therapy is defined as:

> . . . the examination, evaluation, intervention, and prevention of physical disability, movement dysfunction, and pain resulting from injury, disease, disability, or other health-related conditions. Physical therapy includes:
>
> 1. The performance and interpretation of tests and measurements to assess pathophysiologic, pathomechanical, electrophysiologic, ergonomic, and developmental deficits of body systems to determine diagnosis, intervention, prognosis, and prevention
> 2. The planning, administration, and modification of therapeutic interventions that focus on posture, locomotion, strength, endurance, cardiopulmonary function, balance, coordination, joint mobility, flexibility, pain, healing and repair, and functional abilities in daily living skills, including work
> 3. The provision of consultative, educational, research, and other advisory services (University of Tennessee 2010)

Medicare has set up very specific payment rules to determine whether the prescribed physical therapy services are medically necessary. This means that the services must be considered by standards of care to be effective treatment for the condition and that the treatment will cause the patient's condition to improve. Documentation by the physical therapy providers should be sufficient to prove medical necessity and to justify all treatment modalities as well as to show the amount of time and level of supervision required for the services rendered.

Occupational Therapy Services

Occupational therapy is used to help improve functions of the body that have been adversely affected by injury or illness. The goal of occupational therapy is to improve the patient's ability to perform activities of daily living, such as dressing, cooking, or adapting to working conditions. According to Medicare, these services may include:

- The evaluation (and reevaluation as required) of a patient's level of function by administering diagnostic and prognostic tests

- The selection and teaching of task-oriented therapeutic activities designed to restore physical function—for example, use of woodworking activities on an inclined table to restore shoulder, elbow, and wrist range of motion lost as a result of burns

- The planning, implementing, and supervising of individualized therapeutic activity programs as part of an overall "active treatment" program for a patient with a diagnosed psychiatric illness—for example, sewing activities that require following a pattern to reduce confusion and restore reality orientation in a schizophrenic patient

- The planning and implementing of therapeutic tasks and activities to restore sensory-integrative function—for example, providing motor and tactile activities to increase sensory input and improve response for a stroke patient with functional loss resulting in a distorted body image

- The teaching of compensatory technique to improve the level of independence in activities of daily living

- The designing, fabricating, and fitting of orthotic and self-help devices—for example, making a hand splint for a patient with rheumatoid arthritis to maintain the hand in a functional position or constructing a device that would enable an individual to hold a utensil and feed himself or herself independently

Respiratory Therapy Services

Respiratory therapy, or respiratory care, provides both diagnostic and therapeutic services designed to evaluate and treat conditions associated with the patient's respiratory system. Respiratory therapy professionals also participate in the care of the critically ill patient by monitoring life-sustaining equipment such as mechanical ventilators.

According to Medicare's definitions, respiratory therapy services include:

- The application of techniques for support of oxygenation and ventilation in the acutely ill patient. These techniques include, but are not limited to:

  —Establishment and maintenance of artificial airways

  —Ventilator therapy and other means of airway pressure manipulation

  —Precise delivery of oxygen concentration

  —Techniques to aid removal of secretions from the pulmonary tree

- The therapeutic use and monitoring of medical gases (especially oxygen), bland and pharmacologically active mists and aerosols, and equipment such as resuscitators and ventilators

- Bronchial hygiene therapy, including deep breathing and coughing exercises, intermittent positive pressure breathing (IPPB), postural drainage, chest percussion and vibration, and nasotracheal suctioning

- Diagnostic tests for evaluation by a physician, such as pulmonary function tests, spirometry, and blood gas analyses

- Pulmonary rehabilitation techniques, which include:

  —Exercise conditioning

  —Breathing retraining

  —Patient education regarding the management of the patient's respiratory problems

- Periodic assessment and monitoring of acute and chronically ill patients for indications for, and the effectiveness of, respiratory therapy services (CMS 2009a)

Speech Therapy Services

Speech pathology services are necessary for the diagnosis and treatment of conditions regarding language, speech, and the voice. Most insurance companies reimburse only for services directly related to the treatment of disorders that hinder the patient's ability to communicate or for those conditions that impair the swallowing function.

Medical Social Services

Social services are designed to allow for assessment of an individual's emotional and social conditions to determine an appropriate plan of care. This may include evaluation of the individual's capability for self-care as well as the amount and type of care needed to assist the patient with recovery. In the hospital setting, social services are usually involved in discharge planning. This can entail nursing home placement or other types of home services that patients may require after discharge from the hospital.

Case Management Services

Case management in hospital and other healthcare systems is a collaborative practice model that includes patients, nurses, social workers, physicians, other practitioners, caregivers, and the community. The case management process encompasses communication and facilitates care along a continuum through effective resource coordination.

The goals of case management include the achievement of optimal health, access to care, and appropriate utilization of resources, balanced with the patient's right to self-determination. Among their many services to patients, case managers engage in the following activities:

- Working directly with patients and their families to provide information and emotional support
- Helping develop care plans
- Serving as the patient's advocate
- Coordinating medical care among different disciplines and specialties
- Helping patients establish their long- and short-term health goals
- Helping patients and families sort through and prioritize information needed to make decisions
- Helping with aftercare planning to foresee possible needs and coordinate referrals for services and equipment
- Working with insurance providers to ensure maximum coverage of services

Inpatient Accommodations

Most inpatient facilities offer various types of accommodations, including private and semi-private rooms, as well as specialty units such as intensive care and newborn nurseries. As new hospitals are being constructed and existing hospitals renovated, private rooms have become more commonplace.

Medicare, for example, allows a hospital to charge the patient an additional amount for a private room if the hospital has both private and semiprivate rooms available, as long as the private room is not medically necessary and if the patient has requested a private room and was notified of the additional charge.

Some common medically necessary reasons for private rooms include (CMS 2010):

- *Need for isolation:* A private room is medically necessary when isolation of a beneficiary is required to avoid jeopardizing his or her health or recovery or that of other patients who are likely to be alarmed or disturbed by the beneficiary's symptoms or treatment or subjected to infection by the beneficiary's communicable disease. The private room must be ordered by the physician.

- *Admission required and only private rooms available:* A private room is considered to be medically necessary even though the beneficiary's condition does not require isolation if he or she needs immediate hospitalization (that is, his or her medical condition is such that hospitalization cannot be deferred) and the hospital has no semiprivate or ward accommodations available at the time of admission.

- *All-private room providers:* If the patient is admitted to a provider that has only private accommodations and no semiprivate or ward accommodations, medical necessity will be deemed to exist for the accommodations furnished. Beneficiaries may not be subjected to an extra charge for a private room in an all-private room provider.

Special Units

Special units for inpatients are equipped and staffed to provide specialized care that is focused on the specific needs of different patient populations. Among these special units are those for intensive care, coronary care, neonatal intensive care, nursery, and recuperative care.

Intensive Care

The intensive care unit (ICU) or critical care unit (CCU) is designed for the care-intensive patient who has sustained life-threatening illnesses or injury. It may consist of a wardlike atmosphere with multiple patients in a large room, or the patient areas may be divided into individual rooms. Patients in this unit receive intensive monitoring of vital signs and organ functioning by specially trained nursing professionals. Some facilities have special subdivisions of their ICUs, such as coronary care, trauma care, or neonatal intensive care units, to care for specific types of patients.

Coronary Care

The coronary care unit may be included in the hospital's intensive care area or may be a distinct unit. Patients treated in the coronary care unit have heart-related conditions and require intensive cardiac monitoring. Patients recovering from open-heart surgery, such as a coronary artery bypass grafting (CABG), may be placed in either the coronary care or a special post-surgical ICU.

Neonatal Intensive Care Unit

The neonatal intensive care unit (NICU) is a specially designed nursery. Premature and critically ill newborns frequently require time-consuming and resource-intensive medical evaluation and treatment. Because these babies may require a great deal of medical care during and after their recovery, staff in a typical NICU include specially trained nurses and neonatologists, social services representatives, and discharge planning personnel. Hospitals may have several levels of neonatal units, including one that specializes in the treatment of babies recovering from surgery.

Nursery

The nursery is a unit designed to care for newborn babies who do not require the additional services provided in the NICU. Many facilities have a birthing center that allows for care of the mother and baby together, but separate newborn nurseries are still available to care for the healthy newborn for the first few days of life.

Recuperative Care/Swing Bed

Patients in small, rural hospitals may require short-term skilled nursing care following their acute care hospitalization. These facilities are allowed to use beds for acute care and also to provide skilled care. Because the hospital beds can be used as both acute care and skilled care beds, as needed, the term *swing bed* has been utilized. Under these regulations, a patient who meets criteria for skilled care may be discharged from acute care and admitted into swing bed care without physically changing beds. Because this is a discharge from one type of service to another, the physician and staff complete two separate sets of documentation, including a discharge summary from acute care and one from swing bed care.

In larger facilities, a patient needing skilled care would be discharged to a recuperative care unit in the hospital.

Types of Hospitals

Acute care hospitals designated as for-profit or not-for-profit healthcare systems are differentiated on the basis of ownership status. Other types of hospitals, such as Veterans Affairs (VA) healthcare facilities, short-term acute care hospitals, long-term acute care hospitals, children's hospitals, and critical access hospitals (CAHs), provide care for a specific population, duration, or locality and may operate under a unique reimbursement system.

For-Profit Hospitals

For-profit hospitals are usually owned by corporations whose shareholders own a portion of the business. There are several large for-profit hospital corporations in the United States.

Not-for-Profit Hospitals

Not-for-profit hospitals are typically governed by a board of trustees or directors and do not have shareholders. The term *not for profit* is somewhat misleading in that not-for-profit hospitals are allowed to make a profit but do not have shareholders with expectations of specific profits.

Most not-for-profit hospitals are considered to be public hospitals and are owned by a church, community organization, or government agency such as a county. In a county-owned facility, the board of trustees/directors is usually chaired by the county judge or mayor and the board is composed of elected or appointed members of the community.

Veterans Hospitals

The federal government established VA hospitals in 1930 to care for wounded soldiers returning from war. According to the Department of Veterans Affairs, more than five million people received care in VA healthcare facilities in 2008. There are approximately 153 medical centers across the country with more than 1,400 sites of care, including outpatient clinics, nursing homes, home healthcare, and rehabilitation treatment programs. Veterans with service-connected injuries or disabilities are treated at no cost to them. Other veterans may receive treatment at VA hospitals, but their insurance company can be billed for billed for treatment of conditions not related to military service. VA hospitals are commonly located in medical centers where they serve as teaching sites for medical students, residents, and other healthcare professionals (VA 2009).

Short-Term Acute Care Hospitals

Short-term acute care hospitals generally provide services to patients recovering from surgery or being treated for acute illnesses and injuries. Short-term care is usually considered to be less than 30 days.

Long-Term Acute Care Hospitals

Medicare defines long-term acute care hospitals (LTCHs) as hospitals that "have an average inpatient length of stay greater than 25 days. These hospitals typically provide extended medical and rehabilitative care for patients who are clinically complex and may suffer from multiple acute or chronic conditions. Services may include comprehensive rehabilitation, respiratory therapy, cancer treatment, head trauma treatment and pain management" (CMS 2004).

Critical Access Hospitals

Medicare has determined that some hospitals are exempt from prospective payment systems (PPSs). As part of the Balanced Budget Act of 1997, the government established the Medicare Rural Hospital Flexibility Program, which enabled some hospitals to be designated as CAHs. A CAH is a small Medicare acute care hospital or a health clinic or other facility that was a hospital prior to being converted into a clinic. CAH facilities have to be located in a state that has a Medicare Rural Hospital Flexibility Program in place and has been designated by the state as a CAH (CMS 2009a). These facilities must be more than 35 miles from another hospital (15 miles in an area with only secondary roads or in mountainous terrain) unless they were designated as "necessary providers" by the state prior to January 1, 2006. The facilities must provide 24-hour emergency services, have an average length of stay of no more than 96 hours, and be licensed for no more than 25 beds. A unit of the hospital with up to 10 beds for treatment of psychiatric and/or rehabilitation conditions may also be operated. CAHs are paid based on a percentage of reasonable costs for both inpatient acute care and swing bed services. More information about CAHs is available from CMS (2009c).

Summary

When patients are admitted to healthcare facilities as inpatients, the many services they require are provided by a variety of professionals on the healthcare team. Hospitals in the United States vary according to size, type of ownership, types of services offered, governance structure, and even methodology of reimbursement. It is important to recognize these variances in order to understand the complexity of inpatient treatment.

References

American Society of Plastic Surgeons. 2010. What is the difference between cosmetic and reconstructive surgery? http://www.plasticsurgery.org.

Centers for Medicare and Medicaid Services. 2004 (June). Long-term care hospital prospective payment system news. http://www.cms.hhs.gov/LongTermCareHospitalPPS/Downloads/ltch_factsheet_fr.pdf.

Centers for Medicare and Medicaid Services. 2007. Inpatient psychiatric hospital services. Chapter 2 in *Medicare Benefit Policy Manual*. http://www.cms.hhs.gov/manuals/Downloads/bp102c02.pdf.

Centers for Medicare and Medicaid Services. 2009a. Comprehensive outpatient rehabilitation facility (CORF) coverage. Chapter 12 in *Medicare Benefit Policy Manual*. http://www.cms.gov/manuals/Downloads/bp102c12.pdf.

Centers for Medicare and Medicaid Services. 2009b. Covered medical and other health services. Chapter 15 in *Medicare Benefit Policy Manual*. http://www.cms.hhs.gov/manuals/Downloads/bp102c15.pdf.

Centers for Medicare and Medicaid Services. 2009c. Critical access hospitals. http://www.cms.hhs.gov/CertificationandComplianc/04_CAHs.asp.

Centers for Medicare and Medicaid Services. 2010 (Jan. 15). Manual System: Pub 100-02 Medicare Benefit Policy. Transmittal 119, Change Request 6699: Coverage of Inpatient Rehabilitation Services. http://www.cms.hhs.gov/Transmittals/Downloads/R119BP.pdf.

Department of Veteran's Affairs. 2009. Facts about the Department of Veterans Affairs. http://www1.va.gov/opa/publications/factsheets/fs_department_of_veterans_affairs.pdf.

Jonas, S. 1998. *An Introduction to the U.S. Health Care System,* 4th ed. New York: Springer-Verlag.

Southeast Tennessee Legal Services n.d. http://www.selegal.org/glossary.htm.

University of Tennessee. 2010. Physical therapy program. http://www.uthsc.edu/allied/pt/.

Webref.org. n.d. Surgery. http://www.webref.org/cancer/s/surgery.htm.

Chapter 2

Reimbursement Methodologies for Inpatient Services

Over the years, reimbursement for healthcare services has gone through many changes. This chapter focuses on the various types of payment systems used to reimburse hospitals for inpatient services. It also discusses some of the most common payers in the US healthcare system. Currently there is a great deal of discussion regarding healthcare reform; therefore, these options and payers could drastically change over the next few years.

Methods of Payment

Typical reimbursement for medical services is paid using several different methods. Some of the most common of these include capitation, fee for service, case rate, per diem, prospective payment system, and fee schedule.

Capitation

Capitation consists of a fixed fee per patient enrolled in the plan. This is considered to be a risk-sharing arrangement because if the patient is extremely sick and requires extensive services, care must be provided without the incentive of additional payment from the patient or the insurance company. Providers must maintain a high quality of care but have to be cost conscious to remain profitable.

Fee for Service

In the fee-for-service payment system, facilities and practitioners are paid for the services provided to the patient without negotiated rates or other forms of cost containment. This form of reimbursement was very common prior to the managed care era of healthcare payment.

Case Rate

A facility that negotiates a contract based on "case rates" is paid a specific amount that is based on the average cost of caring for a patient with a specific disease or on the service provided.

Per Diem

The term *per diem* means "per day." This form of reimbursement is a fixed rate of payment per day of hospitalization or date of service. It is commonly used in healthcare units such as critical care or skilled nursing units. Usually, a defined list of items is included in the per diem payment rate.

Prospective Payment System

Prospective payment system (PPS) methodology for inpatients involves dividing patients into Medicare severity adjusted diagnosis-related groups, or MS-DRGs. MS-DRGs are used for financial measures but are also a clinical method of dividing patients into groups according to the average cost to care for the patient's condition. These divisions are considered to be both clinically meaningful and statistically valid, meaning that patients in a single group statistically use similar amounts of resources. Although this methodology is used primarily for Medicare inpatient reimbursement (discussed extensively in chapter 3), some other insurance companies have modified the Medicare system for their own payment plans.

Fee Schedule

Physicians and ancillary services such as laboratory and physical therapy services are usually paid based on a fee schedule. A fee schedule is a list of codes and the amount of money the insurance company will pay for each service. If the insurance company pays $3.00 for a urinalysis, for example, that is the total amount the facility will receive regardless of the actual cost of providing the service or the charges submitted.

Reimbursement Arrangements for Healthcare Facilities

The previously discussed methods of payment generally illustrate how facilities are paid; the following paragraphs provide greater detail about the various types of reimbursement arrangements made by insurance carriers. These arrangements typically include fee-based services, managed care payment systems, and diagnosis-related groups (DRG)-type PPSs.

Fee-Based Services

In the past, most payment was based on charges or actual costs of providing a service. Some insurance companies still reimburse on a fee-based system (fee for service), but this method now is much less common. The fee-based system is also known as retrospective payment because it pays based on the actual charges of providing the services determined after the patient is discharged from the facility.

Insurance plans based on the fee-for-service model are known as indemnity plans. This form of payment was very common prior to managed care, and many experts think that it caused many of the current issues in healthcare reimbursement. At times, charges were much higher than actual costs to provide services to the patient. Facilities had no incentive to control costs and, in fact, even seemed to be "rewarded" for expensive medical care. Thus, the price of healthcare increased to the point where the healthcare reimbursement industry had to make major changes in order to remain viable. Even the existing indemnity plans have adopted some

Table 2.1. Differences between traditional insurance and managed care

Traditional Insurance	Managed Care
Places restrictions on choice of providers	Encourages or requires use of selected providers
Offers fee-for-service reimbursement of providers	Pays negotiated rates to providers
Functions apart from the healthcare delivery system	Integrates the finance and delivery system
Assumes all financial risk	Shares risk with providers
Offers few financial incentives to control costs	Creates financial incentives for providers and enrollees to control costs
Takes no interest in measuring quality and appropriateness of services	Participates actively in methods to measure quality and monitor appropriateness of care
Has no real budget for cost of services, simply "pay as you go"	Establishes budget for cost of services, prepayment of a fixed premium in many cases

of the concepts commonly used by the managed care community to help control costs, such as preadmission approval and utilization review of services provided. Table 2.1 presents the differences between traditional insurance and managed care.

Managed Care Payment Systems

Managed care payment systems, or managed care organizations (MCOs), are capitated payment plans in which all services are provided to the patient for a fixed monthly premium. MCOs include health maintenance organizations (HMOs), preferred provider organizations (PPOs), and point-of-service (POS) plans, which are structured differently but share the following characteristics:

- Rigorous utilization review

- Monitoring and analysis of physicians' practice patterns

- Use of primary care physicians as "gatekeepers" and other caregivers to manage patients

- Steering of patients to high-quality, efficient providers

- Quality improvement programs

- Reimbursement systems that make physicians, hospitals, and other providers financially accountable for the cost and quality of medical services (Huntington 1997)

Health Maintenance Organizations

Typical HMO plans share the "risk" with their physicians. In other words, a percentage of the fixed per-patient fee is held back from the physician's payment until the end of the year when the practice can determine how profitable it was. This serves as an incentive plan for the practitioners to exercise greater cost control while maintaining a high-quality level of care for the plan's members. Patients may lose some freedom of choice because the facilities and providers are limited to those in the HMO plan, but they usually have lower premiums than with some other forms of insurance coverage and do not have to worry about individual visit copayments or deductibles.

There are typically five types of HMO models:

1. Group model

2. Independent provider model

3. Network model

4. Staff model

5. Direct contact model (Miller 2010)

Each of these models is discussed in the following subsections.

Group Model

Under the group model, the HMO contracts with a group of physicians and hospitals to provide services to its patients at a specified rate. Physicians are not employees of the HMO and are free to see patients outside the HMO contract. Instead of being paid for each office visit or service, the physician is paid on a fixed (capitated) fee per patient enrolled in the program.

Independent Provider Model

Independent provider models exist with several different meanings for the acronym IPA: individual practice association, independent physician association, independent practice association, and independent provider association. This form of HMO consists of a group of physicians who together form a legal corporation (the IPA) to provide care for the HMO patients. The IPA then contracts with individual physicians to provide services for the patients in their existing practice. Payment for these services may be arranged on a fee-for-service or a per capita basis. The IPA form of HMO is typically less costly to set up because it uses physicians who already have established practice sites.

An IPA where physicians and hospital(s) join together to provide contracted services is known as a physician–hospital organization (PHO). In a PHO, both the hospital and the physician practices share in the risk associated with prepayment of services.

Network Model

The network model HMO works with contracts between the HMO and multiple hospitals and physician groups to provide a "network" of services for its members. These mixed-type HMOs contract with multiple groups, or IPAs, to provide a variety of benefits and allow for greater numbers of affiliated physicians and/or hospitals. Patients enjoy more flexibility and greater freedom to choose providers while staying within their HMO network.

Staff Model

In the staff model HMO, physicians and other healthcare providers are paid employees of the HMO group, which allows for greater cost control over services provided. They typically share office space, medical records, and other services that are provided only to members of the HMO. Most of the physicians and other practitioners are paid on a salary basis, but in some HMOs, they are paid based on established incentive plans.

Direct Contact Model

In a direct contact model, physicians contract with the HMO but may treat patients in their own offices or clinics. Patients choose a "gatekeeper" or primary care physician (PCP). If the patient needs a specialist, the PCP refers him or her to a specialist who is also contracted and approved by the HMO.

In 1973, a federal law, the HMO Act, was passed. This law established standard qualifications for HMOs, including type of structure, financial requirements, marketing specifications, and delivery of healthcare. To achieve the status of being federally qualified, HMOs must meet the requirements set forth in the HMO Act. The HMO Act was supposed to provide for organizational structure and sound financial backing to ensure the protection of patients. In addition, it was set up to encourage the establishment of more HMO plans. Although HMOs are very common in some parts of the country, they did not become the practice standard that was anticipated.

The story of Kaiser Permanente provides a real-world look at how the group model HMO developed. During the Great Depression, Dr. Sidney Garfield had a small practice caring for workers building a huge aqueduct in the middle of the Mojave Desert. A strong believer in preventive care, Dr. Garfield borrowed money to build a small hospital for his patients. An insurance salesman, Harold Hatch, saw that by providing a fixed fee to the hospital per worker on an upfront basis, everyone would benefit. Workers signed up for this plan at the rate of 5 cents per day, thus beginning a new concept of prepayment for medical services. Henry Kaiser heard about this project and hired Dr. Garfield to provide care for his 6,500 workers building the Grand Coulee Dam in Washington State. The project proved so successful that, in 1945, the Permanente Health Plan was opened to the public with huge support from labor unions. Kaiser Permanente currently is the largest nonprofit health plan in the United States, with more than 8 million members in 10 different states. The company owns more than 30 hospitals and more than 400 medical practices and has approximately 14,000 physicians in its network, providing a wide range of benefit choices for its members (Kaiser Permanente n.d.).

Preferred Provider Organizations

The PPO is a plan that is similar to the group HMO model. PPOs are agreements among groups consisting of hospitals, physicians, and other providers who contract with payers to provide healthcare services at a discounted rate for their members. They are not as strict as traditional HMOs in that, for a higher fee, they allow patients to go outside their network of physicians to receive medical care and they do not have as many risk-sharing incentive plans governing pay for their physicians.

Generally, the greater the emphasis on in-network care, the lower the premiums and the more comprehensive the benefits will be. Out-of-pocket expenses will be less if a network provider is used. If the patient receives a covered service from a provider who is not in the network, reimbursement will be at a lower level than if an in-network provider is used. Typically the patient is not required to obtain a referral to see a specialist (AHIP 2007).

Point-of-Service Plans

Some HMOs have expanded their offerings to include more choices for their members, such as the ability to go out of network under certain circumstances. Such plans, known as point-of-service (POS) plans, allow patients to go out of network, but a higher copayment rate and/or higher deductible is required.

Prospective Payment Systems

Laws requiring new payment methodologies have been in place for Medicare systems since the mid-1980s. These systems, PPSs, call for reimbursement based on the average cost to treat patients in a particular category rather than the actual costs incurred in treating the patient.

Patients are divided into groups such as MS-DRGs (as discussed earlier) based on the diagnoses and procedures used to treat their conditions. Medicare is the primary payer that utilizes PPSs, but many other payers reimburse facilities based on a modified method of PPS. (Medicare's PPS systems for inpatient services are discussed in chapters 3 and 4.)

Other Common Methods of Cost Control

Additional methods are used by most of the different types of insurers to help control costs. Some of the most common are pay for performance, preadmission review, utilization review, case management, and retrospective review of services provided.

Pay for Performance/Value-Based Purchasing

Medicare has instituted a "Pay for Performance" (P4P) initiative to encourage:

> . . . improved quality of care in all health care settings where Medicare beneficiaries receive their health care services, including physicians' offices and ambulatory care facilities, hospitals, nursing homes, home health care agencies and dialysis facilities. (CMS 2007b)

The Centers for Medicare and Medicaid Services (CMS) collaborated with a number of organizations including the National Quality Forum, the Joint Commission, the National Committee for Quality Assurance (NCQA), the Agency for Health Care Research and Quality (AHRQ), and the American Medical Association and their Quality Improvement Organizations (QIO) to develop pay-for-performance initiatives to support quality improvement. For example, hospitals must collect and report data on specific quality measures in order to receive full payment update to their Medicare MS-DRG payments (CMS 2007b).

According to CMS:

> The Centers for Medicare and Medicaid Services (CMS) has articulated a vision for health care quality—*the right care for every person every time.* To achieve this vision, CMS is committed to care that is safe, effective, timely, patient-centered, efficient, and equitable. Medicare's current payment systems reward quantity, rather than quality of care, and provide neither incentive nor support to improve quality of care. Value-based purchasing (VBP), which links payment more directly to the quality of care provided, is a strategy that can help to transform the current payment system by rewarding providers for delivering high-quality, efficient clinical care. Through a number of public reporting programs, demonstration projects, pilot programs, and voluntary efforts, CMS has launched VBP initiatives in hospitals, physician offices, nursing homes, home health services, and dialysis facilities. (CMS 2007a)

Preadmission Review

Preadmission review is the practice of reviewing the circumstances for admission before the patient enters the hospital to assess medical necessity and to ensure coverage. Prior to either elective or nonemergent admissions to the hospital, the facility is required to contact the insurance provider to receive verification of coverage. At this time, the insurance provider may review established criteria to see if the patient's condition requires a hospital admission or if another level of service would be more appropriate for the patient's care. During this process, the insurer may specify the number of days that will be covered under the patient's policy. If the patient requires an extended stay, the hospital and/or physician must obtain approval for the additional coverage.

Utilization Review

Utilization review (UR) is another very popular method of cost control for insurance companies as well as an internal hospital control mechanism. UR is performed by either a nursing professional or a health information management (HIM) professional who is skilled in evaluating health record documentation. The UR professional monitors for documentation completeness in the chart and notifies the physician if the patient's condition or treatment is not supported. Because this process is completed while the patient is still an inpatient, any problems can be addressed during the stay. Typically, the reviewer is checking for appropriate level of care, medical necessity of procedures performed, and need for hospitalization.

Case Management

Case managers may perform services similar to those of the utilization reviewer, but they typically manage the care of more problematic patient cases, such as patients recovering from heart surgery. Case managers frequently use critical paths or care plans established by their medical staff to ensure that the patient's recovery is maximized in order to make the best use of the inpatient hospitalization time frame. They also work with social services to arrange for discharge planning, including skilled nursing and home care as needed by the patient.

Retrospective Review

Many carriers review the patient's health record after he or she is discharged from the hospital. This is called a retrospective review. The reviewer often uses established criteria to determine if the patient met certain standards of care for both severity of illness and intensity of service. If the carrier determines that the patient's record does not reflect the need for the acute admission, it may request a refund for payment for the services.

Common Payers

Many different entities pay for healthcare in the United States, and this section discusses some of the most common payers. These include Medicare, Medicaid, military/veterans programs, and commercial carriers.

Medicare

Medicare was initially designed in the 1960s to provide catastrophic coverage for older Americans who had worked and paid into the Social Security system. It was not designed to be the full-coverage insurance plan into which it has evolved. It has changed over the years to include other individuals such as those with disabilities and those with end-stage renal disease. Moreover, it has been modified by Congress to include more preventive care such as cancer screening. CMS is the government agency that oversees the Medicare program. The Medicare Prescription Drug, Improvement, and Modernization Act (MMA) of 2003 was one of the latest significant changes in Medicare.

The Medicare PPS

As recently as the 1980s, the following scenario was not uncommon: A family member (for example, Grandma) was bedridden and living at home. When the family wanted to go on vacation, they dropped Grandma off at the hospital on the way out of town for what was commonly referred to as respite care. Because of the lack of regulations surrounding Medicare payment, this type of scenario occurred even when there was no acute medical condition that would necessitate Grandma being treated in an acute care facility.

When Medicare was first developed, it paid claims to hospitals based on the fee-for-service reimbursement plan. The patient was admitted to the hospital, where tests and other procedures were performed based on physician orders. After the patient went home, the hospital submitted a bill to Medicare, which paid based on a percentage of the total charges.

This type of indemnity plan actually served to reward physicians and hospitals for over-utilization of services. Basically, when the doctor ordered a test, it was performed and Medicare paid the bill with little or no review of the appropriateness or need for the services rendered. After a few years of this type of payment system, it became clear that the Medicare system was in jeopardy of running out of funding. The government soon realized that the Medicare program would not survive unless changes were made to the system. Consequently, the government started searching for ways to maintain better control over the system. It was at this time that the concept of a PPS was first discussed.

Presently, the family in the scenario just described would have multiple options for taking care of Grandma, but if she did not meet criteria that justified an acute-care admission, she would not be placed in the hospital for respite care. Most insurance companies, not just Medicare, currently require a thorough preadmission assessment to allow patients to be cared for in the setting most appropriate for their conditions.

Characteristics of a PPS

Several key components characterize a system based on prospectively set prices, including the following:

- Payment rates are established in advance and fixed for the fiscal period to which they apply.
- Payment rates are not automatically determined by the hospital's past or current actual cost.
- Rates represent full payment for services provided.
- The hospital retains the profit or suffers the loss resulting from the difference between the rate of payment and the hospital's cost of caring for the patient.

Typically, the fiscal period just mentioned refers to the government's fiscal year (FY), which starts October 1 and ends September 30. However, some of the newer payment systems are set up on other FYs, such as July 1 through June 30. At times, because of errors or changes in technology, some modifications are made to the payment systems quarterly or as needed throughout the year.

Under a PPS reimbursement system, there is a strong incentive for the facility to provide high-quality care at the lowest possible cost. There has been an increase in the use of utilization review professionals and case managers to review the charts during the hospital encounter to ensure that the patient's care is being managed effectively. Prospective payment monitoring also has helped facilities to ensure that services provided are necessary for the patient at the acute level of care.

Because of many legislative changes in the Medicare system over the past 20 years, most types of Medicare services now are paid for under some sort of prospective payment methodology. PPSs currently exist in all the following settings:

- Inpatient acute care hospitals
- Outpatient hospitals
- Physician offices
- Skilled nursing facilities
- Long-term care hospitals
- Home healthcare settings
- Inpatient rehabilitation facilities
- Inpatient psychiatric facilities

Chapter 4 contains detailed discussions of the different PPSs and payment groups currently in effect.

Medicare Programs

Medicare enrollees are known as beneficiaries. Beneficiaries typically are patients older than 65 years, but others who may qualify for Medicare benefits, such as the disabled, are specified in the Social Security Act. Medicare is divided into four main parts (Medicare Parts A through D), each covering different services.

Medicare contracts with local insurance companies to provide services for Medicare beneficiaries in the area. These contractors manage the Medicare program for a specific geographic area of the country and must follow national coverage determinations (NCDs) as set forth by Medicare. They also can establish local policies for items not addressed in the federal guidelines. Local coverage determinations (LCDs) document a decision by the contractor whether to cover a particular service. Corporate hospitals and groups that have facilities in multiple regions of the United States may all be assigned to the same contractor.

Medicare Administrative Contractors

Medicare plans to simplify payment structure by discontinuing "carrier" and "fiscal intermediary" designations and designating regional Medicare Administrative Contractors (MACs). According to the *Medicare Benefit Policy Manual*:

> Through implementation of Medicare Contracting Reform, CMS is integrating the administration of Medicare Parts A and B for the fee-for-service benefit to new entities called Medicare Administrative Contractors (MACs). This operational integration will centralize information once held separately, creating a platform for advances in the delivery of comprehensive care to Medicare beneficiaries. (CMS 2009)

Figure 2.1 shows a map of contractors.

Medicare Part A

Medicare Part A pays for inpatient hospitalization and some skilled aftercare services, such as nursing home, home health, and hospice care for covered beneficiaries. Many people

Figure 2.1. A/B Medicare Administrative Contractors

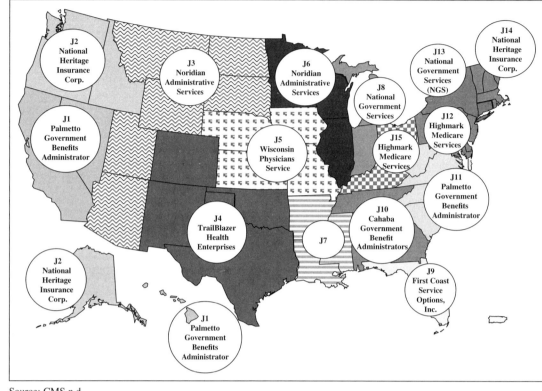

Source: CMS n.d.

automatically receive Part A Medicare starting the first day of the month of their 65th birthday. Benefits are also paid for those younger than 65 years and disabled. Medicare patients have maximum benefit periods of 60 full days plus 30 days of coinsurance coverage. This coverage is renewable after the patient has not been in a hospital or skilled nursing facility for 60 days. Patients also have a lifetime reserve benefit of 60 additional days. Moreover, Medicare patients have a lifetime maximum of 190 inpatient psychiatric days of coverage.

Medicare Part B

Medicare Part B is designed to pay for some medically necessary and preventive physician-related services, some outpatient hospital services, durable medical equipment (DME), and supplies. Medicare beneficiaries must pay an additional monthly premium for this coverage. Certain services normally covered under Part A can be paid under Part B claims when patients have exhausted their Part A benefits.

DME such as wheelchairs, crutches, and other supplies are covered under the jurisdiction of a durable medical equipment Medicare Administrative Contractor (DMEMAC). There are currently four regional MACs for DME. When a hospital provides DME services, it must be certified as a medical equipment provider and must follow special billing rules and regulations as set forth by Medicare and maintained by the regional DMEMAC.

Medicare Part C

Medicare Part C, or Medicare Advantage (MA), is a PPO-type coverage for Medicare beneficiaries provided by private insurance companies that are approved by Medicare. Medicare Advantage plans offer options such as regional PPOs and specialized health plans for certain diagnoses. This plan provides all Part A and Part B coverage, along with emergency and urgent care services, and may also offer additional services such as vision, hearing, dental, and prescription drug services. Medicare pays a fixed amount for care each month for each beneficiary covered by the plan. A statistical model is used to review the costs incurred for the enrollees to determine predictions for future years' healthcare expenses. This model is known as the principal inpatient diagnostic cost group (PIP-DCG) algorithm, a model designed to calculate each beneficiary's relative risk in terms of overall Medicare (CMS 2010).

Medicare Part D

Medicare Part D represents the Medicare Prescription Drug Plan, which provides assistance to Medicare beneficiaries who incur substantial drug expenses. The plan is voluntary and administered by various contractors. The beneficiary is responsible for an annual deductible and copayments, and Medicare reimburses a percentage of drug costs above established thresholds.

Medicaid

Medicaid was established in 1965 by Public Law 89-97 (Title XIX of the Social Security Act) as a jointly funded program between the state and federal governments. The program was set up to care for low-income or indigent patients. However, although it is federally funded, the program is run primarily by the individual states. Eligibility, services provided, and payment rates vary from state to state, but the programs must meet general national guidelines for services. The CMS Medicaid Eligibility Summary defines the following categories of patients as eligible for Medicaid:

- Individuals who meet the requirements for the Aid to Families with Dependent Children (AFDC) program that were in effect in their state on July 16, 1996

- Children younger than 6 years in families whose income is at or below 133 percent of the federal poverty level (FPL)

- Pregnant women whose family income is below 133 percent of the FPL (Services to these women are limited to those related to pregnancy, complications of pregnancy, delivery, and postpartum care.)

- Supplemental Security Income (SSI) recipients in most states (Some states use more restrictive Medicaid eligibility requirements that predate SSI.)

- Recipients of adoption or foster care assistance under Title IV of the Social Security Act

- Special protected groups (typically individuals who lose their cash assistance due to earnings from work or from increased Social Security benefits, but who may keep Medicaid for a period of time)

- All children born after September 30, 1983, who are younger than 19 years, in families with incomes at or below the FPL

- Certain Medicare beneficiaries, such as those with low income

Some states have received permission from the federal government to make modifications to the basic Medicaid plans to include uninsurable individuals, the medically needy, and children.

Military Programs

TRICARE (formerly known as the Civilian Health and Medical Program of the Uniformed Services [CHAMPUS]) provides medical coverage for active-duty and retired service members. This coverage applies to members of the seven uniformed services (Army, Air Force, Navy, Marine Corps, Coast Guard, Public Health Service, and the National Oceanic and Atmospheric Administration) and their dependents, as well as individuals whose spouses were killed in action.

TRICARE pays for coverage in facilities other than military hospitals and offers several options, including an HMO-type of coverage system and a fee-based payment system. The HMO/managed care option is known as TRICARE Prime. TRICARE Extra is a PPO option, and TRICARE Standard is a fee-for-service plan. TRICARE Plus is a variation of the plan used to cover services in military healthcare facilities when available.

For beneficiaries who are Medicare eligible (age 65 years and older), there is also a TRICARE for Life plan option. This plan works as a secondary insurance for those who have Medicare Part B. It covers expenses such as coinsurance and deductible costs after Medicare pays its portion of the bill.

TRICARE for Life uses a DRG-modified system to reimburse facilities for inpatient care. This benefit is available only when the patient is in the hospital for more days than are allowable under the Medicare system. For days 151 and later of a Medicare stay, TRICARE reimburses the hospital the DRG amount minus the patient's additional copayment rate, which is approximately 25 percent of the charges if the hospital is in network. Table 2.2 shows an example of DRG groupings and weights used to determine payment.

The healthcare plan for veterans is the Civilian Health and Medical Program of the Department of Veterans Affairs (CHAMPVA). This plan consists of comprehensive coverage where both the veteran and the Department of Veterans Affairs (VA) pay a portion of covered healthcare expenses.

According to the Department of Veterans Affairs, CHAMPVA is a healthcare benefits program for the spouse or widow(er) and for the children of a veteran who

1. Is rated permanently and totally disabled due to a service-connected disability by a VA regional office, or

2. Was rated permanently and totally disabled due to a service-connected condition at the time of death, or

3. Died from a VA-rated service-connected disability, or

4. Died on active duty (not due to misconduct), and the dependents are not otherwise eligible for DoD TRICARE benefits (VA 2010).

Those who are eligible for TRICARE/CHAMPUS are not eligible for CHAMPVA. In addition, a Medicare secondary plan called CHAMPVA for Life is available for those covered beneficiaries who are age 65 years and older.

Commercial and Nonprofit Group Medical Insurance Plans

Group medical insurance plans are usually purchased through or by an employer. Some patients who cannot qualify for individual insurance plans because of preexisting conditions can obtain insurance through employer-sponsored group plans.

Table 2.2. CHAMPUS weight and threshold summary for FY 2010

DRG Number	Description	CHAMPUS Weight	Arithmetic Mean Length of Stay	Geometric Mean Length of Stay	Short Stay Threshold
1	Heart transplant or implant of heart assist system w MCC	23.1022	36.3	26.6	5
2	Heart transplant or implant of heart assist system w/o MCC	15.8832	28.3	20.3	3
3	ECMO or trach w MV 96+ hrs or PDX exc face, mouth & neck w maj O.R.	18.7853	37.9	30.3	8
4	Trach w MV 96+ hrs or PDX exc face, mouth & neck w/o maj O.R.	12.2743	30.5	23.6	5
5	Liver transplant w MCC or intestinal transplant	15.0007	24.2	16.9	3
6	Liver transplant w/o MCC	5.9473	8.9	8.3	4
7	Lung transplant	11.5348	20.1	17.1	4
8	Simultaneous pancreas/kidney transplant	5.6183*	12.3	10.4	2
9	Bone marrow transplant	7.6374	22.5	19.1	5
10	Pancreas transplant	4.7455*	10.0	8.9	1
11	Tracheostomy for face, mouth & neck diagnoses w MCC	4.8227	15.3	10.5	2
12	Tracheostomy for face, mouth & neck diagnoses w CC	3.1525	7.8	6.4	1
13	Tracheostomy for face, mouth & neck diagnoses w/o CC/MCC	1.9931	5.8	4.8	1
20	Intracranial vascular procedures w PDX hemorrhage w MCC	8.6267	16.7	12.2	1
21	Intracranial vascular procedures w PDX hemorrhage w CC	6.7264	15.2	13.2	4
22	Intracranial vascular procedures w PDX hemorrhage w/o CC/MCC	5.6245	9.9	8.1	1
23	Cranio w major dev impl/acute complex CNS PDX w MCC or chemo implant	6.0551	11.5	7.6	1
24	Cranio w major dev impl/acute complex CNS PDX w/o MCC	4.2286	8.6	6.1	1
25	Craniotomy & endovascular intracranial procedures age >17 w MCC	5.4358	12.2	8.9	1
26	Craniotomy & endovascular intracranial procedures age >17 w CC	3.2170	6.1	4.8	1
27	Craniotomy & endovascular intracranial procedures age >17 w/o CC/MCC	2.4012	3.6	2.9	1
28	Spinal procedures w MCC	4.1648	9.4	6.9	1
29	Spinal procedures w CC or spinal neurostimulators	3.0856	5.8	4.2	1
30	Spinal procedures w/o CC/MCC	1.7646	3.3	2.5	1

Source: TRICARE Management Activity n.d.

Fiscal Year 2010 DRG Weights and Rates for All DRG Numbers
* = low volume DRG with fewer than 10 cases. The Medicare weights and LOS are used for these DRGs.
# = PM-DRGs with fewer than 10 cases. An average weight over the past 5 years were used for these DRGs.
w cc = with Complications and Comorbidities.
w/o cc = without Complications or Comorbidities.

Self-employed individuals or those who work in a group that does not provide group insurance may be eligible to obtain individual medical insurance. These types of policies may cost more than group plans and may contain strict regulations, such as a preexisting clause. Patients who have medical conditions deemed to have existed at the time of coverage do not receive benefits related to those preexisting conditions for a specified time frame after coverage begins.

Insurance companies provide various types of healthcare coverage options and benefits for their customers. For example, a review of a major Blue Cross Blue Shield program shows that it offers the following options:

- *Major medical:* This option is usually a fee-for-service plan as discussed earlier. Although patients enjoy greater flexibility in the types of services and the number of providers to choose from, major medical plans tend to be the most expensive for the patient, with higher deductibles and out-of-pocket expenses.

- *Preferred payment plan:* The preferred payment plan is a PPO-type system in which members have a more limited number of providers to select from based on negotiated contracts with the facilities and physician practices. They may include a POS option, allowing the beneficiary to go out of network for a reduced percentage of reimbursement.

- *Hospital reimbursement program:* The hospital reimbursement program is used for reimbursement for hospital inpatient stays. The hospital agrees to accept a DRG-type payment methodology in which the payment received is considered as payment in full. The beneficiary will incur no costs other than the deductible and copayment amounts. This plan is similar to the DRG system utilized in the Medicare inpatient PPS.

- *COBRA and HIPAA benefits:* Patients who have group insurance and leave their jobs or are laid off are usually eligible to keep their insurance coverage up to 18 months after their employment ends, but are required to pay the premiums in order to keep the coverage intact. These benefits are provided by federal law under the Consolidated Omnibus Budget Reconciliation Act of 1986 (COBRA). Continuation of coverage is only effective under specific circumstances, such as loss of a job or life events such as death or divorce. Typically, COBRA is in effect for employers who offer group healthcare and have 20 or more employees. The Health Insurance Portability and Accountability Act of 1996 (HIPAA) allows for healthcare coverage protection for those who move or change jobs, although the premiums for these policies are often very expensive. HIPAA also prohibits group plans from either denying coverage or charging extra due to current or past medical history. There is usually a limited or no preexisting clause in the HIPAA insurance plan. Patients have to show that they have a minimum of 18 months of credible coverage of previous insurance without significant break (no more than 63 days in a row without insurance) to be eligible for HIPAA insurance.

Summary

Various methods of payment are used to reimburse facilities that provide services to inpatients. Although Medicare's DRG system is probably the most widely studied, other payment methodologies such as HMOs are prevalent in many sections of the country. The wide variety of payment methodologies can be a source of confusion for hospital coders, billers, and other finance personnel, so it is very important to understand these systems and their impact on the financial well-being of the healthcare facility.

References

America's Health Insurance Plans. 2007. Questions and answers about health insurance. http://www.ahip.org/content/default.aspx?bc=411329120888.

Centers for Medicare and Medicaid Services. n.d. A/B Medicare Administrative Contractors. http://www.cms.gov/MedicareContractingReform/downloads/ABMACJurisdictionsMAP.pdf.

Centers for Medicare and Medicaid Services. 2007a (Jan. 17). Hospital pay-for-performance workgroup: Medicare hospital value-based purchasing plan development. Issues paper, 1st public listening session. http://www.cms.hhs.gov/AcuteInpatientPPS/downloads/hospital_VBP_plan_issues_paper.pdf.

Centers for Medicare and Medicaid Services. 2007b (May 14). Office of Public Affairs, Press Release: Medicare pay for performance (P4P) initiatives. http://www.cms.hhs.gov/apps/media/press/release.asp?Counter=1343.

Centers for Medicare and Medicaid Services. 2009. Medicare Administrative Contractor (MAC) jurisdictions fact sheet. http://www.cms.hhs.gov/MedicareContractingReform/Downloads/MACJurisdictionFactSheet.pdf.

Centers for Medicare and Medicaid Services. 2010. Medicare and you 2010. http://www.medicare.gov/Publications/Pubs/pdf/10050.pdf.

Department of Veterans Affairs. 2010. CHAMPVA. http://www4.va.gov/hac/forbeneficiaries/champva/champva.asp.

Huntington, J. 1997 (Jan. 6). Glossary for managed care. *Online Journal of Issues in Nursing* 2(1). http://www.nursingworld.org/MainMenuCategories/ANAMarketplace/ANAPeriodicals/OJIN/TableofContents/Vol21997/No1Jan97/GlossaryforManagedCare.aspx#managedcare.

Kaiser Permanente. n.d. Kaiser Permanente—More than 60 years of quality. http://newsmedia.kaiserpermanente.org/kpweb/historykp/entrypage.do.

Miller, R.C. 2008. What Is an HMO? Kansas City, MO: Monsees, Miller, Mayer, Presley and Amick. http://www.mmmpalaw.com/CM/Articles/articles33.asp.

TRICARE Management Activity n.d. Fiscal year 2010 DRG weights and rates for all DRG numbers. http://www.tricare.mil/drgrates/index.cfm?fuseaction=main.DrgWeights&rangeStart=all&fiscalYear=2010.

Chapter 3

Structure and Organization of the Medicare Inpatient Acute Care Prospective Payment System

The Social Security Act, as amended in 1982 by the Tax Equity and Fiscal Responsibility Act (TEFRA), mandated the use of a prospective payment system (PPS) for inpatient hospital services provided under Part A of Medicare. In the 1970s, a research team at Yale University looked into classifying patients into categories based on the diagnoses that caused them to be admitted to the hospital in order to determine why patients with similar cases differed in their usage of resources. Patients were divided into various categories that were medically meaningful in that all patients in the same category would be expected to respond in a clinically similar manner. The data were averaged statistically to show that patients placed in these categories consumed about equal amounts of the hospital's facilities and resources. The categories became known as diagnosis- (or diagnostic-) related groups (DRGs). In fiscal year (FY) 2008, these DRGs were revised into Medicare severity adjusted DRGs or MS-DRGs. This chapter discusses DRGs, their evolution to MS-DRGs, and their role in the development of the PPS inpatient system.

Diagnosis-Related Groups

DRGs are derived from all the diagnoses and procedures listed in the ICD-9-CM classification system. DRGs are simply numbers signifying into which category the patient best fits. Grouping patients into categories that consume similar amounts of resources reveals typical and atypical patterns of utilization. The researchers who developed the DRG system were trying to define expected lengths of patient stays so that utilization review (UR) activities could be focused on atypical patients. Their design was not established with the intent to use it as the basis for a payment system. However, when the government learned of the study, it became interested and funded a project in New Jersey to see if this type of system would work as a reimbursement system.

Simply defined, a DRG is a group of clinically coherent conditions with a similar pattern of resource intensity determined by the principal diagnosis, significant additional diagnoses (and their present-on-admission status), and procedures as reported on the Uniform Bill-04 (UB-04) (Kennedy 2008).

Development of the Inpatient PPS System

Section 1886(d) of the Social Security Act (the Act) sets forth a system of payment for the operating costs of acute care hospital inpatient stays under Medicare Part A (Hospital Insurance) based on prospectively set rates. Section 1886(g) of the Act requires the Secretary of Health and Human Services to pay for the capital-related costs of hospital inpatient stays under a PPS. Under these PPSs, Medicare payment for hospital inpatient operating and capital-related costs is made at predetermined, specific rates for each hospital discharge (CMS 2009a, 43760). Hospitals subject to the PPS are paid a specific amount for each discharge based on the case's classification into a DRG. Every hospital discharge case fits into a DRG category. A hierarchy has been established to ensure that each case fits into one category group only.

The DRGs provide classification for the complete range of diagnoses represented in the ICD-9-CM codebook.

Because assignment of a case to a particular DRG determines the amount that will be paid for the case, it is important that the assignment be done in a systematic and uniform manner. According to the Centers for Medicare and Medicaid Services (CMS), the following core elements are included in a PPS-type system (CMS 2010a):

- The base payment amount
- A "wage index," which reflects that labor costs vary in different areas of the country
- The standardized weights that are established to compare the average resources needed to care for patients in each DRG
- Additional payments for those hospitals with treatment patterns that fall into specific categories, such as:
  —A large share of low-income or indigent patients
  —Teaching hospitals to reflect the higher cost of providing medical education
  —Additional payment for very high-cost patients, known as outliers

Grouper Software

CMS established the grouper program, which is an automated classification system that uses the prescribed information to assign discharges to their proper DRGs. The fiscal intermediary (FI)/Medicare Administrative Contractor (MAC), which is the organization contracting with Medicare to process hospital inpatient claims for CMS, assigns the proper DRG using the grouper program. Most hospitals assign DRGs for all cases to facilitate quality management activities and estimate revenue, but it is the DRG assigned by the MACs grouper that determines final reimbursement.

Coding instructions for the PPS indicate that the hospital will submit a bill for a particular case using classifications and terminology consistent with ICD-9-CM and the Uniform Hospital Data Discharge Set (UHDDS) prescribed by the National Committee on Vital and Health Statistics (NCVHS).

According to CMS, the updated MS-DRGs and grouper software, used by both the inpatient prospective payment system (IPPS) and the long-term care hospital (LTCH)-MS-DRG system are based on updated ICD-9-CM codes in a manner consistent with current usage and the Health Insurance Portability and Accountability Act of 1996 (HIPAA) regulations. Historically, these codes have been published annually in the IPPS proposed rule and final rule but are also available in *Coding Clinic for ICD-9-CM* published by the American Hospital Association. This brief offers official coding advice for the coder about which ICD-9-CM instructions and UHDDS sequencing guidelines apply when coding for the PPS.

DRG Variables

A patient is assigned to only one DRG group per admission. Because many patients have multiple diagnoses and procedures, a classification hierarchy had to be incorporated into the system. Patients originally were assigned to a DRG based on the following variables:

- Principal diagnosis, if no qualifying surgery is performed
- Secondary diagnoses
- Principal or significant procedure
- Age
- Sex
- Patient status (discharge disposition)

Principal Diagnosis

The principal diagnosis is defined in the UHDDS as "that condition established after study to be chiefly responsible for occasioning the admission of the patient to the hospital for care" (HHS 1985). This helps to establish a standard definition when comparing data from different facilities but causes much confusion in coding. For example, if a patient is admitted with chest pain, and after testing it is determined that the patient is suffering from an acute myocardial infarction (AMI), the AMI qualifies as the principal diagnosis. However, if the patient is admitted for treatment of benign prostate hypertrophy and then after admission has a massive heart attack, even though the focus of the admission has changed, the principal diagnosis is the prostate condition, with the heart attack meeting the definition for additional diagnosis reporting.

It can be confusing for the coder to distinguish between the "principal" diagnosis and the most "significant additional diagnosis." UHDDS defines additional diagnoses as "all conditions that coexist at the time of admission, that develop subsequently, or that affect the treatment received and/or the length of stay" (HHS 1985).

Secondary Diagnoses

According to the UHDDS, secondary diagnoses include all conditions that "coexist at the time of admission, or develop subsequently, which affect the treatment received and/or the length of stay (LOS). Diagnoses that refer to an earlier episode that have no bearing on the current hospital or nursing home stay are to be excluded. Conditions should be coded that affect patient care in terms of requiring clinical evaluation; therapeutic treatment; diagnostic procedures; extended length of hospital or nursing home stay; or increased nursing care and/or monitoring" (HHS 1985). Secondary diagnoses may help to determine the grouping if they qualify as a complication/comorbidity (CC). Originally, a CC was defined as a condition, because of its presence with a specific principal diagnosis, that causes a statistical increase in the LOS by at least 1 day in at least 75 percent of the patients (CMS 2009a, 43792). Complications are those conditions that arise after admission. If a patient is admitted with pneumonia and then has a stroke on the second day of hospitalization, the stroke would be considered a complication according to the UHDDS definition. This definition may not be the same as a complication due to, or caused by, a surgical or medical procedure. Comorbidities are conditions that are present on admission, such as a systemic disease such as Type II diabetes or essential hypertension, or concomitant acute illnesses or injuries. These illnesses may cause a patient to recover at a slower rate than a patient without any additional problems. In the case of paired DRGs, a single CC (complication or comorbid condition) can cause the patient's case to be grouped into the higher-weighted MS-DRG.

For FY 2008, major revisions to the CC list were made according to Medicare and these were divided into CC and MCC (major CC) lists. The definition of CC had not changed since it was first established at the onset of the DRG system. However, there have been many changes impacting the patients that have been admitted to the hospital. In 1983, the average LOS for Medicare patients was 9.8 days, and by 2005 it had dropped to 5.7 days. Changes in practice patterns and an increase in postacute care services as well as a shift to performing more services in the outpatient area has meant that patients who are admitted to the hospital are much sicker than they were in the past. Subsequently, by 2005, approximately 80 percent of Medicare patients admitted to US hospitals had a secondary condition that counted as a CC (CMS 2007, 47153). In FY 2007 there were 115 MS-DRGs split based on the presence or absence of CC, and Medicare began a reevaluation of the types of diagnoses that counted as CCs (CMS 2007).

Chronic Illnesses

The presence of a chronic illness does not automatically extend the patient's hospital stay. Some chronic illnesses do not impact LOS unless they are associated with an acute exacerbation or significant deterioration in the underlying chronic condition. A Medicare-based review of chronic illnesses led to the removal of several of them from the CC list, including congestive heart failure (CHF) and chronic obstructive pulmonary disease (COPD). Another example of a chronic illness is mitral valve disease. Through FY 2007, codes 396.0–396.9 were included on the CC list. Unless these diagnoses are combined with other diagnoses showing acute deterioration such as acute heart failure, acute pulmonary edema, or respiratory failure, they will not necessarily impact the patient's LOS or resources necessary to care for the patient. Therefore, these codes were removed from the revised CC list for FY 2008.

Advanced Chronic Illnesses

For those conditions that are divided into stages of illnesses, only those stages or levels of severity that impact LOS and/or resources used are counted as CCs. For example, a patient with chronic kidney disease is staged according to the glomerular filtration rate. Stages I to III are not counted as CCs, but stages IV, V (kidney failure), or end-stage renal disease are counted as CCs. If morbid obesity is diagnosed in a patient, this condition will count as a CC only if paired with a body mass index of greater than 35.

Codes Where Stage Not Specified

For chronic conditions where the stage is not specified, the conditions were evaluated based on the consistency and intensity of the debility or decompensation associated with the illness.

Quadriplegia, for example, is always considered significant, so it counts as a CC when coded as a secondary diagnosis.

Acute Diagnosis Codes

Acute conditions that always impact LOS and/or amount of resources used remained on the CC list. Examples include:

- AMI (not CC if already impacts MS-DRG assignment)
- Cerebrovascular accident
- Acute respiratory failure
- Pneumonia
- Septicemia

Other acute conditions were included based on their impact on hospital resource usage. If they were found to be comparable to these listed diagnoses, then they were left on the CC list, but if not, they were removed. For example, acute endocarditis remained on the CC list, but urinary tract infection (UTI) was removed.

Revised CC List

In summary, secondary conditions only count as CCs if they have been found to have consistently greater impact on hospital resources and include the following:

- Significant acute diseases
- Acute exacerbation of significant chronic illnesses
- Advanced or end-stage chronic illnesses
- Chronic diseases associated with extensive debility

For FY 2008, this reduced the number of secondary codes that count as CCs from 3,326 to 2,583 and reduced the number of inpatients with CCs to approximately 40.34 percent.

CC Exclusion List

Medicare has a listing of CC exclusions. Some secondary diagnoses may act as CCs with certain diagnoses, but not with others. For example, urinary retention is on the standard CC list, but if present with benign prostatic hyperplasia (BPH), it is excluded as a CC because it is considered to be an integral part of the clinical presentation of BPH. As such, it does not cause an increase in the amount of resources needed to care for the patient. Medicare places codes on the CC exclusion list based on one of these five reasons (CMS 2009a, 43793):

1. Chronic and acute manifestations of the same condition should not be considered CCs for one another.

2. Specific and nonspecific (that is, not otherwise specified [NOS]) diagnosis codes for the same condition should not be considered CCs for one another.

3. Codes for the same condition that cannot coexist, such as partial/total, unilateral/bilateral, obstructed/unobstructed, and benign/malignant, should not be considered CCs for one another.

4. Codes for the same condition in anatomically proximal sites should not be considered CCs for one another.

5. Closely related conditions should not be considered CCs for one another.

Other Factors Influencing DRG Assignment

In some cases in the past, other factors such as age, sex, and discharge status have affected DRG assignment. For example, if patients in one age group tended to use more resources than patients in another age group, the DRGs were split according to age. (This action was eliminated in FY 2008 with the onset of MS-DRGs). Sex is used primarily to indicate a keystroke error, such as a hysterectomy patient classified as a male patient. Discharge status is a factor in the facility obtaining partial DRG payment when the patient is transferred to another facility, or when a certain type of discharge status shows a statistical difference in the amount of resources utilized. Medicare's postacute care transfer policy allows for a decrease in payment if postacute care treatment related to the hospital admission occurs following the patient's discharge. This policy is discussed in detail later in this chapter. Figure 3.1 presents a flowchart of the of DRG process.

Figure 3.1. Flowchart of the MS-DRG process

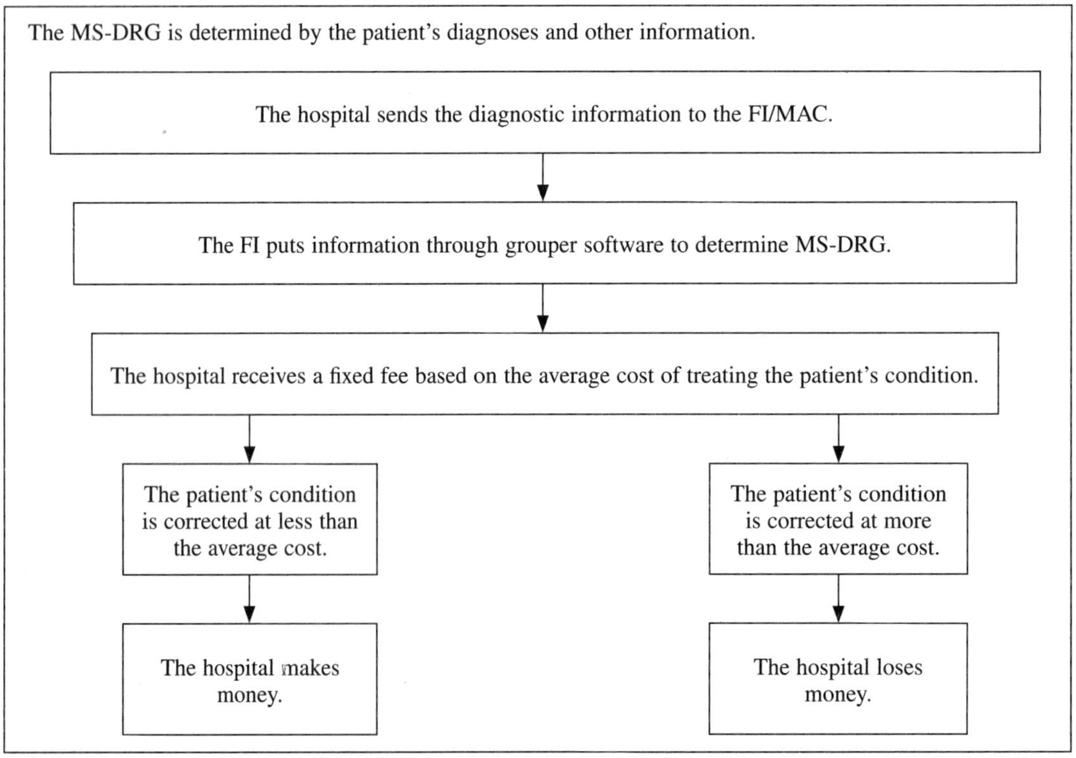

Major Diagnostic Categories and Surgical Hierarchy

Before patients' admissions are divided into DRGs, they are divided into major diagnostic categories (MDCs). Each MDC is based on major body systems and contains multiple DRGs. There were originally 23 MDCs and 470 DRGs. These are reviewed and adjusted each year. As of FY 2010, there are 25 major diagnostic categories and 13 pre-MDCs, composed only of surgical DRGs related primarily to organ transplants. DRGs within each MDC are separated into medical and surgical divisions. When more than one procedure is performed, the DRG that is highest according to the surgical hierarchy in the MDC is assigned. For example, under the MS-DRG system in MDC 5, diseases and disorders of the circulatory system, MS-DRG 242, permanent cardiac pacemaker implant with MCC, takes precedence over MS-DRG 247, percutaneous cardiovascular procedure with drug-eluting stent without MCC. If a patient has both types of procedures during a single admission, he or she would be grouped into MS-DRG 242 according to the surgical hierarchy.

DRG Relative Weight

Each DRG is assigned a relative weight that represents the average resources required to care for a patient assigned to a specific DRG in relation to the national average of resources used to treat all Medicare cases. When DRG groups were first developed, there needed to be a way to compare the different groups according to the amount of resources utilized. To obtain a starting point for comparison, the average cost to treat all Medicare patients was established and assigned a relative weight of 1.0000. All patient cases then were divided into DRGs and ranked in order according to the number of resources utilized. As all other DRGs were compared to the average, they were assigned weights appropriate for their average resources used by patients in that group. For example, if one DRG takes twice as many resources as the average, it would be weighted at 2.0000. Conversely, if a group takes half as many resources as average, it would be weighted at 0.5000. Weights for all DRGs are updated every year and published in the *Federal Register,* with the changes taking effect on October 1 of each year. Relative weights for FY 2010 MS-DRGs range from a high of 24.8548 for MS-DRG 001 (pre-MDC), heart transplant or implant of heart assist system with MCC, to a low of 0.1617 for MS-DRG 795 (MDC 15), normal newborn.

Adjustment to the Facility Payment Rate

Although the DRG weight is the same for all facilities, hospitals may receive different payment rates based on several factors, including labor costs, disproportionate-share hospitals (DSHs), medical education, new technology, and other factors.

Labor Costs

The DRG amount is divided into labor- and nonlabor-related costs. To account for differences in the labor portion, Medicare established wage areas throughout the different regions of the country. In other words, it costs more to hire staff in some areas of the country than in others, so hospitals are compensated for that additional expense. In Alaska and Hawaii, the rate also is adjusted for the area's cost of living. Table 3.1 shows some examples of the wage indexes for FY 2010.

Table 3.1. FY 2010 wage indexes example

CBSA Code	Urban Area	State	Wage Index	GAF
10180	Abilene, TX	TX	0.8336	0.8828
10380	Aguadilla-Isabela-San Sebastián, PR	PR	0.3364	0.4742
10420	Akron, OH	OH	0.8839	0.9190
10500	Albany, GA	GA	0.8931	0.9255
10580	Albany-Schnectady-Troy, NY	NY	0.8805	0.9165
10740	Albuquerque, NM	NM	0.9554	0.9692
10780	Alexandria, LA	LA	0.8152	0.8694
10900	Allentown-Bethlehem-Easton, PA-NJ	NJ	1.1341	1.0900
10900	Allentown-Bethlehem-Easton, PA-NJ	PA	0.9811	0.9870
11020	Altoona, PA	PA	0.8821	0.9177
11100	Amarillo, TX	TX	0.8594	0.9014
11180	Ames, IA	IA	0.9533	0.9678
11260	Anchorage, AK	AK	1.1920	1.1278
11300	Anderson, IN	IN	0.9116	0.9386
11340	Anderson, SC	SC	0.9130	0.9396
11460	Ann Arbor, MI	MI	1.0243	1.0166
11500	Anniston-Oxford, AL	AL	0.7603	0.8289
11540	Appleton, WI	WI	0.9245	0.9477
11700	Asheville, NC	NC	0.9082	0.9362
12020	Athens-Clarke County, GA	GA	0.9205	0.9449
12060	Atlanta-Sandy Springs-Marietta, GA	GA	0.9581	0.9711
12100	Atlantic City-Hammonton, NJ	NJ	1.1341	1.0900
12220	Auburn-Opelika, AL	AL	0.8432	0.8898
12260	Augusta-Richmond County, GA-SC	GA	0.9445	0.9617
12260	Augusta-Richmond County, GA-SC	SC	0.9440	0.9613
12420	Austin-Round Rock, TX	TX	0.9515	0.9665
12540	Bakersfield, CA	CA	1.1745	1.1164
12580	Baltimore-Towson, MD	MD	1.0148	1.0101

Source: CMS 2010b.

Occupational Mix Adjustment

Every 3 years Medicare collects data to determine how occupational mix adjustment impacts wages. According to CMS, "the purpose of the occupational mix adjustment is to control for the effect of hospitals' employment choices on the wage index. For example, hospitals may choose to employ different combinations of registered nurses, licensed practical nurses, nursing aides, and medical assistants for the purpose of providing nursing care to their patients. The varying labor costs associated with these choices reflect hospital management decisions rather than geographic differences in the costs of labor" (CMS 2009a, 43827). Hospitals are required to complete a survey that includes data regarding specific wages, hours, and types of personnel employed in certain job types.

Disproportionate-Share Hospitals

Hospitals that treat a high number of low-income patients may receive an additional amount per case known as their DSH adjustment. Examples of DSH adjustments are shown in table 3.2 (CMS 2009).

This DSH adjustment was enacted by the Consolidated Omnibus Budget Reconciliation Act (COBRA) to impact discharges beginning in May of 1986. There are two ways for hospitals to qualify to receive this additional amount. The more common way to qualify is through a formula determined in COBRA, which determines a DSH patient percentage by adding the Medicare and Medicaid fractions (CMS 2009b). According to CMS, the Medicare fraction is:

. . . computed by dividing the number of the hospital's inpatient days that are furnished to patients who were entitled to both Medicare Part A (including patients who are enrolled in a Medicare Advantage (Part C) plan) and Supplemental Security Income (SSI) benefits by the hospital's total number of patient days furnished to patients entitled to benefits under Medicare Part A (including patients who are enrolled in a Medicare Advantage (Part C) plan). The Medicaid fraction is computed by dividing the hospital's number of inpatient days furnished to

Table 3.2.   Example of DSH adjustments

Name	Total SSI	Total Medicare	SSI Ratio
Southeast Medical Center	8,278	50,829	0.16286
Marshall Medical Center South	1,931	13,401	0.14409
Eliza Coffee Memorial Hospital	5,042	45,345	0.11119
Mizell Memorial Hospital	1,169	6,635	0.17619
Crenshaw Community Hospital	474	2,469	0.19198
Hartselle Medical Center	463	4,218	0.10977
Marshall Medical Center North	1,712	12,495	0.13701
Medical Center East	1,821	27,619	0.06593
Baptist Dekalb	854	6,668	0.12807

patients who, for such days, were eligible for Medicaid, but were not entitled to benefits under Medicare Part A, by the hospital's total number of inpatient days in the same period. (CMS 2009a, 43899)

Because the DSH payment adjustment is part of the IPS, the DSH statutory references to "days" include inpatient only. When the DSH patient percentage is greater than 15 percent, the facility is eligible for an additional payment.

Large urban hospitals also can qualify if their total net inpatient care revenue received from state and local governments for indigent care is more than 30 percent. This percentage does not include funds received from either Medicare or Medicaid. According to CMS, hospitals qualifying through this method are known as "pickle hospitals." Rural hospitals that qualify as rural referral centers or sole community hospitals also may qualify through various formulas established in the law. For rural hospitals with fewer than 500 beds, DSH limits are capped at 12 percent; those that qualify as rural referral centers have no cap. A hospital can qualify as a rural referral center if it has more than 275 beds or if the hospital meets two mandatory prerequisites including a minimum case-mix index (CMI) and discharges in addition to one of three other criteria involving medical staff composition, inpatient sources, and volume of referrals (CMS 2009a, 43897–43899).

Table 3.3 shows the Medicare-defined median CMI per region for FY 2010.

Table 3.3. Medicare-defined median case-mix index per region for FY 2010

Region	States	Case-mix index value
1. New England	CT, ME, MA, NH, RI, VT	1.2612
2. Middle Atlantic	PA, NJ, NY	1.3011
3. South Atlantic	DE, DC, FL, GA, MD, NC, SC, VA, WV	1.4212
4. East North Central	IL, IN, MI, OH, WI	1.3994
5. East South Central	AL, KY, MS, TN	1.3311
6. West North Central	IA, KS, MN, MO, NE, ND, SD	1.4045
7. West South Central	AR, LA, OK, TX	1.4692
8. Mountain	AZ, CO, ID, MT, NV, NM, UT, WY	1.5217
9. Pacific	AK, CA, HI, OR, WA	1.4298

Source: CMS 2009a, 43898.

Medical Education

Teaching hospitals receive an additional payment for their indirect medical education (IME) costs, which are based on a comparison of hospital residents to number of hospital beds. This provision also was set forth in the COBRA law of 1985. The law takes into account direct vs. indirect medical education costs. For direct medical education costs, the hospital's per resident amount (PRA) is determined by dividing its allowable costs for education by the number of residents during the time period. The PRA then is multiplied by the number of full-time equivalent (FTE) residents during the reporting period and the hospital's number of inpatient days for Medicare patients.

When PPS hospitals have residents in an approved graduate medical education (GME) program, the hospital obtains additional payment per Medicare discharge for IME costs. The IME adjustment factor compares the number of residents per number of beds and is multiplied by a rate that is set by Congress. Typically, for each 10 percent increase in resident-to-bed ratio, the facility receives additional funding.

The Balanced Budget Act (BBA), the Balanced Budget Refinement Act (BBRA), and the Benefits Improvement and Protection Act (BIPA) all contained stipulations to allow for modification of the IME multiplier.

New Technology

Another adjustment to the facility's payment rate is based on new technology. At times, Medicare will pay an additional fee for the use of new technology, such as very high-cost medications. According to Medicare (CMS 2009a, 43760):

> A new technology or medical service must demonstrate that it is a substantial clinical improvement over technologies or services otherwise available, and that, absent an add-on payment, it would be inadequately paid under the regular DRG system. This additional payment is designed to protect the hospital from large financial losses due to unusually expensive cases. Any eligible outlier payment is added to the DRG-adjusted base payment rate, plus a DSH, IME, and new technology or medical service add-on adjustment.

There are specific criteria and rules set up to define what is meant by "new" in the language of the law, which includes the provision of paying for the new technology separately until enough time has passed to allow for sufficient data to be collected on the technology. This is defined as at least 2 years, but no longer than 3 years.

For example, for FYs 2009 and 2010, Medicare approved an add-on payment for the new technology of a Temporary Total Artificial Heart System used as a bridge to heart transplant for patients with end-stage biventricular failure. The maximum add-on payment for this technology is $53,000 (CMS 2009a, 43812). Currently, Medicare pays the DRG payment amount plus 50 percent of the costs of the new technology. Makers of new technology are required to formally submit a written proposal to determine if their product will qualify under the new technology regulations.

Other Factors

Other categories of hospitals receive additional payments based on status. Small facilities designated as sole community hospitals (SCHs) and Medicare-dependent rural hospitals (MDHs) are paid based on a formula of DRG rate or on their costs for specific time periods, whichever is higher. When a facility qualifies as an MDH, it is paid 75 percent of the difference between the IPPS rate and the hospital-specific rate when that rate is higher than the IPPS rate for the DRG payment amount. These facilities serve a large Medicare population and are usually located in rural areas. There is no longer a cap on their DSH payment adjustment. SCHs are rural hospitals that must be located at least 15 miles from other like hospitals, among other requirements. MDH hospitals have fewer than 100 beds and are not classified as SCHs.

Facility Base Rate

Each facility is assigned a base rate that takes into account all these factors. The base rate then is multiplied by the DRG weight to determine the actual payment rate for that facility.

Outliers

When the patient's costs exceed a predetermined cost threshold, the facility may be eligible to receive an additional reimbursement added to the DRG base rate. This patient is known as a cost outlier. If the patient qualifies as an outlier, a determination of additional payment is made, which begins at the cost threshold amount. The hospital's cost-to-charge ratios are used to determine whether a patient's costs are greater than the threshold amount. After the threshold limit is reached, the hospital receives a percentage of costs above this amount. The outlier fixed-loss cost threshold for FY 2010 is equal to the PPS rate for the DRG plus any IME and DSH payments and any add-on payments for new technology plus $23,140 (CMS 2009a, 44011).

Hospitals Exempt from Inpatient PPS

These hospitals are paid solely under a reasonable cost-based system. Some facilities are considered to be exempt from the DRG payment system and are paid based on a "reasonable cost-based system" which includes children's hospitals, cancer hospitals, and religious nonmedical healthcare institutions. Other types of facilities that are exempt from the IPPS are now paid based on PPSs specific to their patient populations, such as LTCHs, inpatient psychiatric facilities, and inpatient rehabilitation facilities. The payment methodology for these other systems is discussed in chapter 4.

Transfers

Hospitals must carefully show the patient's discharge status on the billing form because it can have an impact on reimbursement. This is true even of a patient who is transferred from the acute care setting into another unit within the hospital, such as a long-term care or swing bed service.

Because the DRG payment is supposed to pay for all care associated with diagnoses and treatment necessary to care for a patient, when a patient is transferred prior to completion of that care, the DRG payment rate is adjusted to account for the change. For example, when a patient is transferred from one facility that is paid under the IPPS to another facility also paid under the IPPS, the two facilities share the DRG total payment. In the past several years, Medicare has developed a postacute care transfer policy that also adjusts the DRG payment based on incomplete care.

Medicare's postacute care transfer policy distinguishes between discharges and transfers of beneficiaries from inpatient hospitals under the PPS. Consistent with the policy, Medicare pays the full DRG payment to a hospital that discharges an inpatient to home. When a patient is transferred, each transferring hospital is paid a per diem rate for each day of the stay that cannot exceed the full DRG payment that would have been made if the patient had been discharged without being transferred.

In contrast, for specified DRGs, Medicare pays a hospital that transfers an inpatient to certain postacute care settings, such as a skilled nursing facility or home healthcare, a per diem rate for each day of the stay that is not to exceed the full DRG payment for a discharge. Twice the per diem amount is paid for the first day of hospitalization. Only certain DRGs are included in the postacute care payment policy.

The purpose of the IPPS postacute care transfer payment policy is to avoid providing an incentive for a hospital to transfer patients to another hospital early in the patients' stay in order to minimize costs while still receiving the full DRG payment. The transfer policy adjusts the payments to approximate the reduced costs of transfer cases.

Beginning with the FY 2006 IPPS, the regulations specified that a DRG is subject to the postacute care transfer policy if the DRG meets the following criteria:

- The DRG had a geometric mean LOS of at least 3 days;

- The DRG had at least 2,050 postacute care transfer cases;

- At least 5.5 percent of the cases in the DRG were discharged to postacute care prior to the geometric mean LOS for the DRG;

- The total number of discharges to postacute care in the DRG must equal or exceed the 55th percentile for all DRGs; and

- The proportion of short-stay discharges to postacute care to total discharges in the DRG exceeds the 55th percentile for all DRGs. A short-stay discharge is a discharge before the geometric mean LOS for the DRG (CMS 2007, 47187).

Special Payment Methodology

A transfer is subject to the "special payment methodology" if it is in the same base DRG as any other subcategory that qualifies for special payment methodology, in which the patient is transferred early to a postacute care setting. The payment rate for these types of transfers is 50 percent of the total DRG payment plus the average per diem for the first day of the stay plus 50 percent of the per diem for each subsequent day of the stay not to exceed the full DRG payment.

See table 3.4 for an example of FY 2010 MS-DRGs showing which DRGs fall under the postacute care transfer and special payment methodology policies.

Annual Updates

The IPPS was designed to be modified once each year to allow for updates. The largest update occurs because of the creation, revision, or deletion of ICD-9-CM codes. Also, because the IPPS is based on statistical and medical cohesiveness, there are times when changes need to be made, such as a redistribution of codes to different DRG groupings. These changes are published in the *Federal Register* with an effective date of October 1 of each year. The ICD-9-CM coding system may be updated twice per year (October and April) to allow for the addition of codes for new technology, but since this rule has been enacted, very few changes have been made midyear. When new codes are added midyear, they are assigned to current DRG groups until the following October, when the DRG groups are updated as needed.

Severity of Illness

One common criticism of the Medicare DRG system is that the severity of a patient's disease is not always directly reflected in the DRG assignment. In the case of paired DRGs, the presence of a single CC has been shown to significantly add to the resources needed to fully treat the patient. Therefore, patients within one DRG may vary greatly in the number of additional diagnoses they have, meaning that patients in the same DRG could consume quite different quantities of resources. This factor is supposed to be accounted for in the law of averages, as one patient may use fewer resources for his or her care and another may use more, so theoretically the hospital breaks even. However, research is being conducted on variations of the DRG system to attempt to capture severity-of-illness data.

Table 3.4.   Sample of MS-DRGs, relative weighting factors, and geometric and arithmetic mean LOS

MS-DRG	FY 2010 Final Rule Post-Acute DRG	FY 2010 Final Rule Special Pay DRG	MDC	Type	MS-DRG Title	Weights	Geometric mean LOS	Arithmetic mean LOS
038	No	No	01	SURG	Extracranial procedures w CC	1.4783	2.4	3.4
039	No	No	01	SURG	Extracranial procedures w/o CC/MCC	1.0033	1.4	1.7
040	Yes	Yes	01	SURG	Periph/cranial nerve & other nerv syst proc w MCC	3.9518	9.4	12.9
041	Yes	Yes	01	SURG	Periph/cranial nerve & other nerv syst proc w CC or periph neurostim	2.1249	5.2	7.0
042	Yes	Yes	01	SURG	Periph/cranial nerve & other nerv syst proc w/o CC/MCC	1.6448	2.4	3.3
052	No	No	01	MED	Spinal disorders & injuries w CC/MCC	1.4836	4.5	6.3
053	No	No	01	MED	Spinal disorders & injuries w/o CC/MCC	0.8382	3.1	4.0
054	Yes	No	01	MED	Nervous system neoplasms w MCC	1.5637	5.0	6.8
055	Yes	No	01	MED	Nervous system neoplasms w/o MCC	1.0613	3.6	4.9
056	Yes	No	01	MED	Degenerative nervous system disorders w MCC	1.6952	5.7	7.7
057	Yes	No	01	MED	Degenerative nervous system disorders w/o MCC	0.9028	3.9	5.0
058	No	No	01	MED	Multiple sclerosis & cerebellar ataxia w MCC	1.5512	5.8	7.8
059	No	No	01	MED	Multiple sclerosis & cerebellar ataxia w CC	0.9581	4.2	5.1
060	No	No	01	MED	Multiple sclerosis & cerebellar ataxia w/o CC/MCC	0.7083	3.2	3.8
061	No	No	01	MED	Acute ischemic stroke w use of thrombo-lytic agent w MCC	2.9168	6.5	8.7
062	No	No	01	MED	Acute ischemic stroke w use of thrombo-lytic agent w CC	1.9290	5.0	5.9
063	No	No	01	MED	Acute ischemic stroke w use of thrombo-lytic agent w/o CC/MCC	1.5187	3.6	4.2
064	Yes	No	01	MED	Intracranial hemorrhage or cerebral infarc-tion w MCC	1.8258	5.3	7.2
065	Yes	No	01	MED	Intracranial hemorrhage or cerebral infarc-tion w CC	1.1580	4.1	5.0
066	Yes	No	01	MED	Intracranial hemorrhage or cerebral infarc-tion w/o CC/MCC	0.8223	2.9	3.5
067	No	No	01	MED	Nonspecific CVA & precerebral occlusion w/o infarct w MCC	1.3335	4.3	5.5

Table 3.4.   Sample of MS-DRGs, relative weighting factors, and geometric and arithmetic mean LOS *(continued)*

MS-DRG	FY 2010 Final Rule Post-Acute DRG	FY 2010 Final Rule Special Pay DRG	MDC	Type	MS-DRG Title	Weights	Geometric mean LOS	Arithmetic mean LOS
068	No	No	01	MED	Nonspecific CVA & precerebral occlusion w/o infarct w/o MCC	0.8593	2.7	3.4
069	No	No	01	MED	Transient ischemia	0.7289	2.4	2.9
070	Yes	No	01	MED	Nonspecific cerebrovascular disorders w MCC	1.7919	5.7	7.4
071	Yes	No	01	MED	Nonspecific cerebrovascular disorders w CC	1.1027	4.1	5.2
072	Yes	No	01	MED	Nonspecific cerebrovascular disorders w/o CC/MCC	0.7616	2.6	3.3
073	No	No	01	MED	Cranial & peripheral nerve disorders w MCC	1.2939	4.5	6.0
074	No	No	01	MED	Cranial & peripheral nerve disorders w/o MCC	0.8380	3.3	4.1
075	No	No	01	MED	Viral meningitis w CC/MCC	1.6670	5.7	7.3
076	No	No	01	MED	Viral meningitis w/o CC/MCC	0.8336	3.3	3.9
077	No	No	01	MED	Hypertensive encephalopathy w MCC	1.6245	5.3	6.6
078	No	No	01	MED	Hypertensive encephalopathy w MC	0.9822	3.6	4.3
079	No	No	01	MED	Hypertensive encephalopathy w/o CC/MCC	0.7359	2.7	3.2

Source: CMS 2009a, 44126.

MS-DRGs

In FY 2008, Medicare revamped the DRG system to incorporate severity of illness into the DRG payment system. While keeping the core elements and modifications made to DRGs over the years, this update should allow for more accurate payment for patients with multiple diagnoses. The first step in revising the DRG system consisted of consolidating DRGs by combining certain DRGs and eliminating all divisions based on age and divisions between "paired" DRGs, such as those divided based on the presence or absence of secondary conditions.

Three Levels of Severity

Medicare then reviewed all diagnoses on the CC list to determine how each impacted LOS and amount of resources used. The revised CC list was compared with CC lists in the all-patient refined diagnosis-related group (APR-DRG) and all-patient diagnosis-related group (AP-DRG) systems and other severity-based revisions of the DRG system. Conditions were divided into three different levels of severity: non-CC, CC, and MCC.

The lowest level was assigned to those diagnoses that do not significantly affect severity of illness and resource usage and are known as "non-CCs." The diagnoses in the middle level of severity are known as CCs, and the highest level of severity are deemed MCC or major CC.

After this secondary diagnosis analysis, the 311 base MS-DRGs were then subdivided into the three CC subcategories with patients assigned to the subgroup with the most extreme CC present. Each base MS-DRG may be subdivided based on the severity of the patient's secondary diagnoses. These three groups are as follows:

1. Patients with no other secondary diagnoses (dx) or with all other secondary dx that are non-CCs

2. Patients with at least one secondary dx that is a CC, but the patient does not have any MCCs

3. Patients with at least one other secondary dx that is classified as an MCC

For example, in the category of heart failure, code 428.21, Acute systolic heart failure is considered an MCC; 428.1, Left heart failure counts as a CC; and 428.0, Congestive heart failure is a non-CC.

Not all base MS-DRGs are subdivided into three different subcategories. CMS established criteria in order to determine the necessity for division of MS-DRGs into CC and MCC subgroups. Those criteria are as follows:

- Reduction in variance of charges of at least 3 percent
- At least 5 percent of patients in the base MS-DRG fall in CC or MCC subgroup
- At least 500 cases are in the CC or MCC subgroup
- At least a 20-percent difference in average charges between subgroups
- $4,000 difference in average charges between subgroups

For FY 2008, there were a total of 745 MS-DRGs. Fifty-three of those are not subdivided into different subgroups and 456 are base groups divided into three subgroups. One-hundred-twenty-six MS-DRGs consist of base MS-DRGs divided into two subgroups: MCC and CC in one group and non-CCs in another subgroup, while 86 are made up of two subdivisions: non-CC and CC together and MCC in a separate subgroup. Twenty-two consist of mothers and babies in MDC 14, and there are two error MS-DRGs. Hyde and Spencer (2008) provide additional information on the comparisons between the DRG and MS-DRG systems. Some examples are shown in table 3.5.

Hospital-Acquired Conditions (HACs)

Federal law requires Medicare to select at least two conditions that are:

1. High cost, high volume, or both

2. Assigned to a higher-paying MS-DRG when present as a secondary diagnosis (are considered CCs or MCCs)

3. Could reasonably have been prevented through the application of evidence-based guidelines (CMS 2009a, 43782)

As part of Medicare's "pay for performance" policies, hospitals are no longer rewarded with higher reimbursement for conditions that could have been prevented. In order to capture this information, since 2007 hospitals have been required to indicate whether or not each

Table 3.5.   Examples of comparisons between DRG and MS-DRG systems

FY08 MS-DRG V25	FY08 MS-DRG Descriptions	FY08 Weight	FY08 1=Txfer 2=Spl Pay	FY07 CMS DRG V24	FY07 CMS V24 DRG Description	FY07 Weight	FY07 1=Txfer DRG 2=Spl Pay
177	Respiratory infections & inflammations w MCC	1.8444	1	079	Respiratory infections & inflammations age greater 17 w/ CC	1.6268	1
178	Respiratory infections & inflammations w CC	1.5636	1	080	Respiratory infections & inflammations age greater 17 w/o CC	0.8943	1
179	Respiratory infections & inflammations w/o CC/MCC	1.2754	1	081	Respiratory infections & inflammations age 0-17	1.5579	
180	Respiratory neoplasms w MCC	1.5550		082	Respiratory neoplasm	1.4121	1
181	Respiratory neoplasms w CC	1.3126					
182	Respiratory neoplasms w/o CC/MCC	1.1455					
183	Major chest trauma w MCC	1.2664		083	Major chest trauma w CC	1.0308	1
184	Major chest trauma w CC	0.9611		084	Major chest trauma w/o CC	0.6028	1
185	Major chest trauma w/o CC/MCC	0.7298					
186	Pleural effusion w MCC	1.4542	1	085	Pleural effusion w/ CC	1.2459	1
187	Pleural effusion w CC	1.1947	1	086	Pleural effusion w/o CC	0.7132	1
188	Pleural effusion w/o CC/MCC	0.9745	1				
189	Pulmonary edema & respiratory failure	1.3660		087	Pulmonary edema & respiratory failure	1.3838	
190	Chronic obstructive pulmonary disease w MCC	1.1138	1	088	Chronic obstructive pulmonary disease	0.8878	
191	Chronic obstructive pulmonary disease w CC	0.9405	1				
192	Chronic obstructive pulmonary disease w/o CC/MCC	0.8145	1				
193	Simple pneumonia & pleurisy w MCC	1.2505	1	089	Simple pneumonia & pleurisy age greater 17 w/ CC	1.0376	1
194	Simple pneumonia & pleurisy w CC	1.0235	1	090	Simple pneumonia & pleurisy age greater 17 w/o CC	0.6148	1
195	Simple pneumonia & pleurisy w/o CC/MCC	0.8398	1	091	Simple pneumonia age 0-17	0.5598	
196	Interstitial lung disease w MCC	1.3781	1	092	Interstitial lung disease w/ CC	1.1979	1
197	Interstitial lung disease w CC	1.1458	1	093	Interstitial lung disease w/o CC	0.7437	1
198	Interstitial lung disease w/o CC/MCC	0.9654	1				
199	Pneumothorax w MCC	1.4699		094	Pneumothorax w/ CC	1.1474	
200	Pneumothorax w CC	1.0753		095	Pneumothorax w/o CC	0.5871	
201	Pneumothorax w/o CC/MCC	0.8588					
202	Bronchitis & asthma w CC/MCC	0.7841		096	Bronchitis & asthma age greater 17 w/ CC	0.7350	
203	Bronchitis & asthma w/o CC/MCC	0.6252		097	Bronchitis & asthma age greater 17 w/o CC	0.5429	
				098	Bronchitis & asthma age 0-17	0.5870	
204	Respiratory signs & symptoms	0.6658		099	Respiratory signs and symptoms w/ CC	0.7155	
				100	Respiratory signs and symptoms w/o CC	0.5411	

Table available at CMS website: htpp://www.cms.hhs.gov/Medicare/AcuteInpatientPPS/
Inpatient PPS/Acute Inpatient—Files for Download Crosswalk for CMS DRGs to MS-DRGs
Table 5 FY08 and Table 5 FY07 lists DRG weights

Source: Hyde and Spencer 2008, appendix B, 68.

patient's medical conditions were "present on admission" (POA). If a condition on the hospital-acquired condition list was present on the patient's admission, Medicare will continue to assign the patient's discharge to a higher-paying MS-DRG. If a patient acquires a condition that is on the HAC list after admission (not POA), it will be grouped into an MS-DRG as if that condition was not present. For example, if a patient was admitted with secondary condition of a stage III pressure ulcer, this would count as a CC and the patient's case would be grouped into a higher-weighted MS-DRG. However, if this condition occurred after admission then the hospital would be paid as though the pressure ulcer did not exist because this should have been a preventable condition. Figure 3.2 lists the 2010 hospital-acquired conditions (CMS 2009a, 43782–43783).

DRG Modifications

Even though some insurance companies use the DRG methodology for payment purposes, CMS is quick to point out that DRGs are designed to classify the Medicare patient population only. Because of this, revisions have been made over the years to develop systems that group patients of all types. AP-DRGs group patients of all ages, including the pediatric population, into DRGs based on factors such as birth weight, neonatal age, trauma, and substance abuse.

Figure 3.2.   Medicare-defined current Hospital-Acquired Conditions

Hospital-Acquired Conditions	CC/MCC (ICD-9-CM code)
Foreign object retained after surgery	998.4 (CC), 998.7 (CC)
Air embolism	999.1 (MCC)
Blood incompatibility	999.6 (CC)
Pressure ulcer stages III and IV	707.23 (MCC), 707.24 (MCC)
Falls and Trauma: Codes within these ranges on the CC/MCC list: —Fracture —Dislocation —Intracranial injury —Crushing injury —Burn —Electric shock	 800–829 830–839 850–854 925–929 940–949 991–994
Catheter-associated urinary tract infection	996.64 (CC) Also excludes the following from acting as a CC/MCC: 112.2 (CC), 590.10 (CC), 590.11 (MCC), 590.2 (MCC), 590.3 (CC), 590.80 (CC), 590.81 (CC), 595.0 (CC), 597.0 (CC), 599.0 (CC)
Vascular catheter-associated infection	999.31 (CC)
Manifestations of poor glycemic control	250.10–250.13 (MCC), 250.20–250.23 (MCC), 251.0 (CC), 249.10–249.11 (MCC), 249.20–249.21 (MCC)
Surgical Site Infections	
Surgical site infection, mediastinitis, following coronary artery bypass graft	519.2 (MCC) And one of the following procedure codes: 36.10–36.19
Surgical site infection following certain orthopedic procedures	996.67 (CC), 998.59 (CC) And one of the following procedure codes: 81.01–81.08, 81.23–81.24, 81.31–81.38, 81.83, 81.85
Surgical site infection following bariatric surgery for obesity	*Principal Diagnosis*—278.01, 998.59 (CC) And one of the following procedure codes: 44.38, 44.39, or 44.95
Deep vein thrombosis and pulmonary embolism following certain orthopedic procedures	415.11 (MCC), 415.19 (MCC), 453.40–453.42 (CC) And one of the following procedure codes: 00.85–00.87, 81.51–81.52, or 81.54

Source: CMS 2009a, 43783.

The APR-DRG methodology was designed by 3M Healthcare and uses the AP-DRG system as its base. It also uses two other measures to assign patients to categories that include mortality risk and severity of illness factors, assigning patients to subclasses that identify minor, moderate, major, or extreme severity of illness or risk of mortality.

Case-Mix Index

The case-mix index for a hospital is defined as the average MS-DRG weight for all patients over a specified time period. A high case-mix index would signify that the patients treated in the facility were, on average, sicker than those in facilities with a lower case-mix index.

Other Uses of MS-DRGs

Although MS-DRGs are primarily used for payment, the hospital can use the data for many other purposes. One purpose is for utilization review. By examining the MS-DRG data, the facility can examine utilization patterns among similar groups of patients to study variances and problem areas. Hospitals can review differences among physicians to determine reasons for variations in practice patterns or overutilization of ancillary services. Reports can be generated, such as top 10 MS-DRGs, which can provide data that can be reviewed to determine appropriateness of services or provide topics for auditing.

Financial services can use the data for hospital cost analysis with up-to-date information on MS-DRGs for patients being discharged and the costs for treating these patients. Revenue can be monitored in a timely fashion to detect potential problems. Additionally, data can be used to help plan for new services, such as determining whether the facility should expand certain services. Moreover, they can be used for benchmarking best practices with other, similar facilities for epidemiology studies and research. As discussed in chapter 1, Medicare and other third-party payers are utilizing pay-for-performance quality incentives to tie reimbursement to quality of care. The data obtained during MS-DRG assignment are used in part to enable facilities to meet reporting requirements.

Transition to ICD-10

The Department of Health and Human Services published in the *Federal Register* on January 16, 2009, a final rule to establish a timeline for implementation of ICD-10-CM and ICD-10-PCS. These two coding systems will be adopted as the national standards under the HIPAA electronic transactions and coding standards rule to replace the current uses of ICD-9-CM. The effective date for this rule is October 1, 2013 (45 CFR 162).

The transition from ICD-9-CM to ICD-10-CM and ICD-10-PCS will be a tremendous effort. Extensive training sessions and coding materials are being developed to assist coders and facilities with this transition. Because the MS-DRG system is currently based on ICD-9-CM diagnoses and procedure codes, all groups must be "mapped" to the new coding system. General Equivalence Mappings (GEM) documents, also referred to as crosswalks and mappings, are available for diagnoses and procedures and include a reimbursement map that will help with the transition (AHIMA 2009).

CMS has indicated that, initially, PPS case-mix groups that rely on diagnosis and procedure codes including MS-DRGs should not fundamentally change. Mapping methodologies will be used to map the ICD-10-CM and ICD-10-PCS codes to the case-mix group where the corresponding ICD-9-CM code was assigned. In cases when there is no straightforward map, CMS will select the case-mix group that is believed to be the "best fit." Once CMS has collected sufficient claims data coded in ICD-10-CM and ICD-10-PCS, appropriate refinements will be made to the case-mix groups as warranted. CMS is planning to map the new coding systems into its current DRG system. Therefore, hospitals should arrive at the same MS-DRG assignment even though a new coding system is used. There may be a small number of cases where this is not possible because of combination codes within the ICD-10-CM diagnosis system. These cases will be handled on an individual basis, and the most appropriate MS-DRG assignment will be proposed (AHIMA 2009).

Summary

The DRG payment system, which has been in place now for approximately 27 years, just changed to MS-DRGs and is used by Medicare to pay for hospital inpatient admissions. Each year, as the system is updated, it attempts to accurately reflect appropriate payment necessary to treat the changing Medicare population. Medicare is moving ahead in its plans to capture more severity-of-illness information about the Medicare population. The adoption of the MS-DRG system update has brought major changes to this payment system, so coders should familiarize themselves with these updates and various alternatives also being discussed and used by other insurance companies to pay for hospital inpatient care.

References

45 CFR 162: Final Rule. HIPAA administrative simplification: Modifications to medical data code set standards to adopt ICD-10-CM and ICD-10-PCS. 2009 (Jan. 16). http://edocket.access.gpo.gov/2009/pdf/E9-743.pdf.

American Health Information Management Association. 2009. About ICD-10 codes. http://ahima.org/icd10/about.html.

Centers for Medicare and Medicaid Services. 2007 (Aug. 22). 42 CFR Parts 411, 412, 413, and 489. Changes to the hospital inpatient prospective payer systems and fiscal year 2008 rates; Final Rule. *Federal Register* 72(162):47130–48175. http://edocket.access.gpo.gov/2007/pdf/07-3820.pdf.

Centers for Medicare and Medicaid Services. 2009a (Aug. 27). 42 CFR Parts 412, 413, 415, et al. Medicare program; Changes to the hospital inpatient prospective payment systems for acute care hospitals and fiscal year 2010 rates; Changes to the long-term care hospital prospective payment system and rate years 2010 and 2009 rates; Final Rule. *Federal Register* 74(165). http://edocket.access.gpo.gov/2009/pdf/E9-18663.pdf.

Centers for Medicare and Medicaid Services. 2009b. Fact Sheet: Medicare Disproportionate-Share Hospital. http://www.cms.gov/MLNProducts/downloads/2009_mdsh.pdf.

Centers for Medicare and Medicaid Services. 2010a. Acute inpatient PPS overview: Steps in determining a PPS payment. http://www.cms.hhs.gov/AcuteInpatientPPS/02_stepspps.asp.

Centers for Medicare and Medicaid Services. 2010b. Acute Inpatient PPS: Wage Index Files. http://www.cms.gov/AcuteInpatientPPS/downloads/WI_Tables_FY2009_Final.zip.

Health and Human Services. 1985 (July 31). Uniform Hospital Discharge Data Set. *Federal Register* 50(147): 31038–31040.

Hyde, L.A., and C. Spencer. 2008. *Analyzing the Financial Impact of MS-DRGs.* Chicago: AHIMA.

Kennedy, J. 2008. *Severity DRGs and Reimbursement: An MS-DRG Primer.* Chicago: AHIMA.

Chapter 4

Structure and Organization of Other Medicare Inpatient Prospective Payment Systems

Because the federal government considered diagnosis-related groups (DRGs) to be helpful in managing costs and resource consumption in the acute care hospital inpatient setting, over the years legislation has been passed that requires prospective payment–type systems in other healthcare settings. This chapter discusses some of the Medicare systems in place for reimbursement in inpatient settings other than acute care hospitals. These include long-term acute care hospitals (LTCHs), inpatient rehabilitation facilities (IRFs), and inpatient psychiatric facilities (IPFs).

Long-Term Care Prospective Payment System

The Balanced Budget Refinement Act of 1999 (BBRA) and the Benefits Improvement and Protection Act of 2000 established the requirements for a prospective payment system (PPS) for LTCHs, effective with discharges on or after October 1, 2002. Medicare defines LTCHs as hospitals that (CMS Office of Public Affairs 2007):

> . . . have an average inpatient length of stay greater than 25 days. These hospitals typically provide extended medical and rehabilitative care for patients who are clinically complex and may suffer from multiple acute or chronic conditions. Services may include comprehensive rehabilitation, respiratory therapy, cancer treatment, head trauma treatment, and pain management.

LTCHs provide "acute" care and should not be confused with the "long-term care" that is rendered by skilled nursing facilities (SNFs). In addition, although most patients in the LTCH setting receive rehabilitation services, those patients are usually not medically able to tolerate the 3 hours of therapy per day as required by IRFs. The LTCH PPS is based on the inpatient PPS (IPPS) system with modifications made to account for differences in the long-term care patient and was started in 2003. When Medicare updated the Medicare severity adjusted diagnosis-related group (MS-DRG) system in fiscal year (FY) 2008, the long-term care DRG system was also updated to a modified MS-LTC-DRG system. There are also special rules covering occurrences such as short stays, very-high-cost admissions, and interrupted stays. Patients' stays are grouped into categories known as Medicare severity-adjusted long-term care hospital diagnosis-related groups (MS-LTC-DRGs), based on their diagnoses, procedures performed, and discharge status. Like the inpatient MS-DRG system, the MS-LTC-DRG groupings are assigned "an appropriate weight to the MS-LTC-DRGs to account for the difference in resource use by patients exhibiting the case complexity and multiple medical problems characteristic of LTCHs" (CMS 2009b, 43948).

Also like the DRG system, the MS-LTC-DRG system was designed to pay only one amount of reimbursement per hospitalization, which is assigned on a per-discharge basis.

The major elements of the LTCH PPS are described in the following sections.

Classification as an LTCH

To qualify as an LTCH, a provider must have an agreement with Medicare and must have an average Medicare inpatient length of stay (LOS) of greater than 25 days. An alternative classification is applied to providers that were first excluded from PPS in 1986 and can demonstrate that at least 80 percent of their annual Medicare inpatient discharges in the 12-month reporting period ending in FY 1997 have a principal diagnosis of neoplastic disease and an average inpatient LOS for all patients (both Medicare and non-Medicare) of greater than 20 days (CMS 2009b, 43947).

Department of Veterans Affairs (VA) hospitals, hospitals reimbursed under state cost-control systems, and hospitals reimbursed in accordance with demonstration projects are paid under special payment provisions and are not subject to LTCH PPS rules (CMS 2009b, 43947).

MS-LTC-DRGs

Patients are grouped into DRG-type groupings based on the clinical aspects of their disease as well as the amount of resources needed for their care (CMS 2009b, 43947–43948). Each MS-LTC-DRG is weighted, as with the IPPS weights, to reflect patients treated in LTCH-type settings. In a departure from the IPPS, low-volume MS-LTC-DRGs (those with less than 25 LTCH cases) are grouped into five quintiles based on average charge per discharge. These quintiles are then used to develop the relative weights for those MS-LTC-DRGs, because LTCHs do not usually treat the full range of diagnoses that an acute care hospital would treat (CMS 2009b, 43947–43948).

The average LTCH base rate that is multiplied by the relative weight for the MS-LTC-DRG is approximately $39,000, as compared with an average base rate for a short-term acute care hospital of approximately $5,000 (CMS 2009b, 43947–43948).

Payment Adjustments

A 5-year transition period was implemented on October 1, 2002, to phase in the PPS for LTCHs from cost-based reimbursement to 100 percent federal prospective payment. Payment was based on an increasing percentage of the LTCH PPS amount and a decreasing percentage of the cost-based reimbursement rate for each discharge. This phase-in period was typical of that used with the other types of prospective payment methods to prevent undue financial hardship on facilities in the early days of the new systems. According to CMS (CMS 2009b, 43945), "for cost reporting periods beginning on or after October 1, 2006, all LTCHs are paid 100 percent of the adjusted federal rate under the LTCH PPS."

Unlike IPPS, the FY, or rate year (RY), was set to begin on July 1 each year and end on June 30, which would require two updates per year. In July, the federal payment rate was updated, and in October the MS-LTC-DRGs and relative weights would be updated to incorporate the annual October 1 ICD-9-CM and IPPS changes in conjunction with payment adjustments for IPPS. In the May 9, 2008, LTCH PPS Final Rule for RY 2009, the annual update for payment or RY was consolidated, beginning with RY 2010, so that the updates to the rates and relative weights are now effective on October 1 of each year. Although ICD-9-CM codes may be updated twice per year, the groupings and relative weights established in the MS-LTC-DRG system are updated only in October. See table 4.1 for a portion of the MS-LTC-DRG list. Additional information on MS-LTC-DRGs is available from the Centers for Medicare and Medicaid Services (CMS) LTCH PPS overview (CMS 2009b, 43947–43948).

Similar to the IPPS, facility payment is based on a set fee per discharge that takes into account the resources used to care for the patient. Adjustments are made for short-stay cases,

Table 4.1. Portion of the MS-LTC-DRG list

MS-LTC-DRG	MS-DRG Title	FY 2008 LTCH Cases	FY 2010 Relative Weight	Geometric Average Length of Stay	Short Stay Outlier Threshold
1	Heart transplant or implant of heart assist system w MCC	0	0.0000	0.0	0.0
2	Heart transplant or implant of heart assist system w/o MCC	0	0.0000	0.0	0.0
3	ECMO or trach w MV 96+ hrs or PDX exc face, mouth, and neck w maj O.R.	290	4.5845	65.2	54.3
4	Trach w MV 96+ hrs or PDX exc face, mouth, and neck w/o maj O.R.	1,401	3.1040	45.3	37.8
5	Liver transplant w MCC or intestinal transplant	0	0.0000	0.0	0.0
6	Liver transplant w/o MCC	0	0.0000	0.0	0.0
7	Lung transplant	0	0.0000	0.0	0.0
8	Simultaneous pancreas/ kidney transplant	0	0.0000	0.0	0.0
9	Bone marrow transplant	0	1.6608	37.7	31.4
10	Pancreas transplant	0	0.0000	0.0	0.0
11	Tracheostomy for face, mouth, and neck diagnoses w MCC	2	1.6608	37.7	31.4
12	Tracheostomy for face, mouth, and neck diagnoses w CC	0	1.1636	24.1	20.1
13	Tracheostomy for face, mouth, and neck diagnoses w/o CC/MCC	0	1.1636	24.1	20.1
20	Intracranial vascular procedures w PDX hemorrhage w MCC	0	1.6608	37.7	31.4
21	Intracranial vascular procedures w PDX hemorrhage w CC	0	0.6392	21.6	18.0
22	Intracranial vascular procedures w PDX hemorrhage w/o CC/MCC	0	0.6392	21.6	18.0
23	Cranio w major dev impl/ acute complex CNS PDX w MCC	1	0.7552	24.0	20.0

Source: CMS 2009c.

interrupted stays, readmissions within a certain time frame, cost outliers, and geographic wage rate and cost-of-living increases.

Interrupted Stays

Interrupted-stay cases are those in which patients have an "intervening" stay during the time of their long-term care admission. There are two categories of interrupted stays: 3-day or less interrupted stay, and greater than 3-day interrupted stay. The 3-day or less interrupted stay policy provides that only one payment will be made to the LTCH for that patient. Any off-site tests or medical treatment, either inpatient or outpatient delivered at an acute care hospital, IRF, or SNF will be covered by the LTCH "under arrangements" if the patient is readmitted to the LTCH within 3 days. All days of the 3-day or less interruption will be counted in the patient's LOS for the LTCH, as it impacts the 25-day average LOS, unless the patient went home during that interruption (CMS 2007b, 273–275).

The greater than 3-day interrupted stay is defined as when a patient who is discharged from the LTCH to an acute care hospital, an IRF, or a SNF for a period greater than 3 days, but is readmitted to the LTCH within the applicable fixed day period (between 4 to 9 days for acute care, 4 to 27 days for an IRF, and 4 to 45 days for a SNF). The interrupted stay is treated as one discharge from the LTCH and generates only one MS-LTC-DRG payment. However, the acute care hospital, IRF, or SNF bills Medicare separately for treatment or care given to the patient during the interruption (CMS 2007b, 273–275).

LTCH hospitals that are colocated with other Medicare providers, such as hospitals within hospitals, satellite facilities, and on-site SNFs, are subject to the interrupted stay policy. However, if that facility's discharges and readmissions exceed 50 percent for a cost-reporting period, then all readmissions during that cost-reporting period are paid as one discharge regardless of time. CMS defines a hospital within a hospital as part of a hospital that provides inpatient services in a building also used by another hospital or in another building or buildings on the same campus (CMS 2004a; CMS 2005; CMS 2006a).

The day count for purposes of determining the LOS away from the LTCH begins on the day that the patient is first discharged from the LTCH, which is also the day of admission to the other facility (CMS 2004a; CMS 2005; CMS 2006a).

Short-Stay Outliers

Cases where the LOS is between 1 day and up to and including five-sixths of the average geometric mean length of stay (GMLOS) for the respective MS-LTC-DRG are considered short-stay outliers (SSOs).

SSOs are reimbursed in one of four ways:

1. 100 percent of the cost of the case

2. 120 percent of the MS-LTC-DRG per diem (per day) amount

3. The full MS-LTC-DRG amount

4. A blend of the IPPS amount for the DRG and 120 percent of the MS-LTC-DRG per diem amount

This policy was revised for RY 2008 for cases where the LOS is less than or equal to the average LOS for the same MS-LTC-DRG, known as the IPPS comparable threshold. These cases will be paid similarly to other SSOs, except for the IPPS per diem amount, which is multiplied by the LOS. The deciding factor for which payment option is used is determining if the SSO exceeds the IPPS threshold (MLN n.d.).

The Medicare, Medicaid, and State Children's Health Insurance Program (SCHIP) Extension Act of 2007 (MMSEA) included additional policy changes that impact LTCH hospitals. The first provision was a 3-year delay in applying the fourth payment adjustment option just described for SSOs. A second provision was a 3-year moratorium on establishment of new LTCHs and LTCH satellite facilities, and increases in beds in existing LTCHs and LTCH satellite facilities. An additional provision was a 3-year delay in certain payment adjustments for colocated and non-colocated LTCHs and LTCH satellites (CMS 2009b, 43946–43947).

Medicare also removes cases with an LOS of 7 or fewer days from statistical formulas when setting MS-LTC-DRG relative weights because these stays alter the law-of-averages principle on which the DRG system was built (CMS 2009b, 43959).

Hospital-Specific Relative Value Method

LTCHs tend to specialize in treating different groups of patients; for example, ventilator-dependent patients, or those requiring rehabilitation or wound care. As a result, the CMS developed an adjustment method known as the hospital-specific relative value method. This method converts charges for each LTCH into hospital-specific relative values (HSRVs) based on that hospital's average charge (which, by definition, averages 1.0 for each LTCH) that then are adjusted based on the individual hospital's case mix. This average adjusted charge (HSRV) reflects the complexity of the cases treated by a particular hospital relative to the complexity of cases treated by all other LTCHs. The resulting ratio is then multiplied by that LTCH's case-mix index to determine the standardized charge for a particular case (CMS 2009b, 43952–43953).

Other Adjustments

CMS established a policy for determining an LTCH PPS wage index value for core-based statistical areas (CBSAs) where there are no IPPS wage data. The fixed-loss amount for high-cost outlier cases was increased. Estimated aggregate high-cost outlier case payments are limited to 8% of total estimated LTCH payments. CMS also developed a market basket increase, similar to that in IPPS, to account for price increases in services provided. Currently, the market basket increase applied to LTCHs is based on data from IRFs, IPFs, and LTCHs. CMS is moving toward developing separate market baskets for IRFs, IPFs, and LTCHs for the future (CMS 2009b, 43945–43952).

CMS also applies the same methodology to LTCHs as to short-term hospitals for offsetting payment adjustments for changes in case-mix index due to changes in documentation and coding practices rather than increases in patient severity of illness (CMS 2009b, 43945–43952).

Expanded Review of Medical Necessity

The MMSEA of 2007 also included provision for expansion of medical necessity review of LTCH patients for discharges occurring on or after October 1, 2007. The reviews are to occur on an annual basis, and the fiscal intermediary or contractor must "guarantee" that 75 percent of overpayments of medically unnecessary admissions to LTCHs are identified and recovered. The days related to those medically unnecessary admissions will not count toward the average 25-day LOS to qualify as an LTCH.

Documentation of medical necessity must start prior to admission and continue throughout the stay. The law requires a 48-hour validation of medical necessity that is documented in the medical record. LTCHs must develop a process to screen patients prior to admission for appropriateness as an LTCH patient and validation within 48 hours that LTCH admission criteria are met. The criteria to be used are not specified in the statute. The admission criteria (such as InterQual, Milliman, and so on) should be approved by the Medical Executive Committee and Board for the LTCH. In addition to the 48-hour validation, there must be documentation of continued stay review throughout the patient's stay. The statute also requires documentation that there is active physician involvement with patients during their treatment. All services by the treatment team must be physician-directed, with physician on-site availability on a daily basis to review progress. Also, consulting physicians must be "on call" and available to be at the patient's bedside within a reasonable period of time, if needed.

Unique Coding Challenges for LTCHs

Coders must follow the same rules as those used for coding IPPSs, which includes following official coding guidelines and the Uniform Hospital Discharge Data Set (UHDDS) definitions. This includes the definition for principal diagnosis, complications, comorbidities, those conditions that affect treatment, and all procedures performed during the patient's stay. The same grouper software is used for calculating MS-LTC-DRGs as is used for inpatient DRG grouping with relative weights that are reflective of patients in the long-term acute care setting. Payment rates are based on data in the MedPar database consisting of claims previously submitted by LTCHs (Bronnert 2008).

The complexity of coding LTCH cases is based on the fact that many of the conditions have been completely or partially treated in the short-term acute care hospital, prior to transfer to the LTCH. Coders must determine which conditions have been resolved prior to the LTCH admission, which ones are unresolved acute and/or chronic conditions that will continue to be treated in the LTCH, and which ones are late effects of a previously treated condition. Each case must be evaluated on its unique set of circumstances and coded according to the documentation in the medical record. Often the physician documentation on admission to the LTCH includes information and diagnoses applicable to the short-term stay that do not apply to the reason for transfer to the LTCH. Depending on the documentation, either a code reflecting the acute condition(s) responsible for transfer to the LTCH or an Admission for Rehab code would be designated as principal diagnosis. If physician documentation as to the reason for transfer to the LTCH and which conditions still require treatment is unclear, physician queries should be generated for clarification. *Coding Clinic* has published guidelines and coding examples specific to the LTCH setting (AHA 2003; CMS 2005, 24177).

In addition, for cases that meet the guidelines for an interrupted stay, the original claim for the initial portion of the stay should be deleted and a second claim submitted to cover the entire interrupted stay. The principal diagnosis and other conditions coded should be reflective of both portions of the interrupted stay, so that the case can be assigned to the proper MS-LTC-DRG (CMS 2005, 24204).

Inpatient Rehabilitation Facility PPS

Implementation of a per discharge PPS for IRFs was authorized in section 4421 of the Balanced Budget Act of 1997 (Public Law 105-33), as amended by section 125 of the Medicare,

Medicaid, and SCHIP Balanced Budget Refinement Act of 1999 (Public Law 106-113), and by section 305 of the Medicare, Medicaid, and SCHIP Benefits Improvement and Protection Act of 2000 (Public Law 106-554), authorized through new section 1886(j) of the Social Security Act (CMS 2009a, 39763).

In 1995, CMS sponsored a study by the RAND Corporation to develop an IRF per discharge PPS using a system known as functional independence measures–functional-related groups (FIM-FRGs). This study was updated in 1999 to reflect payment information, including facility payment adjustments and the impact of other diagnoses (comorbidities) on patient resource utilization.

To account for the types of patients treated in IRFs, this system uses information from the patient assessment instrument (PAI). The information from the resulting IRF-PAI is entered electronically into grouper software, which determines the health insurance prospective payment system (HIPPS) codes used to establish reimbursement. The software is known as Inpatient Rehabilitation Validation and Entry (IRVEN) and is provided at no cost to facilities (CMS 2009a, 39764).

The HIPPS codes then are grouped into 1 of 100 case-mix groups (CMGs), which determine reimbursement for the hospitalization.

Qualification as an IRF

CMS has one criterion to classify a hospital or distinct unit of a hospital as an IRF. The criterion specifies that a minimum percentage of a facility's total inpatient population must require intensive rehabilitation services for the treatment of certain medical conditions. The original rule specified that to qualify as an IRF, 75 percent of the patients treated must require intensive rehabilitation services for 1 of 13 medical conditions (see Figure 4.1). This is known as the "percent rule" (Casto and Layman 2009, 132–133; CMS 2007a, 26233). Because payment rates for an IRF are substantially higher for providing rehabilitation services than the IPPS rates for similar services, the percent rule (or compliance threshold) would serve to ensure that the patient is treated in the most appropriate facility and that appropriate payments are made to each type of provider.

In the May 2004 Final Rule, the 75 percent compliance threshold was temporarily lowered, with a transition period to allow hospitals to obtain the 75 percent threshold. During this transition period, there was a shift in the types of conditions treated in the IRF setting. The number of strokes, brain injuries, and nervous system complications had risen, whereas the numbers of patients treated for joint replacements, cardiac conditions, osteoarthritis, and pain syndrome had decreased. The 13 conditions that qualify for IRF services include "bilateral" knee or hip joint replacements immediately preceding the IRF stay that also meet one of three additional criteria. However, CMS developed a proposal to reimburse IRFs for unilateral knee, unilateral hip replacements, and unilateral hip fractures at reduced rates based on the average SNF payments for these conditions plus an allowance for higher overhead and patient care costs unique to IRFs. This proposal is intended to focus payment on the needs of the patients, rather than on the setting of the services rendered. This proposal has not yet been adopted (CMS 2007a).

To count in the IRF's percentage rate, several of the conditions require that the patient must have had an acute hospitalization for the condition, and documented evidence must show that the less aggressive treatment (at least twice per week) administered for a 3-week period failed within 20 days following admission. If a facility does not meet the requirements during a 12-month period, the hospital will lose certification as an IRF and will be paid under the methodology for an acute care facility.

During the transition period for the 75 percent compliance threshold and prior to July 1, 2008, patients with the conditions listed in figure 4.1 as either principal or secondary diagnoses would count in the percentage rate. For discharges occurring after July 1, 2008, the condition must be the first-listed principal diagnosis (main reason for the admission) or the patient would not be counted in the overall percentage rate. However, the MMSEA revised the compliance threshold to 60 percent ("the 60 percent rule") and continued the practice of including co-morbidities in the calculation of the compliance percentage (CMS 2009a, 39798).

For rehabilitation hospitals or distinct rehabilitation units of hospitals classified as an IRF after June 3, 2004, failure to meet the IRF requirements specified in subpart B of Part 412 will result in termination of the facility's classification as an IRF. Payment contractors will use

Figure 4.1. IRF qualified medical conditions

- Stroke
- Spinal cord injury
- Congenital deformity
- Amputation
- Major multiple trauma
- Femur fracture (hip fracture)
- Brain injury
- Neurologic disorders, including multiple sclerosis, motor neuron diseases, polyneuropathy, muscular dystrophy, and Parkinson's disease
- Burns
- Active polyarticular rheumatoid arthritis, psoriatic arthritis, and seronegative arthropathies resulting in significant functional impairment of ambulation and other activities of daily living that have not improved after an appropriate, aggressive, and sustained course of outpatient therapy services or services in other, less intensive rehabilitation settings immediately preceding the inpatient rehabilitation admission or that result from a systemic disease activation immediately before admission but have the potential to improve with more intense rehabilitation
- Systemic vasculidities with joint inflammation arthropathies resulting in significant functional impairment of ambulation and other activities of daily living that have not improved after an appropriate, aggressive, and sustained course of outpatient therapy services or services in other, less intensive rehabilitation settings immediately preceding the inpatient rehabilitation admission or that result from a systemic disease activation immediately before admission but have the potential to improve with more intense rehabilitation
- Severe or advanced osteoarthritis (osteoarthrosis or degenerative joint disease) involving two or more major weight-bearing joints (elbows, shoulders, hips, or knees, but not counting a joint with a prosthesis) with joint deformity and substantial loss of range of motion, atrophy of muscles surrounding the joint, significant functional impairment of ambulation and other activities of daily living that have not improved after an appropriate, aggressive, and sustained course of outpatient therapy services or services in other, less intensive rehabilitation settings immediately preceding the inpatient rehabilitation admission or that result from a systemic disease activation immediately before admission but have the potential to improve with more intense rehabilitation. (A joint replaced by a prosthesis is no longer considered to have osteoarthritis or other arthritis, even though this condition was the reason for the replacement.)
- Knee or hip joint replacement, or both, during an acute hospitalization immediately preceding the hospital rehabilitation stay, which also meet one or more of the following specific criteria:
  — The patient underwent bilateral knee or bilateral hip joint replacement surgery during the acute hospital admission immediately preceding the IRF admission.
  — The patient is extremely obese with a body mass index of at least 50 at the time of admission to the IRF.
  — The patient is age 85 or older at the time of admission to the IRF.

Source: CMS 2004a, 25762–25766.

presumptive and medical review methodologies to review claims data and/or medical records to determine that the IRF still meets the compliance threshold (60 percent rule) to maintain its classification as an IRF. The Final Rule for FY 2010 also expands requirements for submission of an IRF-PAI to Medicare Part C (Medicare Advantage) patients for use in meeting the 60 percent compliance threshold, effective for compliance review periods on or after October 1, 2009 (CMS 2009a, 39798).

IRF-PAI and CMGs

The IRF PPS system is based on an 85-item rehabilitation-specific IRF-PAI. CMS developed an IRF-PAI Training Manual for use in completing the PAI (CMS 2009e). The manual was revised in 2004, and the guidelines included in the revised manual are mandatory for performing the assessment and submitting the IRF-PAI data electronically. The IRF-PAI must be completed for each patient on admission and again at discharge, according to specific timetables. Included in the assessment is a Functional Independence Assessment Tool for use in determining the patient's level of functional abilities. The functional abilities are divided into motor and cognitive functioning. The scores of both are totaled. The totals, along with the patient's diagnoses and age, determine the CMG for that patient (Casto and Layman 2009, 132–133).

Rehabilitation Impairment Categories

Prior to placing the patient in one of the CMGs, the patient is grouped into a major group reflective of the primary need for rehabilitation care, which is known as the rehabilitation impairment category (RIC). The primary reason for the patient's admission is coded using an impairment group code (IGC). There are 85 IGCs provided in the IRF-PAI Training Manual, Appendix A (a portion of which is shown in table 4.2). The IGCs determine which RIC the patient will fit into,

Table 4.2. Portion of Appendix A: Impairment group codes

Impairment Group Codes		
Impairment Group	**Code**	**Description**
Stroke	01.1 01.2 01.3 01.4 01.9	Left Body Involvement (Rt Brain) Rt Body Involvement (Left Brain) Bilateral Involvement No Paresis Other Stroke
Brain Dysfunction	02.1 02.21 02.22 02.9	Nontraumatic Traumatic, Open Injury Traumatic, Closed Injury Other Brain
Neurologic Condition	03.1 03.2 03.3 03.4 03.5 03.8 03.9	Multiple Sclerosis Parkinsonism Polyneuropathy Guillain-Barré Syndrome Cerebral Palsy Neuromuscular Disorders Other Neurologic Disorders

Source: CMS 2004b, A-1.

Figure 4.2.   List of RICs for IRFs

01	Stroke	13	Rheumatoid, Other Arthritis
02	Traumatic Brain Injury	14	Cardiac
03	Nontraumatic Brain Injury	15	Pulmonary
04	Traumatic Spinal Cord Injury	16	Pain Syndrome
05	Nontraumatic Spinal Cord Injury	17	Major multiple trauma, no brain injury or
06	Neurological		spinal cord injury
07	Fracture of Lower Extremity	18	Major multiple trauma, with brain or spinal
08	Replacement of Lower Extremity Joint		cord injury
09	Other Orthopedic	19	Guillain-Barré
10	Amputation, Lower Extremity	20	Miscellaneous
11	Amputation, Other	21	Burns
12	Osteoarthritis		

Source: Casto and Layman 2009, 138.

as determined by the pricer (Appendix B of Training Manual). Currently, there are 21 RICs in use in the IRF PPS system, as listed in figure 4.2 (Casto and Layman 2009, 138).

Etiologic Diagnoses

The IRF-PAI includes an ICD-9-CM code for the etiology of the problem that led to the condition requiring the inpatient rehabilitation services. Therefore, the "principal diagnosis" as defined by UHDDS is not reported on the IRF-PAI (see table 4.3).

Complications/Comorbidities

Complications are comorbidities that occur after admission to the IRF. Comorbidities are secondary diagnoses the patient has on admission in conjunction with his or her primary illness or injury. The presence of these comorbidities may impact resources used and the patient's rate of recovery. Therefore, the comorbidities were accounted for in the relative weight of each CMG. Just as in the other PPS systems, the relative weights help to differentiate between resources required to care for patients within the CMG. For instance, a weight of 2 means that, on average, it takes twice as many resources to care for patients than it would in a category with a weight of 1 (CMS 2009a, 39766).

These comorbid conditions are divided into three tiers based on associated costs. The "comorbidity tiers" represent comorbid conditions that have been shown statistically to increase the amount of resources consumed by the patient. For example, a diagnosis of acute myocardial infarction adds cost to the patient's care, so the facility is entitled to greater reimbursement. Some procedures, such as dialysis, also increase the costs associated with the patient's care, so patients undergoing those procedures are placed in tier 1. The comorbidity tiers are included in Appendix C of the IRF-PAI Training Manual. Tier 1 conditions are high-cost, tier 2 conditions are medium-cost, and tier 3 conditions are low-cost. Conditions inherent to a specific RIC are excluded from the relevant comorbidities for that RIC and do not impact the relative weight and payment for that RIC (see table 4.4).

Case-Mix Groups

Within each RIC, there are several CMGs based on established criteria related to the functional independence of the patient. CMS used a statistical method, known as classification and regression trees (CART), to effectively group the patients into the CMGs. The CMGs consist

Table 4.3. Portion of Appendix B: ICD-9-CM codes and etiologic diagnoses for impairment groups

Stroke (01) Includes cases with the diagnosis of cerebral ischemia due to vascular thrombosis, embolism, or hemorrhage.

Note: Do NOT use for cases w/ brain dysfunction secondary to nonvascular causes such as trauma, inflammation, tumor, or degenerative changes. These should be coded under Brain Dysfunction (02) instead.

Impairment Group	Impairment Group Code (Item 21)	RIC	ICD-9-CM Code (Item 22)	Etiologic Diagnosis
Stroke	01.1–01.9	Stroke (01)	430	Subarachnoid hemorrhage, including ruptured cerebral aneurysm
			431	Intracerebral hemorrhage
			432.0–432.9	Other and unspecified intracranial hemorrhage
			433.x1	Occlusion and stenosis precerebral arteries, w/ cerebral infarction
			434.x1	Occlusion cerebral arteries w/ cerebral infarction
			436	Acute, but ill-defined cerebrovascular disease
			438.0–438.9	Late effects of cerebrovascular disease **NOTE: Use only when an inpatient rehabilitation program has been completed for the same stroke prior to the current admission**

Source: CMS 2004b, B-1.

Note: DO NOT use codes 435.0–435.9 Transient cerebral ischemia (TIA).

Table 4.4. Portion of Appendix C: List of comorbidities

ICD-9	ICD-9-CM Label	Tier	RIC Exclusion
478.31	Vocal Paralysis unilateral partial	1	15
478.32	Vocal Paralysis unilateral total	1	15
008.42	Pseudomonas enteritis	2	
008.45	Intestinal infection Clostridium difficile	2	
787.20	Dysphagia NOS	2	01
787.23	Dysphagia pharyngeal	2	01
011.00	TB Lung infiltrate, unspecified	3	15
011.01	TB Lung infiltrate—no exam	3	15

Source: CMS 2004b, C-3.

of five-digit numbers. The first digit represents the comorbidity tier and the last four digits represent the actual case-mix grouping. Table 4.5 provides a sample of current CMGs. Within an RIC, the numbering of the CMG is hierarchical. Therefore, a CMG with a higher number indicates more complex cases requiring greater resources. There are 100 CMGs—95 are clinical and 5 are administrative, including 1 for short-stay cases and 4 for expired patients. These last four are based on the condition and the LOS for the case.

Table 4.5. Portion of relative weights and average LOS for CMGs for FY 2010

CMG	CMG Description (M = Motor, C = Cognitive, A = Age)	Relative Weights				Average Length of Stay			
		Tier 1	Tier 2	Tier 3	None	Tier 1	Tier 2	Tier 3	None
0101	Stroke M > 51.05	0.7547	0.7070	0.6484	0.6128	9	11	9	9
0102	Stroke M > 44.45 and M < 51.05 and C > 18.5	0.9248	0.8663	0.7945	0.7509	11	12	11	10
0103	Stroke M > 44.45 and M < 51.05 and C < 18.5	1.0798	1.0115	0.9277	0.8768	12	14	12	12
0104	Stroke M > 38.85 and M < 44.45	1.1632	1.0897	0.9993	0.9446	13	14	13	13
0105	Stroke M > 34.25 and M < 38.85	1.3697	1.2831	1.1767	1.1122	16	17	15	14

Source: CMS 2009a, 39767–39773.

CMGs are derived using criteria including age, functional status, and RICs. Patients are assigned to a CMG based on their ability to function in categories such as transfer, self-care, sphincter control, and movement, as well as 13 motor tasks and 5 cognitive tasks. New data added to the IRF-PAI also include items such as shortness of breath and presence of ulcers. According to instructions in the *CMS IRF-PAI Instruction Manual,* the cognitive and motor skills are evaluated and assigned a score from 0 to 7, with 7 meaning that the patient is very comfortable in performing the skill (CMS 2009e). A score of 1 indicates the patient requires total assistance in order to complete the task. A score of 0 means the skill was not assessed. Beginning in FY 2006, the motor skills scores were weighted based on the average ability of patients to perform the functions identified. See figure 4.3 for the motor and cognitive tasks that are evaluated to assess patients' functional status.

Each CMG was weighted to account for variation in resource consumption across the IRF patient spectrum, as well as the impact of additional (comorbid) diseases. The CMS software that assigns patients to CMGs is the Pricer. The Pricer uses the IGCs on the PAI to assign to an RIC, which then determines the CMG. There are four payment rates for each of the 95 clinical CMGs. One rate is for cases without a comorbid condition, and three rates for comorbid conditions based on the tier they fit into. Up to 10 comorbid conditions can be reported on the PAI. The Pricer selects the condition that assigns the case to the highest tier, with the highest payment. The base payment rate for FY 2010 is $13,661 (Casto and Layman 2009, 138–139).

Additionally, adjustments were made for a facility with a high percentage of low-income patients, wage variations, and rural location, as well as transfers, interrupted stays, and cost outliers (CMS 2009a, 39773). A new adjustment for teaching facilities was added in 2005. Table 4.6 presents the special CMGs not included in the RIC categories.

Similar to LTCHs, interrupted stays are cases where the patient is discharged from the IRF and returns within 3 calendar days. Only one payment is made, based on the CMG initial patient

Figure 4.3. Motor and cognitive tasks assessed on the IRF-PAI

Eating	Walking/wheelchair use
Grooming	Climbing stairs
Bathing	Cognitive skills:
Dressing upper body	Comprehension
Dressing lower body	Expression
Toileting	Social interaction
Bladder and bowel management	Problem solving
Transfer to:	Memory
Tub/shower, toilet, bed/chair/wheelchair	

Source: CMS 2006b.

Table 4.6. Special CMGs not included in the RIC categories for FY 2010

CMG	Description	Relative Weight	Average LOS
5001	Short-stay cases, LOS 3 days or less	0.1429	3
5101	Expired, Orthopedic, LOS 13 days or less	0.6001	8
5102	Expired, Orthopedic, LOS 14 days or more	1.5188	20
5103	Expired, Not Orthopedic, LOS 15 days or less	0.6998	8
5104	Expired, Not Orthopedic, LOS 16 days or more	1.8258	24

Source: CMS 2009a, 39767–39773.

assessment. A five-digit, alphanumeric HIPPS code is placed on the claim (Uniform Bill [UB]-04). The letter designates the comorbidity tier, and the last four digits reflect the CMG.

Transfers are defined as those patients transferred to another site of care after a stay in the IRF that is less than the average LOS for the CMG that the patient was grouped into. Transfers are paid a per diem case level adjustment (CMS 2007a, 26250–26251).

Coverage Requirements

The Final Rule for FY 2010 also includes new coverage requirements to be applied to individual claims. These coverage requirements are NOT to be confused with the requirements for classification as an IRF. Failure to meet the coverage criteria for a particular claim will only result in denial of that claim, not a change in the classification of the facility as an IRF.

The revised requirements relate to medical necessity and are required, effective with discharges occurring on or after January 1, 2010 (CMS 2009a, 39788–39797). They include the following:

1. Preadmission screening to be conducted by qualified clinicians within 48 hours immediately preceding the IRF admission and documented in the medical record. This comprehensive screening can be conducted earlier than 48 hours prior to IRF admission, as long as an update is performed within 48 hours of IRF admission.

2. Postadmission physician evaluation to be conducted within 24 hours after IRF admission and documented in the medical record.

3. An individualized plan of care developed by the rehabilitation MD, with input from the interdisciplinary team and documented in the medical record by the end of the fourth day after admission.

4. Evaluation of the appropriateness of the IRF admission, to indicate the patient's condition will allow him or her to participate in intensive rehabilitation therapy, usually defined as 3 hours of therapy per day at least 5 days per week, to include at least two therapy disciplines (physical therapy, occupational therapy, speech therapy, or prosthetic-orthotic therapy).

5. A coordinated interdisciplinary team approach, with the first team meeting occurring during the first week after admission, and occurring at least weekly throughout the IRF stay. The rehabilitation MD directing the care would be required to document concurrence with the plan at each meeting.

6. The rehabilitation MD coordinating the care must conduct and document a face-to-face visit with each patient at least 3 days per week throughout the IRF stay.

7. Requirements that therapies (including the initial evaluation) be initiated for each patient within 36 hours from midnight of the day of admission. Group therapies should be considered as adjunct therapies, rather than a replacement for one-on-one therapies offered in an IRF setting (CMS 2009a, 39788–39797).

Unique Coding Challenges for IRFs

There are unique coding guidelines applicable to assignment of diagnoses on the IRF-PAI. Coding guidelines applicable to ICD-9-CM do not address code assignments for the "etiology" reported on the IRF-PAI. Guidelines for coding the Etiology and Comorbidities are included in the IRF-PAI Training Manual. The Etiologic Diagnosis is defined as the condition causing the impairment for which the patient was admitted to the IRF (Item 21—Impairment Group). The CMG assigned for payment depends on the IGC at admission and is NOT affected by the discharge IGC. Assignment of ICD-9 codes for comorbid conditions and/or complications should NOT be made for diagnoses identified the day prior to or the date of discharge from the IRF (AHA 2006, 3–6; CMS 2004b; AHIMA 2006).

There are also some variations in assigning codes for comorbid conditions from the ICD-9 coding guidelines. For example, a patient admitted following a cerebral artery occlusion with infarction with right hemiplegia and dysphagia would have the following assignments:

Impairment Group: Stroke w/ right body involvement		01.2
Etiology: Cerebral artery occlusion w/ infarction		434.91
Comorbidities	Hemiplegia	342.90
	Dysphagia	787.20

The combination late effect code 438.x is not reported, because the stroke is already captured by the etiologic diagnosis. However, the 438.x code would be reported on the UB-04 (AHIMA 2004, 3–6).

Per *Coding Clinic* 1st Quarter 2002 and 3rd Quarter 2006, there are different sets of ICD-9-CM codes assigned on the IRF-PAI, as compared to the UB-04 (AHA 2002, 18; AHA 2006, 3–6). A code from V57x, Care involving use of rehab procedures, should be assigned as the principal diagnosis for all claims for patients admitted to an IRF for services. There are additional examples of coding guidelines for assigning secondary diagnoses on the claim form in 3rd Quarter 2006.

Inpatient Psychiatric Facilities

The BBRA of 1999 required that a PPS be established for licensed inpatient psychiatric hospitals and hospital-based psychiatric units. Because a per-discharge payment such as those used in LTCHs and IRFs did not adequately reflect the cost variations for psychiatric encounters, the BBRA gave CMS 3 years to develop a per-diem system. This IPF PPS was to be phased in over a 3-year period, starting with discharges on or after January 1, 2005. For cost reporting periods beginning on or after January 1, 2008, all IPFs were paid 100 percent of the federal per diem payment amount (CMS 2009f, 20364). Like most of the other PPS systems, this system is based on the inpatient DRG system with modifications to account for differences unique to the patients needing intensive psychiatric treatment. Updates to the IPF PPS are effective on July 1 of each year to allow for a yearly cycle to begin in July, making the RY different than for LTCHs and IRFs.

IPF MS-DRG Categories

Although psychiatric facilities are accustomed to using the *Diagnostic and Statistical Manual of Mental Disorders,* Fourth Edition (DSM-IV) coding system, the PPS is based on codes found in ICD-9-CM (CMS 2009f, 20368–20369).

Facilities are required to use the UHDDS definition of principal diagnosis for selection of the first code to list on the billing form. IPF facilities also may code up to eight additional diagnosis codes, as well as one principal procedure code and up to five additional procedure codes.

IPF Payment Adjustments

Like most of the PPS systems, Medicare included a stop-loss provision to prevent hospitals from sustaining large losses in funds during the transition to the new system. The IPF system consists of a per diem payment. The per diem amount represents the average daily operational, ancillary, and capital costs expended for Medicare beneficiaries. Facility- and patient-level adjustments are made to cover the cost variations among IPFs. Beginning on January 1, 2008, the stop-loss period ended, and payments are based 100 percent on the IRF PPS payment rates.

Patient-Level Payment Adjustments

The inpatient MS-DRG system is used to group IPF patients into 17 psychiatric MS-DRG categories, although the inpatient payment methodology is not used in the psychiatric payment system. The IPF PPS payment is based on IPFs admitting "only patients whose admission to the unit is required for active treatment, of an intensity that can be provided only in an inpatient hospital setting, of a psychiatric principal diagnosis that is listed in Chapter 5 (Mental Disorders) of ICD-9-CM or in the Fourth Edition, Text Revision of the American Psychiatric Association's Diagnostic and Statistical Manual (DSM-IV-TR)" (CMS 2009f, 20368). (See table 4.7 for a list of psychiatric MS-DRGs.)

Principal Diagnosis Adjustments

When a patient has a principal diagnosis as outlined in chapter 5 of ICD-9-CM or the DSM-IV-TR and groups to 1 of the 17 specified psychiatric MS-DRGs, the IPF receives the federal per diem base rate plus additional adjustment amounts, including any applicable

Table 4.7. Psychiatric MS-DRGs

V 24 DRG	V 25 MS-DRG	MS-DRG Description	Adjustment Factor
12	056 057	Degenerative nervous system disorders w/ MCC Degenerative nervous system disorders w/o MCC	1.05
023	080 081	Nontraumatic stupor and coma w/ MCC Nontraumatic stupor and coma w/o MCC	1.07
424	876	O.R. Procedure w/ principal dx of mental illness	1.22
425	880	Acute Adjustment reaction & psychosocial dysfunction	1.05
426	881	Depressive neuroses	0.99
427	882	Neuroses except Depressive	1.02
428	883	Disorders of personality and impulse control	1.02
429	884	Organic disturbances and mental retardation	1.03
430	885	Psychoses	1.00
431	886	Behavioral and developmental disorders	0.99
432	887	Other mental disorder diagnoses	0.92
433	894	Alcohol/drug abuse or dependence, left AMA	0.97
521–522	895	Alcohol/drug abuse or dependence w/ rehab therapy	1.02
523	896 897	Alcohol/drug abuse or dependence w/o rehab therapy w/ MCC Alcohol/drug abuse or dependence w/o rehab w/o MCC	0.88

Source: CMS 2009f, 20369.

MS-DRG adjustment. Psychiatric principal diagnoses that do not group to 1 of the 17 designated MS-DRGs receive the per diem rate and other applicable adjustments, but do not receive an MS-DRG adjustment.

Comorbidity Adjustments

Comorbidities are those secondary conditions that affect the patient's ability to recover and benefit from treatment. Seventeen groups of comorbid conditions generate an additional payment under the IPF PPS system. Table 4.8 shows the comorbidity groupings. The comorbidity groupings include those conditions that were found to be more costly to treat for psychiatric patients in IPFs. For each claim submitted, only one comorbidity adjustment per category may be made, but the provider may receive an adjustment for more than one comorbidity category (CMS 2009f, 20369–20372).

Patient Age Adjustments

Data indicate that the cost per day increases with age. The older patient age groups are more costly to treat than the patient group younger than 45 years. As a result, there are nine age group adjustments made for patients younger than 45 years and 45 years and older, as listed in table 4.9 (CMS 2009f, 20372).

Table 4.8. IPF PPS comorbidity groups

Description of Comorbidity	ICD-9-CM Code	Adjustment Factor
Developmental Disabilities	317, 318.0, 318.1, 318.2, and 319	1.04
Coagulation Factor Deficits	2860 through 2864	1.13
Tracheotomy	51900 through 51909 and V440	1.06
Renal Failure, Acute	5845 through 5849, 63630, 63631, 63632, 63730, 63731, 63732, 6383, 6393, 66932, 66934, 9585	1.11
Renal Failure, Chronic	40301, 40311, 40391, 40402, 40403, 40412, 40413, 40492, 40493, 585, 586, V451, V560, V561, and V562	1.11
Oncology Treatment	1400 through 2399 WITH a radiation therapy code 92.21–92.29 or chemotherapy code 99.25	1.07
Uncontrolled Diabetes Mellitus, with or without complications	25002, 25003, 25012, 25013, 25022, 25023, 25032, 25033, 25042, 25043, 25052, 25053, 25062, 25063, 25072, 25073, 25082, 25083, 25092, and 25093	1.05
Severe Protein Calorie Malnutrition	260 through 262	1.13
Eating and Conduct Disorders	3071, 30750, 31203, 31233, and 31234	1.12
Infectious Disease	01000 through 04110, 042, 04500 through 05319, 05440 through 05449, 0550 through 0770, 0782 through 07889, and 07950 through 07959	1.07
Drug and/or Alcohol Induced Mental Disorders	2910, 2920, 29212, 2922, 30300, and 30400	1.03
Cardiac Conditions	3910, 3911, 3912, 40201, 40403, 4160, 4210, 4211, and 4219	1.11
Gangrene	44024 and 7854	1.10
Chronic Obstructive Pulmonary Disease	49121, 4941, 5100, 51883, 51884, and V4611 and V4612	1.12
Artificial Openings—Digestive and Urinary	56960 through 56969, 9975, and V441 through V446	1.08
Severe Musculoskeletal and Connective Tissue Diseases	6960, 7100, 73000 through 73009, 73010 through 73019, and 73020 through 73029	1.09
Poisoning	96500 through 96509, 9654, 9670 through 9699, 9770, 9800 through 9809, 9830 through 9839, 986, 9890 through 9897	1.11

Source: CMS 2009f, 20372.

Table 4.9. Age groupings and adjustment factors

Age	Adjustment Factor
Younger than 45	1.00
45 and younger than 50	1.01
50 and younger than 55	1.02
55 and younger than 60	1.04
60 and younger than 65	1.07
65 and younger than 70	1.10
70 and younger than 75	1.13
75 and younger than 80	1.15
80 and older	1.17

Source: CMS 2009f, 20373.

LOS Adjustments

Data indicate that the cost per day decreases as the LOS increases. Variable per diem adjustments were developed to account for higher ancillary and administrative costs that occur in the first days after admission to the IPF. The adjustments begin on day 1 and decline gradually until day 21 of the patient's stay. For day 22 and beyond, the per diem adjustment remains the same each day for the rest of the patient's stay. However the adjustment on day 1 depends on whether the IPF has a qualifying emergency department. If it does, the adjustment is a 1.31 adjustment factor for day 1; if not, the IPF receives a 1.19 adjustment factor for day 1 of the stay (CMS 2009f, 20373).

Electroconvulsive Therapy Adjustments

Data indicate that costs are doubled for IPF stays that include electroconvulsive therapy (ECT). Therefore, an additional payment is made to the IPF for each ECT session performed. When patients receive ECT during an IPF admission, the facility should bill ICD-9-CM code 94.27 under revenue code 0901 to receive the additional payment. The total number of ECT treatments received should be indicated in the "service units" category on the same line item on the bill. The per diem base rate for RY 2010 is $651.76, with an additional ECT rate of $280.60 (CMS 2009f, 20364).

Facility-Level Payment Adjustments

CMS also has allowed for facility-level adjustments to account for teaching facilities, wage index variations, cost of living, rural location, high-cost outliers, and for IPFs with a fully functioning emergency department. The IPF PPS wage index adjustment is not based on the newly reclassified CBSA values that are used for IPPS (CMS 2009f, 20373).

Interrupted Stays

Inpatients who have to be transferred to other types of facilities for treatment not performed in the IPF facility, such as dialysis, are still considered inpatients. However, when the patient is discharged and readmitted to the same or another IPF prior to midnight on the third day (that is, the length of the interruption is 3 or fewer days), the IPF stay is paid as one episode of care rather than two. When the patient is not officially discharged, the IPF retains responsibility for care during the interruption. This policy was developed to prevent facilities from discharging and readmitting patients to receive the higher per diem rate associated with the early days of new IPF admissions. CMS has instructed IPFs to hold claims for 3 days to check for readmissions prior to billing (CMS 2009d).

Medical Necessity Provision

Medical necessity must be established for each patient upon admission to the IPF. Physician recertification to establish continued need for inpatient psychiatric care is required on the 18th day following admission. Inpatient psychiatric care is needed when intensive multimodalities are required, such as 24-hour supervision, safety concerns, diagnostic evaluations, monitoring adverse effects of drug therapy, and evaluation of behavior. Many substance abuse admissions may not meet medical necessity for an inpatient psychiatric admission (Casto and Layman 2009, 151).

Unique Coding Challenges for IPFs

As stated earlier, psychiatric principal diagnoses that do not group to 1 of the 17 designated MS-DRGs receive the per diem rate and other applicable adjustments, but do not receive an MS-DRG adjustment. The exception to this is for cases where the "code first" ICD-9-CM instructions require that the psychiatric diagnosis not be sequenced as principal diagnosis. When a nonpsychiatric diagnosis must be sequenced as principal, the grouper will search the secondary diagnosis fields for a psychiatric code from the "code first" list to determine if an MS-DRG adjustment should be made. It is also important that any condition meeting the official coding guidelines for reporting additional diagnoses should be coded, even if that condition is not in a comorbidity category (CMS 2009f, 20368–20369).

Summary

PPSs have been adapted successfully for a number of patient care settings other than acute short-term care hospitals. LTCHs, IRFs, and IPFs all currently operate under unique prospective payment requirements and modifications, with an increasing emphasis on review and documentation to ensure that medical necessity requirements have been met for each of these resource-intensive inpatient settings.

References

American Hospital Association. 2002. *Coding Clinic,* 1st Quarter 2002.

American Hospital Association. 2003. *Coding Clinic,* 4th Quarter 2003.

American Hospital Association. 2006. *Coding Clinic,* 3rd Quarter 2006.

American Health Information Management Association. 2004 (Feb. 4). Guidelines for assignment of codes for IRF-PAI. Posted to AHIMA Communities of Practice. http://cop.ahima.org/Portals/0/SynNet_CoP_Files/topic_resources/4301/Guidelines%20for%20assignment%20of%20codes%20for%20the%20IRF.doc.

American Health Information Management Association. 2006 (Sept. 28). Audioseminar: Coding for IP rehab services.

Bronnert, J. 2008. Coding in long-term care hospitals: How Medicare distinguishes LTCHs from other providers. *Journal of AHIMA* 79(4):74–76.

Casto, A. and E. Layman. 2009. *Principles of Healthcare Reimbursement,* 2nd ed. Chicago: AHIMA.

Centers for Medicare and Medicaid Services. 2004a (May 7). 42 CFR Part 412. Medicare program; Prospective payment system for long-term care hospitals: Annual payment rate updates and policy changes; Final Rule. *Federal Register* 69(89).

Centers for Medicare and Medicaid Services. 2004b. Inpatient Rehabilitation Facility—Patient Assessment Instrument (IRF-PAI) Training Manual: Effective 4/01/04. http://www.cms.hhs.gov/InpatientRehabFacPPS/downloads/irfpaimanual040104.pdf.

Centers for Medicare and Medicaid Services. 2005 (May 6). 42 CFR Part 412. Medicare program; Prospective payment system for long-term care hospitals: Annual payment rate updates, policy changes, and clarification; Final Rule. *Federal Register* 70(87).

Centers for Medicare and Medicaid Services. 2006a (May 12). 42 CFR Part 412. Medicare program; Prospective payment system for long-term care hospitals RY 2007: Annual payment rate updates, policy changes, and clarification; Final Rule.

Centers for Medicare and Medicaid Services. 2006b. Form CMS-10036. Inpatient Rehabilitation Facility—Patient Assessment Instrument. http://www.cms.hhs.gov/InpatientRehabFacPPS/downloads/CMS-10036.pdf.

Centers for Medicare and Medicaid Services. 2007a (June 8). Inpatient Rehabilitation Facility PPS and the 75 Percent Rule. http://www.cms.hhs.gov/InpatientRehabFacPPS/Downloads/IRF_PPS_75_percent_Rule_060807.pdf.

Centers for Medicare and Medicaid Services. 2007b. Medicare Claims Processing Manual. http://www.cms.hhs.gov/manuals/downloads/clm104c03.pdf.

Centers for Medicare and Medicaid Services. 2009a (Aug. 27). 42 CFR Parts 412, 413, 415, et al. Medicare program; Changes to hospital inpatient prospective payment systems for acute care hospitals and fiscal year 2010 rates; Changes to the long-term care hospital prospective payment system and rate years 2010 and 2009 rates; Final Rule. *Federal Register* 74(165).

Centers for Medicare and Medicaid Services. 2009b (Aug. 7). 42 CFR Part 412. Medicare program; inpatient rehabilitation facility prospective payment system for federal fiscal year; Final Rule. *Federal Register* 74(151).

Centers for Medicare and Medicaid Services. 2009c. FY 2010 MS-LTC-DRG file (effective 10/1/2009–9/30/2010). http://www.cms.hhs.gov/LongTermCareHospitalPPS/Downloads/Table11_FR10.zip.

Centers for Medicare and Medicaid Services. 2009d. Inpatient psychiatric facilities: Overview—Frequently asked questions. http://www.cms.hhs.gov/InpatientPsychFacilPPS/01_overview.asp.

Centers for Medicare and Medicaid Services. 2009e. Inpatient rehabilitation facility PPS: IRF patient assessment instrument. http://www.cms.hhs.gov/InpatientRehabFacPPS/04_IRFPAI.asp.

Centers for Medicare and Medicaid Services. 2009f (May 1). Medicare program; Inpatient psychiatric facilities prospective payment system payment update for rate year beginning July 1, 2009 (RY 2010); Notice. *Federal Register* 74(83).

Centers for Medicare and Medicaid Services Office of Public Affairs. 2007 (Jan. 25). Medicare proposes payment changes for long-term care hospitals for rate year 2008 and for Medicare graduate medical education. http://www.cms.hhs.gov/apps/media/press/release.asp?Counter=2075.

Medical Learning Network. n.d. Update—Long Term Care Hospital Prospective Payment System (LTCH PPS) Rate Year (RY) 2008. http://www.cms.hhs.gov/MLNMattersArticles/downloads/MM5652.pdf.

Medicare, Medicaid, and SCHIP Extension Act of 2007 (MMSEA). 2007. Public Law 110-173. http://frwebgate.access.gpo.gov/cgi-bin/getdoc.cgi?dbname=110_cong_public_laws&docid=f:publ173.110.pdf.

Part II

Coding for Inpatient Services

Chapter 5

Diagnostic and Procedural Coding for Inpatient Services

Clinical coding, the process of transforming verbal descriptions of diseases, injuries, conditions, and procedures into numeric designations, has been a health information management (HIM) function since the health record profession was established. It has enabled healthcare facilities and associated agencies to tabulate, store, and retrieve disease-, injury-, and procedure-related data. With the passage of numerous pieces of legislation over the years that have required code assignment as a condition for reimbursement, coding has taken on increased significance.

Under prospective payment systems (PPSs), coding is linked directly to the healthcare facility's financial viability, and ICD-9-CM codes are the primary element of many of the PPSs. Billing cannot be done until documentation is sufficient to allow for complete coding.

The inpatient PPS marked the beginning of a new era for the health information service, and the update of the system to account for severity of illness has yet again brought the coding process under increased scrutiny. As more healthcare areas have migrated to some form of prospective payment, the need for effectively managing coded data has increased and there is a high demand for the expertise of credentialed coding professionals. Coded information is reported to state and national databases and used for facility report cards, quality reporting, and benchmarking. As stated in *Top 200 Coding Hospitals*:

> The health care industry's increasing reliance on code-based prospective payment systems, such as diagnosis-related groups and ambulatory payment classifications, underscores the critical impact of clinical documentation and coding on hospital revenues. The primary purpose is to use data to benchmark coding performance, improve revenue management and quality reporting. (Ingenix 2008)

This chapter discusses general coding rules and guidelines and how they are implemented in facility coding policies.

Ethical Coding

As health information services face the pressures of deadlines and outside review agencies, adoption of ethical practice standards becomes increasingly important. Recognizing the increased responsibility of coding professionals, the board of directors of the American Health Information Management Association (AHIMA) developed a Code of Ethics. The Code of Ethics and the Standards for Ethical Coding are intended to serve as guides to ethical practice for coders and health information services by which departmental coding practices can be measured. Appendix A contains both of these documents.

Coding Conventions, Rules, and Guidelines

Although many rules are involved in the coding process, in some cases, code selection is based on several different sets of rules within the coding hierarchy. Coders first must understand and utilize the rules in the ICD-9-CM coding book. This includes following all sequencing and cross-reference instructions found in the book. For example, when a patient has the diagnosis of diabetic retinopathy, the coder would find the following notations:

Retinopathy: Diabetic 250.5 *[362.01]*

When ICD-9-CM shows two codes listed in such a fashion, the coder should assign both codes to fully identify the patient's condition and must list them in the order in which they are printed in the book. In other words, the book is giving a sequencing rule: code the underlying disease (in this case, the diabetes [250.5x]) first, followed by the code for the manifestation (the retinopathy [362.01]). Manifestation codes are printed in italics and can never be sequenced as the first-listed diagnosis, nor may they stand alone as a diagnosis. All other sequencing rules are superseded by this codebook instruction. After following the codebook rules, the coding professional must adhere to any Official Coding Guidelines, and third in the hierarchy includes the official guidance provided in the *Coding Clinic for ICD-9-CM*.

The Cooperating Parties

The four agencies that have responsibility for maintaining and updating the ICD-9-CM coding system are known as the Cooperating Parties. These agencies are:

- The American Hospital Association (AHA), which maintains the Central Office on ICD-9-CM to answer case-specific questions from coders and publishes the *Coding Clinic for ICD-9-CM*

- The National Center for Health Statistics (NCHS), a branch of the Centers for Disease Control and Prevention, which maintains and updates the diagnosis portion of ICD-9-CM (Volumes 1 and 2) and releases the *ICD-9-CM Official Guidelines for Coding and Reporting,* available on its website

- The Centers for Medicare and Medicaid Services (CMS), which maintains and updates the procedure portion of ICD-9-CM, Volume 3

- AHIMA, which provides training and coding resources and certifications for coding professionals

ICD-9-CM Official Guidelines for Coding and Reporting

One of the main duties of the Cooperating Parties is to develop the official coding guidelines to provide detailed and official rules for the use of ICD-9-CM coding.

Health Insurance Portability and Accountability Act of 1996

In 2000, the Department of Health and Human Services (HHS) set forth regulations for electronic transactions and coding standards as mandated by the Health Insurance Portability and Accountability Act of 1996 (HIPAA). HIPAA designated ICD-9-CM diagnosis codes as the official standard for coding diagnoses in all facilities and ICD-9-CM procedure codes as the standard for coding procedures for hospital inpatients. The *ICD-9-CM Official Guidelines for Coding and Reporting* also were named in the rulings, establishing that in order to be in compliance with HIPAA, all entities must use and follow the official guidelines (Schraffenberger and Kuehn 2010, 16).

Many publishers have included references to specific official coding guidelines in their coding publications.

Coding Clinic for ICD-9-CM

Coding Clinic for ICD-9-CM is a quarterly publication of AHA. According to the September 3, 1986, *Federal Register* (as quoted in AHIMA 2010):

> Coding guidelines are clarified through unanimous agreement by the Cooperating Parties of the ICD-9-CM Coding Clinic.

The Cooperating Parties achieve this by serving as the only voting members of the editorial advisory board of *Coding Clinic for ICD-9-CM*. *Coding Clinic* addresses questions from across the country and publishes official coding advice and includes the *ICD-9-CM Official Guidelines for Coding and Reporting* in their publication. The Editorial Review Board, made up of members representing the Cooperating Parties, review articles, responses to questions, and answers in *Coding Clinic* prior to publication. The advice given is to be followed by coders in all settings, including physician office, clinic, outpatient, and hospital inpatient coding. Coders should review this publication regularly for updated information regarding ICD-9-CM coding.

ICD-9-CM Coordination and Maintenance Committee

In 1985, the ICD-9-CM Coordination and Maintenance Committee was established to provide a public forum for discussion of revisions to the *International Classification of Diseases, 9th Revision, Clinical Modification* (ICD-9-CM) codebook. This federal committee is co-chaired by representatives from NCHS and CMS and meets twice a year in Baltimore. Both the public and private sectors are encouraged to comment on the suggested modifications and to recommend changes to the ICD-9-CM codes. Decisions are not made at this meeting; however, comments are reviewed by the appropriate agency. The final modifications are published in the *Federal Register* and the *Official Authorized Addendum to the ICD-9-CM* (CDC 2010). Minutes and additional information can be obtained on the committee's website noted in this chapter's reference list.

Uniform Bill-04 (UB-04)

To standardize billing forms with the standardized systematized terminology required by the Uniform Hospital Discharge Data Set (UHDDS), the National Uniform Billing Committee (NUBC) developed Uniform Bill-82 (UB-82). This single, uniform bill consolidated the numerous forms that hospitals were using to submit bills to third-party payers. A revision of UB-82 was approved in 1992, and another revision became effective in March 2007. This revision, named UB-04, permits hospitals to report 18 diagnosis codes and 6 procedure codes, although CMS only processes 9 diagnosis codes and 6 procedure codes. UB-04 contains an admitting diagnosis field in addition to three fields for reason for visit on outpatient claims. Medicare and most other third-party payers require use of UB-04 for inpatient billing in hospitals. Although much of the data on the form are collected by the admission and financial services departments, the health information service supplies the clinical coded data that are placed on the form and must ensure their accuracy. Each state has a UB committee that incorporates specific requirements unique to that state.

The UB-04 billing form was also designed to accommodate changes brought about by new transaction standards for the electronic exchange of data and the eventual adoption of ICD-10-CM. The UB-04 form reflects increased emphasis now placed on the clinical coding components. More information on the UB-04 can be found on the NUBC website at http://www.nubc.org/new.html.

Coding Policies

Each hospital's health information service must identify its requirements for coded data and establish coding policies and procedures based on its health information needs. These should reflect the standard usage of the definitions as set forth by the UHDDS, the *ICD-9-CM Official Guidelines for Coding and Reporting,* and *Coding Clinic,* as overseen by the Cooperating Parties. Policies and procedures ensure that data are consistently reported for analysis and reporting purposes. These requirements should be initiated by the director of the health information service in consultation with the administration, medical staff, and other healthcare professionals. Coded data may be needed for reimbursement, marketing, planning, utilization management, quality of care assessment, and research. New initiatives such as pay for performance, benchmarking, and quality reporting requirements are also based on coded data, so it is imperative that data are reported on a consistent basis.

At a minimum, coding policies should clarify how coding professionals should address issues such as the assignment of optional evaluation (E) codes and management (M) code assignment "history of" diagnoses, not reporting incidental x-ray and laboratory findings, and informing which procedures should be coded by the coding professional. Facility-based coding guidelines should be developed for those areas that have not been addressed by the official sources for coding advice or that have been addressed but require expansion or definition for an individual facility. Policies should address the physician query process for coding clarification and how to handle inconsistent diagnoses by a single physician in chart documentation, as well as conflicting diagnoses among physicians. See appendix B for a sample physician query form. Some corporations have developed coding policies that are being used consistently by all the hospitals in their organizations.

Written coding policies may be helpful in resolving coding disputes with outside reviewers. However, such policies must adhere to UHDDS definitions and sequencing guidelines, as well as be applicable to ICD-9-CM coding principles and official ICD-9-CM coding guidelines.

Complete, accurate, and consistent coding of all diagnoses and procedures documented is required for compliant coding. The number of codes to be assigned depends on the statistical and retrieval needs of the health information service, including data needs for utilization management, quality management activities, hospital planning, research, pay for performance, and benchmarking. See appendix C for the *Journal of AHIMA* article, "Managing Coding Compliance: Leadership, Collaboration Keep Processes from Derailing" (Bodnar and Willard 2009). Sample coding policies are available online from HCA Management Services (2010).

Uniform Hospital Discharge Data Set

In 1974, the Department of Health, Education, and Welfare developed what has become known as the Uniform Hospital Discharge Data Set (UHDDS). The UHDDS is defined as:

> . . . a minimum, common core of data on individual acute care short-term hospital discharges in Medicare and Medicaid programs. It sought to improve the uniformity and comparability of hospital discharge data. (Schraffenberger 2010, 47–48)

Over the years, the definitions have been refined and updated as changes in healthcare continued. In its latest revision, it includes all "nonoutpatient" settings, which include long-term acute care hospitals, psychiatric hospitals, home health agencies, and nursing homes. The PPSs use the UHDDS definitions as the basis for making some payment decisions.

The UHDDS includes definitions for demographic information such as identification, race, and residence; encounter information such as admission and discharge dates, physician identification, and disposition of patient; and reimbursement information such as expected payer, diagnoses, and procedure definitions. With regard to prospective payment, the most important of these definitions include the definitions of principal diagnosis, selection of other diagnoses, and procedures.

Diagnoses

All diagnoses that affect the current hospital stay must be reported as part of the UHDDS. The *principal diagnosis* is designated and defined in the UHDDS as "the condition established after study to be chiefly responsible for occasioning the admission of the patient to the hospital for care" (NCVHS 1996). The words "after study" in this definition are most significant and cannot be ignored when selecting the principal diagnosis. Patients with symptoms that require further study before a definitive diagnosis can be identified are frequently admitted to hospitals. See table 5.1 for examples of such symptoms.

Other diagnoses are designated and defined as "all conditions that coexist at the time of admission, that develop subsequently, or that affect the treatment received and/or the length of stay" (NCVHS 1996). Diagnoses that relate to an earlier episode and that have no bearing on the current hospital stay are to be excluded. In addition, it is not appropriate for coding professionals to refer to previous admissions to obtain documentation to support coding of diagnoses for the current admission.

A *complication* is an *additional* diagnosis describing a condition arising after the beginning of hospital observation and treatment that modifies the course of the patient's illness or the medical care required. Complications prolong the patient's length of stay (LOS) by at least 1 day in 75 percent of cases. Progress notations by physicians, nurses, and other healthcare providers often describe signs and symptoms that represent possible complications. Before assigning a code, however, the coder should make sure that the attending physician has documented such notations appropriately and that no conflicting documentation is found in the patient's health information. Examples of notations that provide possible clues to the actual condition are found in table 5.2.

Comorbidity is a preexisting condition that will, because of its presence with a specific principal diagnosis, cause an increase in the patient's LOS by at least 1 day in 75 percent of cases. Health record documentation must substantiate that the patient's management and care were affected by the conditions that coexisted at admission or that developed subsequently. In other words, the documentation should indicate that the patient received medication, other therapy, or diagnostic evaluation for each condition entered on the claim. For example, if diabetes mellitus is listed, the documentation should reflect either type I or type II diabetes and should also show that the patient was administered insulin or oral antidiabetic medication such

Table 5.1.   Examples of symptoms requiring further study before a definitive diagnosis can be identified

Admitting Diagnosis	Diagnosis after Study
Severe abdominal pain	Diverticulitis with perforation
Severe abdominal pain	Ruptured ectopic pregnancy
Severe abdominal pain	Gastric ulcer with obstruction
Unexplained convulsions	Metastatic carcinoma of brain
Unexplained convulsions	Primary astrocytoma of brain
Unexplained convulsions	Convulsions NOS
Ascites	Cirrhosis of liver
Ascites	Metastatic carcinoma from breast to peritoneum with malignant ascites
Jaundice	Obstruction of common duct
Jaundice	Acute hepatitis A
Chest pain	Acute myocardial infarction
Chest pain	Gastroesophageal reflux disease

Table 5.2.   Examples of notations that could indicate complicating conditions

Condition	Possible Clues
Wound disruption	Gaping postoperative wound with resuturing or other closure
Urinary tract infection	Symptoms of dysuria and frequency with orders for urine cultures
Myocardial infarction	Complaints of chest pain, orders for EKGs and cardiac enzyme/troponin studies

as Diabinese, Orinase, or Tolinase. Additionally, the results of at least one blood glucose determination should be recorded. If a patient with type II diabetes receives insulin, the coder should also assign V58.67, long-term (current) use of insulin.

Principal Diagnosis Selection

The principal diagnosis is the key to appropriate reimbursement because it determines DRG assignment in most cases. However, errors in selecting the principal diagnosis are common.

At times, it seems that both physicians and coders have difficulty distinguishing between the principal diagnosis and the "most significant" diagnosis. The most significant diagnosis is the condition that has the most impact on the patient's health, LOS, and resource consumption. This diagnosis may or may not be the principal diagnosis. Each year the Office of the Inspector General chooses problem-prone areas to study, and the hospital inpatient DRG system is always high on the list.

Example: A patient is admitted with a fractured hip because of an accident. The fracture is reduced and the patient is discharged. After further study, the principal diagnosis is the fractured hip. If this same patient suffers a myocardial infarction during hospitalization, the myocardial infarction is a complication of the admission and should be coded as an additional diagnosis. The principal diagnosis remains the fractured hip.

In the example above, the myocardial infarction might be the most significant diagnosis in terms of the patient's health and resource consumption. After study, however, it is not found to be the reason for the patient's admission and thus is not the principal diagnosis.

Examples of common problem areas are discussed further in chapter 9.

Procedures and Date

All significant procedures must be reported. For significant procedures, the identity (by unique number within the hospital) of the person performing the procedure and the date the procedure was performed should be reported. Surgery includes incision, excision, amputation, introduction, endoscopy, repair, destruction, suture, and manipulation.

A *significant procedure* is one that:

- Is surgical in nature
- Carries a procedural risk
- Carries an anesthetic risk
- Requires specialized training

Procedural Risk

The term *procedural risk* refers to a professionally recognized risk that a given procedure may induce some functional impairment, injury, morbidity, or even death. This risk may arise from direct trauma, physiologic disturbances, interference with natural defense mechanisms, or exposure of the body to infection or other harmful agents. Traumatic procedures are those that are invasive (including nonsurgical procedures that use cutdowns), cause tissue damage (such as irradiation), or introduce some toxic or noxious substance (such as caustic test reagents).

Physiologic risk is associated with the use of virtually any pharmacologic or physical agent that can affect homeostasis (for example, those that alter fluid distribution, electrolyte balance, or blood pressure levels, and stress or tolerance tests).

Any procedure in which it is obligatory (or usual) to use preprocedure or postprocedure medications associated with physiologic or pharmacologic risk should be considered as having a procedural risk. For example, some procedures require heavy sedation using drugs selected for their systemic effects (such as alteration of metabolism, blood pressure, or cardiac function).

Some procedures may involve harmful exposures, such as cardiac catheterization, which may introduce bacteria into the bloodstream. Other procedures that carry an exposure risk include those capable of suppressing the immune system, those that can precipitate idiosyncratic reactions (such as anaphylaxis after the use of contrast materials), and those involving substances with known systemic toxicity (such as digitoxin).

Long-life radioisotopes, such as carbon 14, pose a special type of exposure risk to other persons as well as to the patient. These substances require special precautionary measures, and the procedures for using them carry procedural risk.

Anesthetic Risk

Any procedure that requires or is regularly performed under general anesthesia carries anesthetic risk. This risk also occurs in procedures performed under local, regional, or other forms of anesthesia that induce sufficient functional impairment, necessitating special precautions to protect the patient from harm.

Specialized Training

This criterion is important for procedures that are performed exclusively or appropriately by specialized professionals, qualified technicians, or clinical teams either specifically trained for this purpose or whose services are dedicated principally to performing these procedures. Whenever specially trained staff resources are necessary or are customarily employed in the performance of a procedure, it is considered significant.

Although procedural risks, anesthetic risk, and specialized training are defined in the UHDDS, it may be difficult for the coder to determine exactly which procedures require coding. Traditionally, however, healthcare facilities and third-party payers have not expected coders to code routine x-rays and laboratory tests. The coding policies of each hospital should be consulted to determine the procedures coded at that facility.

Principal Procedure

The term *principal procedure* is used to describe a procedure that was performed for definitive treatment, rather than one performed for diagnostic or exploratory purposes or to treat a complication.

> **Example:** A patient admitted for hemoptysis undergoes a bronchoscopy with biopsy that reveals epidermoid carcinoma. Therefore, a left lower lobectomy is performed. The principal procedure is the left lower lobectomy because it was performed for definitive treatment; the bronchoscopy with biopsy was performed for diagnostic purposes.

When two procedures appear to be principal, the one most related to the principal diagnosis should be selected as the principal procedure.

> **Example:** Following an automobile accident, a patient was admitted with an open fracture of the neck of the femur, for which an open reduction with internal fixation was performed. During the hospitalization, the patient's inguinal hernia became strangulated, requiring an inguinal herniorrhaphy to be performed. The reduction with internal fixation is the principal procedure because it is most related to the principal diagnosis of open fracture of the neck of the femur.

Many payers do not require that the principal procedure be sequenced first because they use computer software to select the highest-paying surgical procedure. However, for correct data quality, it is important for the coder to select both the correct principal diagnosis and the correct principal procedure.

Medicare Code Editor

CMS provides Medicare Administrative Contractors (MACs) with a Medicare Code Editor (MCE) to detect and report errors in the coding of claims data. This software is designed to detect the errors listed in figure 5.1.

Figure 5.1. Examples of errors that MCEs are designed to detect

- *Invalid diagnosis or procedure codes:* Each diagnosis or procedure code is checked against a listing of codes included in ICD-9-CM volume 1 (Diseases) and volume 3 (Procedures) to ensure its validity.

- *Invalid fourth or fifth digit:* Any diagnosis (including the admitting diagnosis) or procedure requiring a fourth or fifth digit that is either missing or not valid for the code in question.

- *E code as principal diagnosis:* An E code describes the circumstance that caused an injury, not the nature of the injury. Therefore, an E code should not be used as a principal diagnosis.

- *Duplicate diagnosis:* The MCE detects when the principal diagnosis is duplicated as a secondary diagnosis. For example, a coder assigns 800.12 twice because a patient has a closed frontal bone fracture with cerebral laceration and a closed parietal bone fracture with cerebral laceration and contusion. Because both fractures are assigned the same number, only one code is required. This edit was included because the duplicate code may be considered a significant complication or comorbidity that may result in assignment to an inappropriate DRG.

- *Age conflicts:* Age conflicts are inconsistencies between a patient's age and any diagnosis on the patient's claim. For example, code 779.0, Convulsions in newborn, should not appear on the record of an elderly patient. Four age categories are evaluated:

  —Diagnoses intended only for newborns and neonates with an age of 0, such as 775.1, Neonatal diabetes mellitus

  —Diagnoses considered reasonable only for children between 0 and 17 years, such as 331.81, Reye's syndrome

  —Maternity diagnoses that are usually valid only for patients between the ages of 12 and 55 years, such as 646.60, Infections of genitourinary tract in pregnancy

  —Diagnostic codes considered valid only for patients over the age of 14 years, such as 600.00, Hypertrophy (benign) of the prostate without urinary obstruction and other lower urinary tract symptoms

- *Sex conflicts:* Sex conflicts are inconsistencies between a diagnosis or procedure on the claim and the patient's sex. For example, a male patient is reported with uterine cancer or an oophorectomy. In both instances, the codes conflict with the stated sex. Therefore, the patient's diagnosis, procedure, or sex is presumed to be incorrect.

- *Manifestation code as a principal diagnosis:* These codes describe the manifestation of an underlying disease, not the disease itself. Therefore, they cannot be used as the principal diagnosis. Claims with these diagnoses will be returned to the healthcare facility. In volume 1 of the ICD-9-CM codebook, these codes have been italicized. A partial listing of the most common etiology codes that should be listed appropriately before a given italicized code also is provided. Because there are so many underlying causes for a given manifestation code, other etiological codes also may be used.

- *Nonspecific principal diagnoses:* Although unspecified diagnosis codes (particularly those designated as "not otherwise specified") are valid ICD-9-CM codes, a more precise code should be used, when possible, for the principal diagnosis. However, unspecified codes may be necessary on the claims of deceased patients because a patient who died may not have received a complete diagnostic workup. The Medicare contractor reviews bills submitted by providers for this exception type and determine whether provider education is necessary. Some intermediaries reject such claims for payment; others release them and then review them on a postpayment basis. To help educate physicians on this issue, the MCE generates a report for nonspecific principal diagnosis claims. The code editor program considers these valid ICD-9-CM codes insufficient for making Medicare coverage determinations.

- *Questionable admission:* The code edit detects diagnoses that do not usually provide sufficient justification for admission to an acute care hospital. Quality improvement organizations (QIOs), which are responsible for ensuring that appropriate care is rendered to Medicare beneficiaries in the appropriate setting, review questionable admission cases on a postpayment basis. Examples of a diagnosis that might precipitate a questionable admission flag would be benign hypertension or uncomplicated diabetes.

- *Unacceptable principal diagnoses:* Certain codes describe a circumstance that influences an individual's overall health status but has no specific bearing on a current illness or injury. For example, code V16.6, Family history of leukemia, does not specifically explain why a patient was admitted. CMS considers such codes "unacceptable" for use as a principal diagnosis. If a provider files a claim using an "unacceptable principal diagnosis" code, that claim is returned with a request for a principal diagnosis describing the illness or injury. Some unacceptable principal diagnoses, such as benign hypertension, also are included on the questionable admission list.

CMS considers some codes (such as V57.0, V57.4, V58.2, and V58.62) unacceptable for use as a principal diagnosis unless they carry a secondary diagnosis code describing the origin of the impairment. If the provider submits a claim that reports one of these codes as principal diagnosis without the necessary secondary diagnosis, the claim will be returned with a request for a secondary diagnosis code. See figure 5.2 for examples.

When an invalid discharge status is reported, the patient is presumed (for the purpose of performing the nonspecific principal diagnosis check) to have been discharged alive.

Figure 5.2.   Codes that CMS considers <u>unacceptable for principal diagnosis</u> unless they carry a secondary diagnosis code

- *Nonspecific operating room procedures:* These procedures include a set of operating room (OR) procedure codes, particularly those described as "not otherwise specified." Although these codes are valid according to the ICD-9-CM coding scheme, more precise codes should be used. For example, rather than use 79.20, Open reduction of fracture without internal fixation, unspecified site, a code specifying the site should be used.

- *Noncovered operating room procedures:* The Medicare program does not provide payment for certain procedures. When one of these procedure codes is reported, the fiscal intermediary (FI) that pays for Medicare will return the bill as a no pay and request either a correction in the procedure code or a bill that identifies the covered and noncovered procedures. Included in the noncovered OR procedures are those procedures that Medicare has determined are not proven to be efficacious. Code 37.35, Partial ventriculectomy (ventricular reduction surgery), performed for treatment of end-stage heart failure due to cardiomyopathy, is an example of a noncovered OR procedure, as is code 37.52, Implantation of total replacement heart system (artificial heart).

- *Open-biopsy check:* Biopsies can be performed as open, percutaneous, or endoscopic procedures. The DRG definitions assign patients to different DRGs depending on whether the biopsy was open. In general, open biopsies are performed infrequently for most organ systems. There are specific ICD-9-CM codes for open and closed biopsies. Because the distinction made by the different biopsy codes is not applied uniformly, the MCE identifies all biopsies that are coded as open. When an open biopsy appears as either the principal or the secondary procedure, the FI may contact the hospital prior to payment to verify the procedure and obtain an operative report. If the operative report substantiates an open biopsy, the claim is processed. If the operative report reveals that the biopsy was performed percutaneously, by punch, or scope, the procedure code on the bill is changed to the corresponding closed-biopsy code before processing.

- *Medicare secondary payer alert:* The code editor will help contractors identify patients who may be covered under automobile insurance, workers' compensation, or other liability insurance. In such instances, Medicare should be the secondary payer. Claims with trauma codes are checked to determine which payer has primary responsibility for the claim.

- *Invalid age:* A patient's age is usually necessary for DRG determination. If the age reported is not between 0 and 124 years, the MCE will assume the age is in error.

- *Invalid sex:* A patient's sex is sometimes necessary for appropriate DRG determination. The sex code reported must be either 1 (male) or 2 (female).

- *Invalid patient status (discharge disposition):* A patient's discharge status is necessary for appropriate DRG determination. Patient status must be coded according to UB-04 definitions and conventions, for example:

  01   Discharged to home or self-care (routine discharge)

  02   Discharged/transferred to another short-term general hospital for inpatient care

  03   Discharged/transferred to Medicare-certified skilled nursing facility (SNF) (For hospitals with an approved swing bed arrangement, use code 61, Swing bed. For reporting discharges/transfers to a noncertified SNF, use code 04-ICF.)

  04   Discharged/transferred to an intermediate care facility (ICF)

  05   Discharged/transferred to another type of institution (including distinct parts)

  06   Discharged/transferred to home under care of organized home health service organization

  07   Left against medical advice or discontinued care

  08   Discharged/transferred to home under care of home IV drug therapy provider

  09   Admitted as an inpatient to this hospital

(continued on next page)

Figure 5.2.   Codes that CMS considers unacceptable for principal diagnosis unless they carry a secondary diagnosis code *(continued)*

10–19	Discharge to be defined at state level, if necessary
20	Expired (or did not recover—Christian Science patient)
30	Still patient
40	Expired at home (hospice claims only)
41	Expired in a medical facility, such as a hospital, SNF, ICF, or freestanding hospice (hospice claims only)
42	Expired—place unknown (hospice claims only)
43	Discharged/transferred to a federal hospital (effective 10/1/03)
50	Hospice—home
51	Hospice—medical facility
61	Discharged/transferred within this institution to a hospital-based Medicare-approved swing bed
62	Discharged/transferred to an inpatient rehabilitation facility (IRF), including rehabilitation-distinct parts of a hospital
63	Discharged/transferred to a Medicare-certified long-term care hospital (LTCH)
64	Discharged/transferred to a nursing facility certified under Medicaid, but not certified under Medicare
71	Discharged/transferred/referred to another institution for outpatient services as specified by the discharge plan of care
72	Discharged/transferred/referred to this institution for outpatient services as specified by the discharge plan of care

How the Rules Relate to Legislation to Combat Fraud and Abuse

As part of the ongoing fraud and abuse prevention legislation, penalties can be assessed against anyone who engages in a "pattern of presenting a claim for an item or service based on a code the person knows or should know will result in greater payment than appropriate" (OIG n.d.). The phrase "knows or should know" is interpreted to mean if the guideline was published in *ICD-9-CM Official Guidelines for Coding and Reporting* or published and disseminated by the federal government or MAC through provider bulletins or memoranda. Coders must have access to these publications on a regular basis in order to remain current on all regulations and guidelines as published. Moreover, coding staff should have regular meetings to share the content of these publications to ensure that all coders are following the same rules, as these rules may change frequently.

Key Resources for the Clinical Coding Specialist

Each hospital should have at least a minimal set of references for coders, such as those listed in the annotated bibliography. The library should include a subscription to *Coding Clinic,* medical disease references, laboratory references, a medical dictionary, and drug references. If the facility uses an encoder tool, most of these references are included. As rules change, coders are advised to check frequently for updated guidance and information.

Summary

Because coding currently is tied directly to reimbursement of the facility, coders must understand many rules, regulations, and laws. This knowledge must be combined with clinical knowledge and skill to interpret clinical documentation and apply coding rules and guidelines to make accurate code assignment. Moreover, facilities must provide the training and resources necessary to ensure that coders maintain competency and stay abreast of changes that affect appropriate coding and billing.

References

American Health Information Management Association. 2010. Coding resources. http://www.ahima.org/coding/coding_resources.asp.

Bodnar, C., and D. Willard. 2009. Managing coding compliance: Leadership, collaboration keep processes from derailing. *Journal of AHIMA* 80(4):74–75.

Centers for Disease Control and Prevention. 2010. ICD-9-CM Coordination and Maintenance Committee. http://www.cdc.gov/nchs/icd/icd9cm_maintenance.htm.

HCA Management Services. 2010. Policies and procedures. http://hcaethics.icu.ehc.com/CustomPage.asp?PageName=Policies-Procedures..

Health and Human Services. 2000 (Oct. 5). OIG compliance program for individual and small group physician practices. *Federal Register* 65(194):59434–59452. http://www.oig.hhs.gov/authorities/docs/physician.pdf.

Ingenix. 2008. Ingenix top 200 hospitals report. http://go.ingenix.com/top200/attachments/Top200FastFacts2008.pdf.

National Committee on Vital and Health Statistics. 1996 (August). Core health data elements. http://ncvhs.hhs.gov/ncvhsr1.htm.

Office of the Inspector General. n.d. Civil monetary penalties. http://oig.hhs.gov/fraud/enforcement/cmp/index.asp.

Schraffenberger, L.A. 2010. *Basic ICD-9-CM Coding,* 2010 Edition. Chicago: AHIMA.

Schraffenberger, L.A., and L. Kuehn. 2010. *Effective Management of Coding Services,* 4th ed. Chicago: AHIMA.

Chapter 6

Coding and DRG Assignment

All coders must be ready to make decisions. The ICD-9-CM codebook contains approximately 13,000 diagnostic terms, but the Alphabetic Index recognizes more than 120,000 such terms. Additionally, physicians use thousands of terms not included in the Alphabetic Index and the coder must decide how to translate them into numeric designations. Although some coding discrepancies will inevitably occur, errors can be kept to a minimum if coders adhere to recommendations and guidelines found in American Health Information Management Association's (AHIMA's) Standards of Ethical Coding (AHIMA HOD 2008) and the practice brief entitled "Developing a Coding Compliance Policy Document" (Bielby et al. 2010). Some of those recommendations include the following:

- Use the complete health record as the coding source document.
- Employ qualified coding professionals with ongoing education and training in coding systems.
- Develop written coding policies that conform to the Uniform Hospital Discharge Data Set (UHDDS) definitions and the Cooperating Parties' official coding guidelines.
- Establish quality control procedures to monitor the consistency and completeness of code assignment.

Finally, persons who assign and report codes should always remember that it is unethical to manipulate codes to maximize reimbursement in ways that do not conform to the UHDDS definitions or guidelines.

The ability to review a health record and accurately assign the appropriate ICD-9-CM codes is a skill developed over an extended period of time. To become an expert at coding, one must have an understanding of disease processes and treatment. For accuracy and compliance in coding, the coder must rely on the documentation provided by physicians involved with the care of the patient, including both the attending physician and any consultants he or she deems necessary to assist with patient care. This chapter discusses the basic parts of a health record, what the coder should look for in each part, and the steps in a record review that coders should follow to determine principal diagnosis.

Circumstances of Admission

The guidelines indicate that the circumstances of inpatient admission always govern the selection of the principal diagnosis. The circumstances of the admission are determined by reviewing the documentation contained in the health record.

The health record entries made at the time of admission should be reviewed carefully to identify why the patient was admitted. For patients admitted through the emergency department, the coder should identify the symptoms, findings, and/or diagnoses recorded in the emergency department record. Often the emergency department record will clearly identify the diagnosis necessitating admission. In other health records, however, the documentation may not be so clear and it may be necessary to review additional sources of information, such as:

- The admitting diagnosis listed on the face sheet

- The physician's conclusions recorded in the history and physical examination

- The patient's chief complaint as recorded on the nursing assessment, history, and physical examination

- The initial and subsequent progress notes

- Reports by consultants who saw the patient soon after admission

- The initial orders to identify the focus of treatment. (Most hospitals require that the admission diagnosis be recorded as part of the admission order, although this diagnosis may be quite vague.)

Progress note documentation is especially relevant for patients admitted with symptoms or physical findings that require further study to identify underlying causes. In the progress notes, the physician records the results of studies being performed, assesses the patient's status, and draws the conclusion when all studies are performed.

Data recorded at or near the time of admission are more useful in identifying the circumstances of the admission than the discharge summary or final progress notes because these documents contain information related to the patient's condition at the time of discharge. Thus, the physician may focus on the most significant diagnosis in terms of implications for the patient's health, medical care, and use of the hospital. If death occurs, the physician may record the cause of death instead of identifying why the patient was admitted.

In most instances, it is possible to identify the principal diagnosis with a high degree of certainty after carefully reviewing health record documentation. However, there may be problems with ambiguous, incomplete, or conflicting documentation. In such instances, documentation deficiencies should be queried, according to facility policy, with the physician or the appropriate medical staff committee.

Identifying the Sections of the Health Record

Every health record is composed of five basic sections:

1. An initial database
2. Consultations

3. Diagnostic tests
4. Therapeutic procedures
5. Daily documentation

Initial Database

The initial database consists of the emergency department record (if applicable) and the patient's history and physical examination. This initial information will provide a key to the potential principal diagnosis.

History and Physical Examination

The history and the physical examination need to be reviewed for two types of information. The first type of information can influence identification of the principal diagnosis and includes the following:

- The chief complaint
- The history of present illness
- Current medications
- Presenting physical signs and symptoms

The second type of information can influence the number and types of additional diagnoses, which are considered secondary diagnoses. This information may include identification of potential complications to the principal diagnosis. For example, a review of the patient's current medications may make it possible to identify stable conditions that are presently under treatment and that should be reported as secondary diagnoses, such as acute diastolic heart failure, acute exacerbation of chronic obstructive pulmonary disease (COPD), type I or type II diabetes, hypertension, or peptic ulcer disease. Any diagnosis identified in this review must be confirmed by physician documentation in the final diagnostic statement. If questions arise about whether a diagnosis should be reported, the physician should be consulted for confirmation.

Although not all-encompassing, the list in table 6.1 represents common medications associated with typical secondary diagnoses.

Table 6.1. Examples of common medications associated with secondary diagnoses

Diagnoses	Common Medications
Hypertension	Dyazide, Propranolol, Captopril
COPD	Theophylline, Aminophylline, Theo-Dur
Angina	Nitrostat, Nitro Paste, Nitro-Bid
Congestive heart failure	Lasix, Digoxin, Lanoxin
Peptic ulcer disease	Zantac, Tagamet, Pepcid

Diabetes mellitus
   Type I
   Type II
	
	Novolin, NPH, Humulin
	Orinase, Dymelor, Diabinese, Glucotrol

Consultations

If the attending physician requests consultations from specialists, their reports should be reviewed for support of the potential principal diagnosis, as well as significant secondary diagnoses. In some hospitals, diagnoses that are identified and treated by consultants are added routinely to the final list of diagnoses. However, the attending physician retains control of the patient's care throughout the hospital visit and is responsible for reviewing the documentation provided by the consulting physician(s) and assessing its significance for the patient. Hospital coding guidelines should address this issue. The attending physician reviews the reports provided by the consulting physician and assesses and documents the significance of the findings.

When a patient is admitted for surgery, a medical consultation report for "surgery clearance" may be present. Frequently, this type of consultation identifies significant medical conditions for which the patient is undergoing treatment that may influence the surgical outcome or length of stay (LOS). Such conditions should be added to the diagnostic statement when documented by the attending physician. When a condition is identified, but not documented, a query process should be started.

Diagnostic Tests

This section of the health record may help justify a principal diagnosis or support the coding of a secondary diagnosis. For example, in the case of a patient with suspected sepsis, a positive blood culture present on admission or within several hours after admission will usually support sepsis as a principal diagnosis, particularly when the record identifies the focus of treatment as such. Negative or inconclusive blood cultures, however, do not preclude a diagnosis of sepsis in a patient with clinical evidence of the condition.

Repeated monitoring of laboratory values or abnormal values followed by a treatment order may suggest the presence of a significant secondary diagnosis that also may be a complication or comorbidity. For example, repeated tests for potassium levels followed by orders for a potassium supplement would suggest hypokalemia as a secondary diagnosis, if verified by the attending physician. However, coders should always be cautious in reviewing diagnostic tests. Even though a value may be abnormal, an additional diagnosis should not be added unless the related condition is treated or meets the criteria for inclusion as a secondary diagnosis. In unclear cases, the coder is obligated to consult the attending physician. The *ICD-9-CM Official Guidelines for Coding and Reporting* (section III, B) explain:

Abnormal findings (laboratory, x-ray, pathologic, and other diagnostic results) are not coded and reported unless the physician indicates their clinical significance. If the findings are outside the normal range and the attending physician has ordered other tests to evaluate the condition or prescribed treatment, it is appropriate to ask the physician whether the abnormal finding should be added (NCHS 2009, 94).

Any cultures of body fluids also should be reviewed because they may assist in identifying bacterial infections that would influence the patient's treatment. When these diagnostic tests indicate that a secondary condition may be present, the coder should review the progress notes for the attending or consulting physician's comments for documentation of possible additional diagnoses. (Refer to the discussion of progress in the section below on daily documentation.)

Therapeutic Procedures

As the treatment pattern begins to emerge, therapeutic procedures may be used to correct particular problems. These procedures may or may not influence MS-DRG assignment. For example, a case of angina with a cardiac catheterization and subsequent coronary artery bypass graft (CABG) procedure will be assigned to a different DRG than a case of angina with only a cardiac catheterization.

Therapeutic procedures may be performed in an operating room or at the patient's bedside and still have an impact on the DRG assignment. For example, different DRGs would be assigned for the following two patients:

> **Example:** Patient A is admitted with decubitus ulcers. The ulcers are conservatively treated with intravenous antibiotics, repeat scrubbing, and topical medications.
>
> Patient B is admitted with the same diagnosis, but the ulcers are débrided with a scalpel at the bedside.

Procedures such as the sharp débridement of skin ulcers using a scalpel to "bleeding" tissue at the patient's bedside require close review of the progress notes because that may be the only method of identifying that the procedure was performed. Of course, these procedures also may be performed in the operating room.

Daily Documentation

One of the most important sections of the health record, daily documentation, usually includes the physician and allied health progress notes, physician orders, flow sheets for critical care, ventilator support, and ancillary records.

The physician orders will help identify the focus of treatment and support selection of the principal diagnosis. Here, the coordination of care can be located. It is important to coordinate the review of diagnostic tests and consultations to appropriately identify not only the principal diagnosis, but also significant secondary conditions. This is the place to find the patient's current medications for "stable" types of chronic problems that might still affect patient management in the current episode of care.

The progress notes provided by the physician and allied health team will document the patient's response to treatments. Moreover, they serve as backup documentation for various diagnostic and therapeutic procedures until a dictated report is provided. The coder should review the notes carefully to determine whether LOS was affected by secondary diagnoses or whether a complication developed postoperatively. For example, it may be possible to identify a postoperative complication of urinary retention by noting whether the patient had to be recatheterized or whether he or she received diuretics to restart the passage of urine after surgery. The complication must be documented by the physician or the coder may query for the cause-and-effect relationship.

Reviewing the Health Record

Each section of the health record serves a separate purpose. When reviewed correctly by the clinical coding professional, the sections taken together will support or justify the principal diagnosis and any secondary conditions that might affect reimbursement. It is important to remember that, in order to be coded, these conditions must be appropriately documented by the physician. When the documentation is incomplete, ambiguous, or conflicting, a physician query is in order. See appendix B for a sample physician query form.

A suggested sequence of review follows. The coder should:

1. Determine if an *emergency department record* is attached and, if so, review physician documentation and any comments from the ambulance report for pertinent information.

2. Review the *admission orders* to confirm any suspected principal diagnosis and/or to support the admitting diagnosis.

3. Read the *history and physical examination* to determine admitting diagnoses that may be categorized as the principal diagnosis and to identify potentially codeable secondary diagnoses.

4. Read the *consultation reports* from specialists that may further support or refute the potential principal diagnosis and/or potentially codeable secondary diagnoses.

5. Read all *progress notes* and develop a sense of the focus of treatment, progression of signs, and symptoms to diagnoses.

6. Verify any potential secondary diagnoses with *laboratory, radiology,* or *other ancillary tests, progress notes,* and *physician orders* and identify need to query.

7. Read the *operative reports, pathology reports, discharge summary,* and/or *special procedures or reports* to confirm primary and secondary diagnoses and procedures and identify need to query.

8. Identify the *principal diagnosis* and, when necessary, confirm appropriateness with the attending physician.

9. Develop a *list of secondary diagnoses* to be reported and, when needed, verify with the attending physician to ensure accuracy.

10. *Code all relevant diagnoses* following ethical coding standards and the UHDDS official guidelines.

Querying the Physician

As stated throughout this chapter, there are times when documentation is incomplete or insufficient to support the diagnoses found in the chart. It is for this reason that facilities should establish a physician query policy. Coders and physicians need to be familiar with the policy and procedures to ensure that this process works as smoothly as possible. The most common way of querying the physician is through the use of a query form.

Query Forms

Query forms should be developed and used with care and should only be used as tools to facilitate communication between coder and physician. The facility should develop a standardized form with input from both coders and physicians. Usually, the query form is not considered part of the official legal medical record. AHIMA recommends that facilities choosing to incorporate the form into their medical record should do so only under guidance from legal counsel and the compliance department in order to avoid problems.

The coder should keep to factual/clinical information (clinical indicators) and should not "lead" the physician toward a particular answer. Questions asked should remain open-ended to allow the physician to improve documentation. The physician should be guided toward clarifying any discrepancies in the body of the documentation, rather than just replying on the query form. This can be accomplished through use of an addendum to the discharge summary or progress notes.

According to Sue Bowman, AHIMA's director of coding policy and compliance, organizations should establish a process for "ensuring that the physician documents in the health record any clarification or additional information resulting from communication with coding staff. Communication tools between coding personnel and physicians, such as coding summary sheets, attestation forms, or coding clarification forms (e.g., physician query forms), should never be used as a substitute for appropriate physician documentation in the health record (Prophet 2002)."

See appendix B for AHIMA's practice brief on Managing an Effective Query Process (2008).

The facility should ensure that its query policy follows Medicare, Joint Commission, and facility documentation guidelines, as well as official coding guidelines. Coders should be encouraged to query the physician when the documentation is unclear or ambiguous; however, coders should not use the process to diagnose or question the physician's medical judgment.

Clinical Documentation Improvement Program

Over the years, many facilities have struggled over when to begin the coding process. Traditionally, the chart is coded after the patient's encounter or episode of care is complete. If documentation is clear and complete, then the coder should have all the information needed to accurately assign codes to the patient's diagnoses and procedures. However, if information is missing or ambiguous, obtaining answers to coding queries is difficult and time-consuming once the patient has been discharged and the clinician has moved on to treating other patients. As Medicare and other payers look to improve patient care and provide more accurate payment based on the patient's documented severity of illness, organizations are retooling their coding process.

One such alternative to the retrospective querying process is commonly known as a Clinical Documentation Improvement (CDI) program. Coders work together with nursing staff and/or case managers to help ensure that clinical documentation is sufficient to support the patient's medical care. This process is designed to enhance patient care through better documentation. It also allows for a smoother coding process because any documentation issues are identified in real time instead of days or weeks after the patient has been treated.

Clinical documentation specialists (CDSs) are coding professionals and nurses who work on the patient floors or alongside the physicians in the clinic setting. Although some facilities may choose nursing staff for this position, coding professionals also are excellent candidates. It is imperative that the CDS has a mixture of coding and clinical knowledge and possesses the communication skills necessary to query physicians and other clinicians when questions arise regarding the medical documentation. In the physician clinic setting, the CDS may also review inpatient chart documentation to facilitate correct coding for the physician's professional services. This task also requires a strong working relationship between the hospital and physician practice (Scott 2008).

Present on Admission

Portions of this section are adapted from *Present on Admission* (Garrett 2007).

With the implementation of the Uniform Bill-04 (UB-04) billing form in 2007, an additional field was added to allow for indication of whether each diagnosis was present on admission (POA). Reasons for the addition of the POA indicator are included in the MEDPAC Report to the Congress (2005, 191):

> Currently, a diagnosis recorded on the discharge summary that may have been present on admission cannot be distinguished from one that developed during the hospital stay. This additional information would significantly enhance the ability to identify which complications are avoidable. It would improve risk-adjustment of mortality and complications measures. Several quality organizations have supported this concept, and it should not significantly increase hospital burden.

The POA indicator is required to be addressed on all short-term inpatient admission claims. It is designed to identify conditions that are diagnosed prior to admission and conditions diagnosed during admission that were clearly present but not diagnosed until after admission occurred. Any condition that was present at the time the order for inpatient admission occurs, including conditions that develop during an outpatient encounter, such as in an emergency department, during observation, or in outpatient surgery, are considered as POA.

The POA indicator is assigned to the principal and secondary diagnoses and the external cause of injury codes except where exempt from reporting. Appendix I was added to the Official Coding Guidelines to define and explain proper usage of the POA indicator (NCHS 2009, 100–112). According to these guidelines, POA is *not* intended to replace any coding guidelines in the main body of ICD-9-CM *Official Guidelines for Coding and Reporting* and is *not* to provide guidance on when a condition should be coded.

Short-term acute care hospitals began reporting the POA for each diagnosis code on October 1, 2007, by using one of four indicators:

1. Y = Yes, the condition was POA
2. N = No, the condition was not POA
3. W = Clinically undetermined (the provider is unable to clinically determine if the condition was POA)
4. U = Unknown. This indicator shows that the chart documentation is insufficient to determine whether or not the condition was POA. The U indicator should not be used much because it should serve to prompt the coder to query the physician for additional information.

To further facilities down the path of pay for performance (P4P), CMS was required by law to select at least two conditions that will be excluded from the payment calculations if they are acquired during the hospitalization. These hospital-acquired conditions (HACs) will result in a decrease in reimbursement to hospitals if the condition is a complication or comorbidity (CC) or major complication or comorbidity (MCC) and occurred after the patient was admitted to the hospital.

> Section 1886(d)(4)(D) of the Act addresses certain hospital-acquired conditions (HACs), including infections. By October 1, 2007, the Secretary was required to select, in consultation with the Centers for Disease Control [and Prevention] (CDC), at least two conditions that: (a)

are high cost, high volume, or both; (b) are assigned to a higher paying MS-DRG when present as a secondary diagnosis (that is, conditions under the MS-DRG system that are CCs or MCCs); and (c) could reasonably have been prevented through the application of evidence-based guidelines. The list of conditions can be revised, again in consultation with CDC, from time to time as long as the list contains at least two conditions (CMS 2009, 43782).

The following criteria were applied to select the final list of conditions:

1. **Coding:** Easily identified by unique ICD-9-CM codes

2. **Burden:** High cost, high volume, or both

3. **Prevention guidelines:** Could reasonably have been prevented through the application of evidence-based guidelines

4. **CC/MCC:** Assignment of a case to an MS-DRG that has a higher payment when the code is present as a CC or MCC

5. **Considerations:** How condition meets statutory criteria in light of potential difficulties that CMS would face if the condition were selected

Beginning in FY 2009 (Oct. 1, 2008), cases with the following conditions were not paid at a higher rate unless the conditions were POA:

- Catheter-associated urinary tract infection

- Pressure ulcers

- Object left in body during surgery

- Air embolism

- Delivery of ABO-incompatible blood products

- Vascular catheter-associated infections

- Mediastinitis after CABG surgery

- Falls and fractures, dislocations, intracranial and crushing injury, and burns

Although these CMS requirements have shifted the focus of attention to assigning these indicators to Medicare claims, it is important to note that the POA requirement is described in the Official Coding Guidelines, as stated earlier. POA is not just to be addressed for Medicare patients only. The POA indicator should be added to all claims for all diagnoses that meet the criteria as established in the Official Coding Guidelines.

Other Guidelines for Reporting Diagnoses

When patients have multiple diagnoses, it is sometimes difficult for the coding professional to find clear evidence of the one that best meets the definition of principal diagnosis. When questions arise, the Official Coding Guidelines provide examples and instructions to assist in the appropriate selection of principal diagnosis. There are also specific instructions found to assist the coding professional in assignment of secondary codes.

Symptoms, Signs, and Ill-Defined Conditions

Manifestations are characteristic signs or symptoms of an illness. Signs and symptoms that pertain to a given diagnosis and primarily affect a specific body system are assigned to categories in chapters 1 through 15 of the Tabular List in the ICD-9-CM codebook.

Examples: 276.2 Acidosis
578.0 Hematemesis

ICD-9-CM chapter 16 (categories 780–799) includes symptoms and signs that point to two or more diseases or two or more systems of the body, abnormal results of laboratory or other investigative procedures, and ill-defined conditions in which no diagnosis classifiable elsewhere is recorded. These codes should not be used to identify a principal diagnosis when a related definitive diagnosis is available.

A sign or symptom code may be used instead of a diagnosis code and may possibly constitute the principal diagnosis in the following instances:

- No more specific diagnosis can be made at the time of discharge or outpatient encounter.
- The transient nature of the signs and symptoms makes it impossible to identify the cause.
- The patient does not return or expires before evaluation permits complete workup.
- The patient is referred elsewhere before a diagnosis is made.
- A more precise diagnosis is unavailable.
- The adverse reaction a patient experiences to a drug is a symptom code.
- The symptom or sign is a sequela related to a late effect of an illness or injury.

When the cause of a symptom or sign is stated in the diagnosis, the coder should report the code identifying the cause. An additional code may be assigned to further identify the symptom or sign when it represents an important problem in medical care on which data may need to be tracked.

Example: Brain metastasis, 198.3
Coma, 780.01

Comatose patients require extra care, so this symptom is reported in addition to the cause.

Example: Leukocytosis, nausea, and vomiting due to acute appendicitis

Only the acute appendicitis would be coded (540.9) because the symptoms specified are signs and symptoms of appendicitis. There is no need to maintain data on these signs and symptoms unless they persist following surgery.

In some circumstances, the symptom may be the sole reason for admission. When a patient is admitted for the purpose of treating the symptom, and there is no treatment or further evaluation of the underlying disease, the symptom can be designated as the principal diagnosis. Often the symptom represents an acute problem caused by a long-standing chronic condition that does not justify hospital admission. In all cases, sequencing of the diagnoses depends on the circumstances of the current admission or encounter.

> **Example:** Back pain management due to chronic lumbosacral strain
>
> Because the treatment is specifically for back pain, it would be coded as the principal diagnosis, even though the pain is a symptom of a chronic condition.

Reporting of Other (Additional) Diagnoses

A joint effort between the attending physician and coding professional is essential to achieve complete and accurate documentation, code assignment, and diagnosis and procedure reporting. To assist both the physician and coder, the Cooperating Parties developed and approved specific guidelines for identifying which diagnoses to report in addition to the principal diagnosis. Hospitals may record other diagnoses, as needed, for internal data use.

UHDDS definitions are used by short-term acute care hospitals to report inpatient data elements in a standardized manner. These data elements and their definitions can be found in the July 31, 1985 *Federal Register* (HHS 1985).

UHDDS item #II-b defines "other diagnoses" as (HHS 1985):

> All conditions that coexist at the time of admission, that develop subsequently, or that affect the treatment received and/or the length of stay. Diagnoses that relate to an earlier episode which have no bearing on the current hospital stay are to be excluded.

General Rule

For reporting purposes, the definition of "other diagnoses" is interpreted as additional conditions that affect patient care by requiring any of the following:

- Evaluation
- Therapeutic treatment or diagnostic procedures
- Extended LOS
- Increased nursing care, increased monitoring, or both

The following guidelines are to be applied in designating other diagnoses when neither the Alphabetic Index nor the Tabular List in the ICD-9-CM codebook provides direction.

Previous Conditions

According to the *ICD-9-CM Official Guidelines for Coding and Reporting:*

> If the provider has included a diagnosis in the final diagnostic statement, such as the discharge summary or the face sheet, it should ordinarily be coded. Some providers include in the diagnostic statement resolved conditions or diagnoses and status-post procedures from previous admission that have no bearing on the current stay. Such conditions are not to be reported and are coded only if required by hospital policy (NCHS 2009, 94).
>
> However, history codes (V10–V19) may be used as secondary codes if the historical condition or family history has an impact on current care or influences treatment (NCHS 2009, 94).

Diagnoses Not Listed in the Final Diagnostic Statement

When the physician has documented what appears to be a current diagnosis in the body of the record but has not included it in the final diagnostic statement, the coding professional should ask the physician to add the current diagnosis. However, according to guidance found in *Coding Clinic,* coders are allowed to code diagnoses from the body of the record (AHA 2000, 17–18):

> When the documentation in the medical record is clear and consistent, coders may assign and report codes. If there is evidence of a diagnosis within the medical record, and the coder is uncertain whether it is a valid diagnosis because the documentation is incomplete, vague, or contradictory, it is the coder's responsibility to query the attending physician to determine if this diagnosis should be included in the final diagnostic statement. *All diagnoses should be supported by physician documentation. Documentation is not limited to the face sheet, discharge summary, progress notes, history and physical, or other report designed to capture diagnostic information. This advice refers only to inpatient coding.*

Conditions That Are an Integral Part of a Disease Process

Conditions that are an integral part of a disease process should not be assigned as additional codes.

Conditions That Are Not an Integral Part of a Disease Process

Additional conditions that may not be associated routinely with a disease process should be coded when present. For example, when a patient is admitted with chest pain, but it is found after study that the patient had referred chest pain due to gastroesophageal reflux disease (GERD), the chest pain would be coded separately to justify the tests performed to evaluate the cause of this symptom, such as electrocardiograms (EKGs) and troponin levels.

Abnormal Findings

Abnormal findings (laboratory, x-ray, pathologic, and other diagnostic results) are not assigned or reported unless the physician indicates their clinical significance. If the findings are outside the normal range and the attending physician has ordered other tests to evaluate the condition or prescribed treatment, it is appropriate for the coder to ask the physician whether the diagnosis should be added.

Angina

When a patient is admitted for another reason but is taking medication for angina, the angina is reportable as an additional diagnosis. It is considered to be under treatment even though the condition is stable and the patient has no episodes during the current stay. The condition is reportable if the physician includes angina in the diagnostic statement. The physician may state that the condition is compensated or stable.

Congestive Heart Failure

When a patient with a history of congestive heart failure (CHF) is admitted for another reason and is currently taking medication for CHF (such as Digoxin and Lasix with a potassium supplement), the CHF should be reported. The patient would continue on the medications during the current stay even if no signs of cardiac decompensation are present. The physician may describe this type of CHF as compensated, stable, or history of CHF. It is still reportable as an additional diagnosis. The coding professional should also review the medical documentation to determine if the heart failure is specified as acute vs. chronic and diastolic, systolic, or both diastolic and systolic. This specificity will impact the selection of the correct coding assignment and the MS-DRG assignment impacting reimbursement because CHF no longer counts as a CC.

Frequently Overlooked Diagnoses

Coders should examine the entire health record carefully for conditions and statements that may indicate additional diagnoses. Remember that in order to code these conditions, they need to be documented by the physician or the potential diagnosis should be queried. The following list is an example of clues for diagnoses that are frequently overlooked in reporting:

- Anemia
    - Faintness, dizziness, pallor, fatigue, thirst, sweating, blood loss (for instance, ulcer, trauma, hematemesis, or melena)
    - Low hemoglobin or hematocrit level
    - Administration of iron or blood components
- Cardiac arrhythmias (especially in patients with acute myocardial infarctions)
    - Palpitations, near-syncope, pallor, nausea, weakness, lightheadedness, fatigue
    - EKG findings confirmed by a physician as clinically significant
    - Cardioversion, digitalis, verapamil therapy, beta- or calcium blockers, pacemaker insertion
- Dehydration (especially in patients with gastroenteritis or those who are eating poorly)
    - History of diarrhea or vomiting, dry mucous membranes, poor skin turgor, weakness
    - Elevated blood urea nitrogen (BUN) level, electrolyte imbalance
    - Force fluids, intravenous rehydration (for instance, greater than 125 cc/hr)
- Urinary tract infection (especially in postoperative patients and those admitted from nursing homes)
    - Dysuria, urinary urgency and frequency, flank pain or tenderness, possible fever, chills, and general malaise
    - White blood cells, red blood cells, and bacteria on urinalysis; urine culture positive for organism causing infection (colony count greater than 100,000)
    - Antibiotic therapy, force fluids
- Heart failure (especially in patients with respiratory disease or other cardiac conditions)
    - Dyspnea, orthopnea, peripheral edema, rales
    - Positive chest x-ray (pulmonary venous congestion)
    - Lasix, Digoxin, low-salt diet, oxygen administration

- Gastrointestinal bleeding (especially in patients with severe gastritis or those taking large quantities of anti-inflammatory drugs)

    —Fatigue, pallor, dizziness, hematemesis, or melena

    —Low hemoglobin/hematocrit level, stool positive for occult blood, endoscopy confirmation, upper and lower gastrointestinal series

    —Blood replacement, nasogastric tube, special diet, antacid prescribed

- Chronic obstructive pulmonary disease

    —Shortness of breath on exertion, dyspnea, chronic intermittent cough or wheezing

    —Positive chest x-ray, increased residual volume and decreased vital capacity on pulmonary function tests, abnormal blood gases, low theophylline levels

    —Treatment focuses on relieving symptoms and preventing exacerbations

    —Chest physiotherapy, bronchodilator, oxygen therapy, corticosteroids

    —Chronic condition vs. an (acute) exacerbation of the COPD

- Malnutrition (especially in patients admitted from nursing homes)

    —Low weight, lethargy

    —Poor appetite

    —Insertion of feeding tube, total parenteral nutrition, nutritional supplements

- Status or disabilities

    —Blindness, deafness, absence of limb, presence of colostomy requiring extra nursing time, pacemaker status, aortocoronary bypass status, transplant status (may require extra testing or increase the risk associated with other diseases and procedures)

Frequently Overlooked Procedures

Following is a list of tips for identifying procedures that are frequently overlooked by physicians and coders:

- *Excisional débridement:* The coder should look for pressure ulcers, diabetic foot ulcers, and/or cellulitis. Nursing and physical therapy notes also should be reviewed for documentation. Bedside procedures, such as excisional débridement, are frequently documented in the nursing notes. Moreover, physicians may perform this procedure during physical therapy. When this is the case, physical therapy notes should be reviewed to verify that the physician visited the patient during a session in the whirlpool and performed the débridement.

- *Adhesiolysis:* The coder should look for abdominal surgery on a patient with a history of previous abdominal procedures, hernia procedures on patients with a previous hernia procedure or a previous lower abdominal procedure, cholecystectomy procedures where the patient has a history of prior appendectomy, and/or a previous history of peritonitis or internal bleeding and ulceration. *Coding Clinic* requires documentation that the adhesiolysis was required in order to access the organ or site of the procedure.

- *Common bile duct exploration with cholecystectomy:* The coder should review the procedure dictation to find documentation that states the surgeon needed to explore the common bile duct for stones. This may be performed with open cholecystectomy procedures. An intraoperative cholangiogram is a diagnostic radiologic procedure to assess the bile ducts. Dye is injected into the bile ducts to assess for the presence of stones or other abnormalities. This is not the same as a common bile duct exploration; a common duct exploration can be performed open, transendoscopically via ERCP (endoscopic retrograde cholangiopancreatography) with endoscopic sphincterotomy, or laparoscopically, but it always requires an incision into the common bile duct and manipulation of the common bile duct to some extent.

- *Bone graft harvesting:* For certain spinal fusions or bone procedures for fracture nonunions, it may be necessary to harvest bone from one anatomic site for use in another. Frequently, the bone (or bone marrow) is harvested from the iliac crest. The bone graft harvesting is included with some ICD-9-CM codes, such as limb-lengthening procedures, but not with others. The coder must review the codebook carefully prior to assigning an additional code.

- *Repair of inadvertent lacerations:* The coder should review operative notes carefully to identify the repair of accidental lacerations. If the surgeon must repair the inadvertent tear, the additional code for the suture of the site of the tear should be added.

- *Pacemaker insertions:* The coder should review progress notes and emergency department notes for insertions of pacemakers. Insertion of both the device and the lead or leads is coded.

- *Mechanical ventilation:* The coder should review progress notes and emergency department notes to determine the start time of mechanical ventilation. Ventilator flow sheets usually accompany the health record of a patient on mechanical ventilation. In some facilities, coding professionals are responsible for calculating total hours of mechanical ventilation based on documentation in the patient's record. Great care should be taken to follow ICD-9-CM instructions for counting both start time and stop time of mechanical ventilation.

- *Biopsies:* During the course of a major procedure, the surgeon may elect to take an unplanned biopsy of other structures. The coder should review the operative notes carefully to identify the additional procedure.

Applying the Guidelines

The following case examples are designed to increase the understanding of, and ability to select, appropriate UHDDS principal and secondary diagnoses. The correct answers can be found at the end of the chapter.

Case 6.1

Patient A was admitted with shortness of breath and chest pain. He has a history of adenocarcinoma of the colon 5 years ago. At that time, he had a colonoscopy and biopsy with removal of malignant lesion, with no disease found in the resected colon. A chest x-ray revealed a large pleural effusion. A thoracentesis was performed to remove a large amount of fluid, after which the patient's breathing and chest pain improved. Cytology revealed metastatic adenocarcinoma of the pleura. An oncology consultant examined the patient and thought that he was a candidate for chemotherapy. Initial treatment of 5-fluorouracil, methotrexate, and Cytoxan was given. The patient was discharged with a diagnosis of pleural effusion due to metastatic adenocarcinoma of the pleura.

Answer:

Principal Diagnosis: _metastatic adenocarcinoma of the Pleura_

Secondary Diagnoses: _HX of adenocarcinoma colon_

Case 6.2

Patient B, an elderly female, was admitted from a nursing home with a history of poor appetite and marked weakness with lethargy for 2 days prior to admission. There was no history of diarrhea or vomiting. Mucous membranes were very dry and skin turgor was poor. The patient had no shortness of breath, chills, or fever. The nursing home BUN level was 65. Intravenous therapy was started for hydration and nutrition. With hydration, the BUN decreased to 30. The patient became more alert and responsive to stimuli, and began eating. She was discharged to the nursing home clinically stable with diagnoses of dehydration, mild malnutrition causing weakness, and elevated BUN.

Answer:

Principal Diagnosis: _dehydration_

Secondary Diagnoses: _malnutrition_

Case 6.3

Patient C is admitted with acute bronchopneumonia unresponsive to outpatient treatment. She has been on chemotherapy for previously resected breast carcinoma of the upper-inner quadrant. She has been on an 8-week regimen that started after her breast surgery. In addition, she has axillary and lung metastases. The pneumonia responded slowly to intravenous antibiotic therapy, but when her lungs cleared, the patient was discharged to resume antineoplastic therapy in 1 week.

Answer:

Principal Diagnosis: _Acute Bronchopneumonia_

Secondary Diagnoses: _metastatic axillary + lung, breast cancer_

Summary

The practice of clinical coding requires a unique blend of coding and clinical knowledge, skill, and judgment. Responsible coding professionals are able to read and interpret documentation in health records, clarify questions with physicians, and apply official coding guidelines accurately, consistently, and completely in assigning principal and secondary diagnoses, procedures, and other applicable codes. The expert coder is one who is aware of and respects the ethical issues in coding compliance.

References

AHIMA House of Delegates. 2008 (Sept.). AHIMA Standards of Ethical Coding.

American Health Information Management Association. 2008. Practice brief: managing an effective query process. *Journal of AHIMA* 79(10):83–88. http://library.ahima.org/xpedio/groups/public/documents/ahima/bok1_040394.hcsp?dDocName=bok1_040394.

American Hospital Association. 2000. *Coding Clinic,* 2nd quarter 2000.

Bielby, J.A., et al. 2010. Developing a coding compliance policy document. *Journal of AHIMA* (Updated Mar. 2010).

Centers for Medicare and Medicaid Services. 2009 (Aug. 27). 42 CFR Parts 412, 413, 415, et al. *Medicare Program; Changes to the Hospital Inpatient Prospective Payment Systems for Acute Care Hospitals and Fiscal Year 2010 Rates; and Changes to the Long Term Care Hospital Prospective Payment System and Rate Years 2010 and 2009 Rates; Final Rule. Federal Register* 74(165). http://edocket.access.gpo.gov/2009/pdf/E9-18663.pdf.

Department of Health and Human Services. 1985 (July 31). Uniform Hospital Discharge Data Set. *Federal Register* 50(147):31038–31040.

Garrett, G. 2007. *Present on Admission.* Chicago: AHIMA.

Medicare Payment Advisory Commission. 2005 (Mar.). Report to the Congress: Medicare Payment Policy. Washington, DC: MEDPAC. http://www.medpac.gov/documents/Mar05_EntireReport.pdf.

National Center for Health Statistics. 2009 (Oct. 1). *ICD-9-CM Official Guidelines for Coding and Reporting.* http://www.cdc.gov/nchs/data/icd9/icdguide09.pdf.

Prophet, S. 2002. *Health Information Management Compliance: A Model Program for Healthcare Organizations,* 2nd ed. Chicago: AHIMA.

Scott, K.S. 2008. *Medical Coding for Non-Coders: Understanding Coding and Reimbursement for Today's Healthcare Industry.* Chicago: AHIMA.

Answers to Case Studies

Case 6.1

Principal Diagnosis: 197.2, Secondary malignant neoplasm of pleura. After study, the principal diagnosis of malignant pleural effusion was found to have been the cause of the shortness of breath and chest pain. These symptoms are not coded because a definitive diagnosis was found.

Secondary Diagnoses: V10.05, History of colon cancer. The history of colon cancer is used because there is documentation that the colon cancer was resected and without evidence of recurrence.

Case 6.2

Principal Diagnosis: 276.51, Dehydration. The principal diagnosis is dehydration because, after study, that is what was identified as the underlying cause of the weakness, lethargy, and increased BUN. Her appetite improved when she became more alert.

Secondary Diagnoses: 263.1, Malnutrition of mild degree should be reported as a secondary diagnosis.

Case 6.3

Principal Diagnosis: 485, Bronchopneumonia, organism unspecified. The principal diagnosis is acute broncho-pneumonia because therapy focused on this condition. The patient's stay was complicated by the metastatic carcinoma, as antineoplastic therapy exerts a suppressive action on the immune mechanisms, thus making the pneumonia more difficult to treat and extending the stay.

Secondary Diagnoses: 174.2, Malignant neoplasm of upper-inner quadrant.

197.0, Secondary malignant neoplasm of lung.

196.3, Secondary neoplasm of axillary lymph nodes.

The breast cancer is reported as current even though it has been surgically excised because it appears that the patient has been on chemotherapy since the surgery and, therefore, it is currently being treated. The metastatic sites of the lymph nodes and lung should be reported.

Part III

Processes Related to Coding and Reimbursement for Inpatient Services

Chapter 7

Data Quality Management

The need for clinical information in the form of coded data has been magnified dramatically since the beginning of the prospective payment system (PPS). Quality improvement organizations (QIOs), third-party administrators, Medicare Administrative Contractors (MACs), employers, and commercial insurance groups rely on the data that health information management (HIM) professionals provide to make financial decisions and to validate quality of care. Because reimbursement is directly tied to quality with the value-based purchasing and pay for performance initiatives, the need for accurate and complete information has resulted in a close examination of the coding process within HIM services. This chapter focuses on the processes for evaluating, controlling, and monitoring the quality of healthcare data.

Coding and Data Quality Evaluation

Critical elements in the data quality evaluation process include:

- Coding practices and policies

- Staff qualifications

- Training

- Types of quality control programs

Coding managers play an important role in the data quality evaluation process. They are responsible for the following types of activities:

- Preparation of specific coding criteria

- Planning of coder educational sessions

- Evaluation and monitoring of educational action plans for individual coders

- Monitoring of ethical coding practices

- Evaluation and monitoring of coding quality

- Preparation of performance evaluations

Quality, as it applies to coded data, means that the performance of the coding function within an HIM department is accomplished at the highest levels of accuracy and consistency possible for the coded data. Likewise, quality is expressed most appropriately in terms of the needs of the customers. That is, the definition of quality implies that optimal reimbursement is provided to the hospital, patients' illnesses and treatments are reported accurately, and payers can identify all the resources required to treat one of their beneficiaries.

Because multiple transitions are encountered in the reimbursement system for government programs, an accurate database for planning is critical. The data that healthcare organizations provide now will have a profound impact on the future reimbursement they may expect. Large-scale data warehousing by organizations such as HealthGrades allows for greater data comparison and benchmarking. By describing the resources used for a patient completely and accurately, HIM professionals ensure that the database for reimbursement decisions is as detailed as possible.

AHIMA's Data Quality Management Model

Because the data in the health record must be of the highest quality to accomplish all the purposes required of it, in 1998 the American Health Information Management Association (AHIMA) developed a task force on the subject of data quality management. This group developed a data quality management model based on four domains and the basic characteristics that apply to them (Cassidy et al. 1998).

Quality Management Domains

Each of the four domains that form the framework of AHIMA's data quality management model represents a set of processes. These domains, with their associated processes, include:

- Data applications, or the purposes for which data are collected
- Data collection, or the processes by which data are collected
- Data warehousing, or the processes and systems by which data are archived or saved for future use
- Data analysis, or the processes by which data are translated into information that can be used for the designated application

Required Characteristics

The processes that result in high-quality data require certain characteristics, ranging from accuracy and accessibility to relevancy and consistency. The characteristics that are applied to the four quality management domains in the AHIMA model are described in the following sections (adapted from Homan 2007, 36–41).

Accuracy — *data is correct – accurate*

Data accuracy refers to the correctness of data. The data should represent what was intended or defined by their original source. For example, the patient's emergency contact information recorded in a paper record or a database should be the same as what the patient said it was. The results of laboratory testing for a particular patient should reflect the results generated by the laboratory equipment. Data related to the medication provided to a particular patient should reflect the actual date, time, and medication administered. The accuracy of the data placed in the health record depends on a number of factors, including:

- The patient's physical health and emotional state at the time the data were collected

- The provider's interviewing skills

- The provider's recording skills

- The availability of the patient's clinical history

- The dependability of the automated equipment

- The reliability of the electronic communications media

Accessibility *data is obtainable - available*

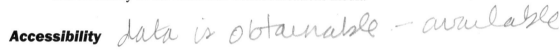

Data accessibility means that the data are easily obtainable. The following factors affect the accessibility of health record data and information:

- Whether previous health records are available when and where they are needed

- Whether dictation equipment is accessible and working properly

- Whether transcription of dictation is accurate, timely, and readily available to health-care providers

- Whether computer data-entry devices are working properly and readily available to healthcare providers

Comprehensiveness *- record is complete*

Data comprehensiveness refers to the fact that all the required data elements are included in the health record. In essence, comprehensiveness means that the record is complete. In both paper- and computer-based systems, having a complete health record is critical to the organization's ability to provide excellent patient care and to meet all regulatory, legal, and reimbursement requirements. In general, the health record must include the following data elements:

- Patient identification

- Consents for treatment

- Problem list

- Diagnoses

- Clinical history

- Diagnostic test results

- Treatments and outcomes

- Conclusions and follow-up requirements

Consistency *- data is reliable*

Data consistency refers to the reliability of the data. Reliable data do not change no matter how many times or in how many ways they are stored, processed, or displayed. Data values are consistent when the value of any given data element is the same across applications and systems. Related data items also should be reliable. For example, the clinical history for a male patient would never include a hysterectomy as a past surgical procedure.

Legitimate documentation inconsistencies do occur in health records. Any given health record may contain numerous references to the patient's diagnosis in terms of:

- The admitting diagnosis
- The diagnostic impression upon physical examination
- The postoperative diagnosis
- The pathology diagnosis
- The discharge diagnosis

Any inconsistencies among the various types of diagnoses would be legitimate. The different diagnoses incorporate the results of tests and findings unavailable at the time the previous documentation took place.

In other instances, however, data inconsistencies in the health record are unacceptable. For example, a nursing assessment might indicate that the patient is deaf when there is no documentation by the physician that the patient's hearing is compromised. Another unacceptable inconsistency occurs when different healthcare providers use different terminology. For example, different providers might use the words *cyst*, *lesion*, and *abscess* interchangeably in documenting a skin condition for the same patient. Such inconsistencies create difficulties for other caregivers and can be very confusing to external users of the health record.

Currency *data is up to date and recorded near time of event or observation*

Data currency and data timeliness refer to the requirement that healthcare data be up-to-date and recorded at or near the time of the event or observation. Because care and treatment rely on accurate and current data, an essential characteristic of data quality is the timeliness of the documentation or data entry.

Definition *users understand meaning of data*

Data definition refers to the meaning of the data and information documented in the health record. For information to be meaningful, it must be pertinent. Further, users of the data must understand what the data mean and represent. Every data element should have a clear definition and a range of acceptable values.

Granularity *attributes and data correct level of detail*

Data granularity is another data quality characteristic that needs to be considered when establishing data definitions. It requires that the attributes and values of data be defined at the correct level of detail. For example, numeric values for laboratory results should be recorded to the appropriate decimal place as required for the meaningful interpretation of test results.

Precision

describe expected data values

Data precision is the term used to describe expected data values. As part of data definition, the acceptable values or value ranges for each data element must be defined. For example, a precise data definition related to gender would include three values: male, female, and unknown. Precise data definition yields accurate data collection. In paper-based health records, much of the documentation and data are collected in narrative format and it is difficult to apply the concept of data precision to narrative text. The movement toward computer-based patient records provides the perfect opportunity to improve data precision in health records.

Relevancy

usefulness of the data

Data relevancy refers to the usefulness of the data in the health record. The reason for collecting the data element must be clear to ensure the relevancy of the data collected. Additionally, the collection instrument should be tested to validate its use (Teslow 2007, 145). For example, nursing documentation is often lengthy, and physicians and other caregivers may not have sufficient time to review it. Therefore, data users may request changes to ensure that the data are useful to them.

Approaches to Controlling Data Quality

There are many approaches to managing the quality of care in the current healthcare environment. Over the years, quality monitoring has taken on many names and methodologies. Different terms and methodologies have been used to attempt to assess and manage data quality. The term *quality assurance (QA) monitoring* has been used and typically consisted of quarterly studies performed on existing problems and issues. Although this approach was a good start, later variations such as total quality improvement attempted to view quality improvement as an ongoing process. Occurrence screens were used to identify a set number of happenings, such as deaths within 24 hours of admission or single blood transfusions, which triggered an audit by a quality committee. More recent approaches to healthcare quality management include programs such as Six Sigma and the clinical value compass.

Six Sigma

The Six Sigma process focuses on overall improvement of a service or process by eliminating variables to obtain a more concise standard product or output. This differs from other quality initiatives in several essential ways. It is a business philosophy, which becomes an integral part of the organization's business strategy, unlike programs that are instituted in just one business unit or department. Because the entire organization is involved, high-level management must assume leadership roles for a Six Sigma program. Six Sigma principles are used as a means to discover performance issues in an existing process and make recommendations for changes. The overall philosophy is to eliminate performance-affecting variation in the end product or service while leaving the process itself intact. A five-phase methodology known as DMAIC (define, measure, analyze, improve, and control) is at the heart of Six Sigma process improvement. When used effectively, it can produce significant success in process change and control (Lambrecht and Wilson 2007).

Clinical Value Compass

The clinical value compass is another data quality methodology. It is designed to link the various components, or indicators, of a process to the directions on a compass. Each point of the compass represents a different indicator, as follows:

North   Health status or function
South   Costs of care
East   Patient satisfaction
West   Clinical outcomes

The relationship between these indicators of quality can be expressed as the following equation:

$$\frac{Clinical\ Outcomes + Functional\ Status\ Outcomes + Satisfaction}{Costs\ of\ Care}$$

As a result, each involved area, such as patient care, billing, and coding, can focus on the possible solutions from a systems approach. In other words, the problem and solutions are viewed from the vantage point of how the entire process is affected rather than just looking at one or two aspects.

The diagram in figure 7.1 shows how one team used the compass approach to reduce cardiac death in postoperative patients.

Appendix D contains an article on improving coding quality measurement written by the AHIMA Work Group on Benchmark Standards for Clinical Coding Performance Measurement quality subgroup. Appendix E contains an article discussing establishment of standard coding workflow and benchmarks.

ICD-10 Implementation

The transition to ICD-10-CM and ICD-10-PCS over the coming years will have an impact on quality reporting. Data and systems used to collect quality performance measures for all provider types will be revised to accommodate ICD-10-CM and ICD-10-PCS codes. The ICD-10 coded data will permit a better assessment of patient severity, the intensity and complexity of services provided to patients, and the resources used in caring for patients (AHIMA 2009). It is anticipated that these data will inform future program and payment policies. Current quality measures would be replaced with codes from the new coding systems. The ICD-10-CM system consists of more than 68,000 diagnosis codes, compared to approximately 13,000 ICD-9-CM diagnosis codes. ICD-10-PCS consists of 87,000 procedure codes. Together the ICD-10-CM and ICD-10-PCS codes have the potential to reveal more about quality of care, so that data can be used in a more meaningful way to better understand complications, better design clinically robust algorithms, and better track the outcomes of care. ICD-10-CM and PCS incorporate greater specificity and clinical detail to provide information for clinical decision making and outcomes research.

Figure 7.1.   The compass approach

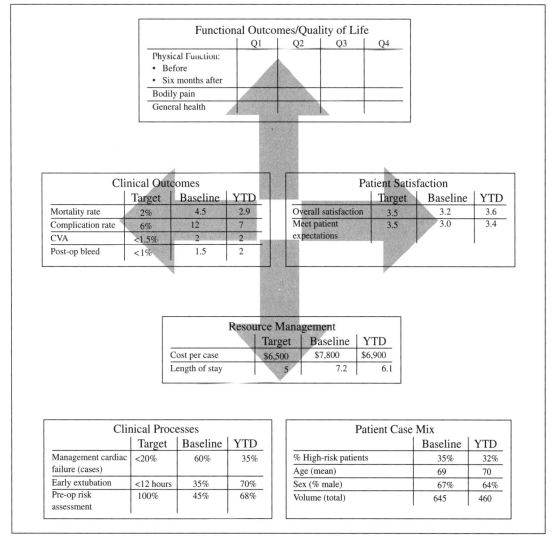

Source: Buff and Hohmann 1999, 46.

Understanding HACs and SREs for Quality Reporting and Reimbursement

This section was originally published in the Journal of AHIMA *(AHIMA Practice Councils 2009).*

The focus on the delivery, measurement, and provision of quality patient care has led to several initiatives in the last few years that link reimbursement to quality care. These initiatives are often referred to as value-based purchasing, and they include present on admission (POA) indicators, hospital-acquired conditions (HACs), and serious reportable events (SREs). These terms are often mistakenly used interchangeably. While they do overlap and can be interrelated, each has a distinct definition and purpose.

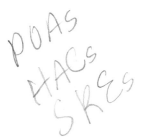

The POA indicator and its terminology were introduced in the Deficit Reduction Act of 2005. The POA indicator identifies conditions present at the time the order for an inpatient admission occurs, including conditions that develop during an outpatient encounter such as an emergency department visit, observation, or outpatient surgery. A POA indicator is assigned to each principal and secondary diagnosis code according to the ICD-9-CM Official Guidelines for Coding and Reporting.

HACs were also developed as a result of the Deficit Reduction Act of 2005. HACs are diagnoses determined by Medicare to be reasonably preventable. The conditions targeted by the Centers for Medicare and Medicaid Services (CMS) are high in cost, high in volume, or both; would result in assignment to a higher-paying DRG when present as a secondary diagnosis; and could reasonably have been prevented through the application of evidence-based guidelines.

Medicare selected specific reasonably preventable conditions that have the potential to increase reimbursement under MS-DRGs. When these conditions are not reported as POA, payment may be reduced for the Medicare claim.

In 2002 the National Quality Forum issued a list of SREs that include "wrong" surgical, device, patient protection, care management, environment, and criminal events. SREs can occur as a result of injury or error from care management or failure to follow standard care or institutional practices and policies. These events can cause serious injury or death. SREs are frequently referred to as "never events," as these events should never occur in a healthcare facility.

Several of CMS's designated HACs are included on the National Quality Forum list of SREs. Overlap occurs between never events and HACs due to the fact that the condition or event must occur or be acquired in the facility to be considered a never event.

However, it is important to recognize distinct differences between the SRE and HAC lists. These include several SREs that are situations that cannot be represented using coded data; for example, patient death or serious disability associated with the use of contaminated drugs, devices, or biologics provided by the healthcare facility or abduction of a patient of any age.

There is never a valid reason for a coder to purposefully omit a code when the physician documentation clearly supports a codeable condition. Organizations' coding policies should reiterate compliant and ethical coding and reference the ICD-9-CM Official Guidelines for Coding and Reporting as well as the AHIMA Standards of Ethical Coding and interpretation section. The same standards apply to the POA indicator. It is not acceptable to falsely report the POA indicator Y when the condition was not present on admission.

The HIM Role

HIM professionals have specialized knowledge of data capture, data analysis, and reimbursement methodologies. This expertise will be essential in contract negotiations with payers. HIM professionals must understand the provisions in contract negotiations regarding HACs and SREs. They should review the following questions to help in their discussions with external payers:

- Will the contract address claim processing requirements or claims adjustments or a broader reporting requirement for all events, including those that are not represented in ICD-9-CM codes?

- Does the hospital collect the POA indicator for non-Medicare claims? Can the payer accept POA indicators? The POA indicator is essential in communicating whether a condition occurred during the hospitalization.

- Will the agreement address conditions identified as HACs for claim adjudication? If so, what payment methodology does the payer use? How will the reimbursement be affected? For example, if DRG-based, will the CMS HAC payment provision be followed? Or if percent of charges, will charges representing the HAC be removed from the claim?

- Is the payer including the "wrong" surgery SREs in the contract? If so, how will these claims be identified and processed and will the reimbursement be affected? Does the payer plan to include any SREs in the contract?

- How will SREs be reported that are not identified by ICD-9-CM code assignment? Are there other requirements being discussed as part of the contract, such as incorporating the Leapfrog Group's recommendation of reporting the occurrence of the SRE, apologizing to the patient and/or family, and performing a root-cause analysis?

- What appeal rights does the hospital have?

It is imperative that payer contracts adhere to ethical coding practices. The following excerpts provide examples of contract terms that address payment policies and are consistent with official coding and reporting guidelines.

- When an SRE is not defined by ICD-9-CM codes, there will be no changes in the codes that are submitted.

- For payers that reimburse on a DRG basis, if an inpatient experiences a HAC, the POA assignment is N (was not POA) or U (documentation is insufficient to determine if the HAC was POA), and the HAC is the only complication or comorbidity on the claim, the hospital will be paid the applicable DRG amount, as if the HAC secondary diagnosis was not present.

- For payers that reimburse on a percent-of-charges or per diem basis, the charges or days that are the direct result of the HAC will be billed as noncovered, so appropriate reduction in payment will be made and there will be no changes made to the coded data.

- In accordance with AHIMA's Standards of Ethical Coding, an HIM professional will refuse to delete the SRE from the claim even at the insistence of the payer.

In the unlikely event that the payer insists that the code be deleted, the provider organization should make an effort to work with the payer to change the payer's policy. For example, it can write a letter explaining why it is important to retain the code for a complete clinical picture of the patient's care, data analysis, statistics, and related uses. If the payer refuses to change its policy, this should be obtained in writing. In this situation, the code should not be deleted from the patient database or from other external data reporting processes.

Other internal processes and policies that organizations must consider include:

- Who determines that a HAC or SRE has occurred and how? Once determined, organizations must outline the steps to take.

- Who determines if a charge is removed from a bill?

- How will the event be reported when submitting the claim?

HAC or SRE cases should be flagged so that no bill is prepared for the case until it is investigated. The patient's bill should be reviewed to determine which, if any, charges should be removed based on the payer requirements.

Internal Uses of Coded Data

The POA indicator provides meaningful information for an organization's internal performance improvement initiatives. HIM professionals should reach out to leaders in quality, risk management, patient safety, infection control, case management, nursing, medical staff, finance, decision support, administration, and the board to ensure they are aware of the data and know how to interpret them.

Coded data allow the reporting and stratification of HACs and certain SREs by service area, DRG, provider, and any other data item available in the organization's healthcare information system. This information is useful for monitoring outcomes, generating quality dashboards and provider profiles, and targeting cases for individual case review or root-cause analysis.

Coded data also reduce time needed for medical record review by quality, infection control, and risk management staff solely to identify HAC and certain SREs. The data may be used to supplement and validate current systems for event reporting and infection surveillance.

Finance may use the information in predicting reimbursement and preparing for contract negotiations with third-party payers. The use of the U indicator can be analyzed to identify opportunities for clinical documentation improvement and to evaluate the physician query process.

The organization can examine the interfaces between the healthcare information system and other internal systems to determine the appropriateness of and ability to include the POA indicator with other coded data. HIM professionals should be strong advocates for the use and understanding of this valuable information.

SRE or HAC?

Table 7.1 was developed by one facility to capture appropriate data to assist in reporting serious reportable events and hospital-acquired condition data. It is not intended to be all-inclusive or involve all regulatory reporting.

Table 7.1

NQF Serious Reportable Events	ICD-9 Codes	CMS-Defined Hospital-Acquired Condition	Hospital Staff Responsible for Data Collection	Potential Party Reported To
Surgical Events				
Unintended retention of a foreign object in a patient after surgery or other procedure	998.4, 998.7	Yes	Quality management, risk management, HIM coding	Voluntary reporting to the Joint Commission, patient accounts, risk management
Surgery performed on the wrong body part (CMS National Coverage Determination)	E876.7 (new code for FY 2010)	No	Quality management, risk management, HIM coding	Centers for Medicare and Medicaid Services (CMS), patient accounts, risk management
Surgery performed on the wrong patient (CMS National Coverage Determination)	E876.6 (new code for FY 2010)	No	Quality management, risk management, HIM coding	CMS, patient accounts, risk management
Wrong surgical procedure performed on a patient (CMS National Coverage Determination)	E876.5 (revised title)	No	Quality management, risk management, HIM coding	CMS, patient accounts, risk management
Intraoperative or immediately postoperative death in an ASA Class I patient	—	No	Quality management, risk management, HIM coding	Patient accounts, risk management
Product or Device Events				
Patient death or serious disability associated with the use of contaminated drugs, devices, or biologics provided by the healthcare facility	—	No	Clinical Engineering Quality management, risk management	FDA, voluntary reporting to the Joint Commission, possibly patient accounts, risk management
Patient death or serious disability associated with the use or function of a device in patient care, in which the device is used or functions other than as intended	—	No	Clinical Engineering Quality management, risk management	FDA, voluntary reporting to the Joint Commission, possibly patient accounts, risk management
Patient death or serious disability associated with intravascular air embolism that occurs while being cared for in a healthcare facility	999.1	Yes	Clinical Engineering Quality management, risk management	FDA, voluntary reporting to the Joint Commission, possibly patient accounts, risk management
Patient Protection Events				
Infant discharged to wrong person	—	No	Clinical Engineering Quality management, risk management	Local law enforcement, voluntary reporting to the Joint Commission, risk management
Patient death or serious disability associated with patient elopements (disappearance)	—	No	Clinical Engineering Quality management, risk management	Local law enforcement, voluntary reporting to the Joint Commission, state department of health, risk management
Patient suicide or attempted suicide resulting in serious disability, while being cared for in a healthcare facility	—	No	Clinical Engineering Quality management, risk management	Local law enforcement, voluntary reporting to the Joint Commission, state department of health, risk management

(continued on next page)

Table 7.1 *(continued)*

NQF Serious Reportable Events	ICD-9 Codes	CMS-Defined Hospital-Acquired Condition	Hospital Staff Responsible for Data Collection	Potential Party Reported To
Care Management Events				
Artificial insemination with the wrong sperm or donor egg	—	No	Incident report	Quality management, risk management, patient
Patient death or serious disability associated with a medication error (e.g., errors involving the wrong drug, wrong dose, wrong patient, wrong time, wrong rate, wrong preparation or wrong route of administration)	—	No	Quality management, risk management, HIM coding	Voluntary reporting to the Joint Commission, possibly state board of pharmacy, state board of nursing, state medical board, risk management
Patient death or serious disability associated with a hemolytic reaction due to the administration of ABO/HLA-incompatible blood or blood products	999.6	Yes	Quality management, risk management, HIM coding, patient discharge (expired status)	Red Cross, risk management
Maternal death or serious disability associated with labor or delivery in a low-risk pregnancy while being cared for in a healthcare facility	—	No	Quality management, risk management, HIM coding	Voluntary reporting to the Joint Commission, risk management
Patient death or serious disability associated with hypoglycemia, the onset of which occurs while the patient is being cared for in a healthcare facility	All applicable codes	Yes	Quality management, risk management, HIM coding, patient discharge (expired status)	CMS, patient accounts, risk management
Death or serious disability (kernicterus) associated with failure to identify and treat hyperbilirubinemia in neonates	—	No	Quality management, risk management, HIM coding	Voluntary reporting to the Joint Commission, risk management
Stage 3 or 4 pressure ulcers acquired after admission to a healthcare facility	707.23, 707.24	Yes	Quality management, risk management, HIM coding	CMS, patient accounts, risk management
Patient death or serious disability due to spinal manipulative therapy	—	No	Quality management, risk management	Risk management
Environment Events				
Patient death or serious disability associated with a fall while being cared for in a healthcare facility	• 800–829 Fracture • 830–839 Dislocation • 850–854 Intracranial Injury • 925–929 Crushing Injury	Yes	Quality management, risk management, HIM coding, patient discharge (expired status)	Voluntary reporting to the Joint Commission, CMS, patient accounts, risk management
Any incident in which a line designated for oxygen or other gas to be delivered to a patient contains the wrong gas or is contaminated by toxic substances	—	No	Quality management, risk management	Risk management

(continued on next page)

Table 7.1 *(continued)*

NQF Serious Reportable Events	ICD-9 Codes	CMS-Defined Hospital-Acquired Condition	Hospital Staff Responsible for Data Collection	Potential Party Reported To
Environment Events (continued)				
Patient death or serious disability associated with a burn incurred from any source while being cared for in a healthcare facility	940–949	Yes	Quality management, risk management, HIM coding	Voluntary reporting to the Joint Commission, CMS, patient accounts, risk management
Patient death or serious disability associated with an electric shock or elective cardioversion while being cared for in a healthcare facility	994.8	Yes	Quality management, risk management, HIM coding	Voluntary reporting to the Joint Commission, CMS, patient accounts, risk management
Patient death or serious disability associated with the use of restraints or bedrails while being cared for in a healthcare facility	—	No	Quality management, risk management	State department of health, CMS, voluntary reporting to the Joint Commission, risk management
Criminal Events				
Any instance of care ordered by or provided by someone impersonating a physician, nurse, pharmacist, or other licensed healthcare provider	—	No	Administration, security, risk management, quality management	Respective licensing board, local law enforcement, risk management
Abduction of a patient of any age	—	No	Administration, security, risk management, quality management	Local law enforcement, risk management
Sexual assault on a patient within or on the grounds of a healthcare facility	—	No	Administration, security, risk management, quality management	Local law enforcement, risk management
Death or significant injury of a patient or staff member resulting from a physical assault (ie, battery) that occurs within or on the grounds of a healthcare facility	—	No	Administration, security, risk management, quality management	Local law enforcement, risk management

Summary

Accurate and complete information is both the goal and the outcome of carefully applied processes for evaluating, controlling, and monitoring the quality of healthcare data. Quality healthcare data are driving the healthcare delivery system as it is now being used in models such as CMS's "pay for performance" initiatives and directly impacts payment for services.

Data quality is a complex issue that is difficult to discuss in isolation because it is so closely connected to other areas such as compliance, quality improvement, and the audit process. Chapter 8 provides further in-depth discussion of data quality and compliance issues, and chapter 9 presents a detailed explanation of the audit process.

References

AHIMA Practice Councils (Clinical Terminology/Classification, Quality Initiatives/Secondary Data). Understanding HACs and SREs for quality reporting and reimbursement. *Journal of AHIMA* 80(9):60–65.

American Health Information Management Association. 2009. About ICD-10 Codes. http://www.ahima.org/icd10/about.aspx.

Buff, E.L. and S. Hohmann. 1999. Navigating from data to excellence. *Journal of AHIMA* 70(5):44–48.

Cassidy, B., et al. 1998. Practice brief: Data quality management model. *Journal of AHIMA* 69(6).

Homan, C. 2007. Functions of the health record. Chapter 2 in *Health Information Technology: An Applied Approach,* 2nd ed. Edited by Johns, M. Chicago: AHIMA.

Lambrecht, J. and P.S. Wilson. 2007. Use of Six Sigma in Data Mapping. AHIMA's 79th National Convention and Exhibit Proceedings, October 2007.

Teslow, M.S. 2007. Health data concepts. Chapter 4 in *Health Information: Management of a Strategic Resource,* 3rd ed. Edited by Abdelhak, M., et al. Philadelphia: Saunders.

Chapter 8

Coding Compliance

The US government has established a defined group, with oversight by the Office of the Inspector General (OIG) of the Department of Health and Human Services (HHS), to investigate areas of fraud and abuse in the healthcare industry. The OIG works with the US Department of Justice, which includes the Federal Bureau of Investigation (FBI) and the US Attorneys' Offices, to investigate and prosecute violations of the law. These groups also work at the individual state level with private insurance carriers, states' attorneys general, state Medicaid fraud units, fiscal intermediaries (FIs), and Medicare Part B carriers to evaluate allegations of fraud and abuse.

According to the OIG, facilities should participate voluntarily in programs designed to maintain compliance with all billing and coding regulations. To assist with this process, the OIG has published compliance program guidance for several different types of healthcare entities, including hospitals. In conjunction with the Centers for Medicare and Medicaid Services (CMS), the FBI, and other federal and state agencies, the OIG works to detect fraud and abuse in the healthcare industry.

This chapter examines the programs and policies involved in ensuring coding compliance. It also describes the components of a facility compliance plan.

See appendix F for details on how to develop an effective compliance audit process and appendix G for sample audit worksheets specific to inpatient settings. Appendix H contains an article discussing development of a coding compliance policy.

Recovery Audit Contractors

One of the newest initiatives by the government to eliminate fraud and abuse and recoup incorrect payments is found in the usage of Recovery Audit Contractors (RACs). These contractors audit charts to identify Medicare overpayments and underpayments and return incorrect payments to the government. These RACs are paid based on a percentage of money they identify and collect on behalf of the government. RACs are working to identify incorrect past Medicare payments and helping to prevent future overpayments to providers (CMS 2010).

RACs primarily review areas such as medical necessity, excessive/duplicate payments, and Medicare as secondary payer issues. Additional review areas will be added as RACs become nationwide in scope.

The RAC demonstration program was successful in returning dollars to the Medicare Trust Fund and identifying monies that need to be returned to providers. It provided CMS with a new mechanism for detecting improper payments made in the past and has also given CMS a valuable new tool for preventing future inappropriate payments.

Therefore, section 302 of the Tax Relief and Health Care Act of 2006 makes the RAC program permanent and requires the HHS Secretary to expand the program to all 50 states by no later than January 1, 2010 (CMS 2010). Each RAC will be responsible for identifying overpayments and underpayments in approximately a quarter of the country. The new RAC jurisdictions match the durable medical equipment Medicare Administrative Contractor (DME MAC) jurisdictions. The CMS website http://www.cms.hhs.gov/RAC/ contains updated information on the RAC jurisdiction map, schedule, and contractor information.

Initial Targets: Hospitals and Diagnosis-Related Groups/ Medicare Severity Diagnosis-Related Groups

RACs are initially focusing on diagnosis-related group (DRG) payment errors prior to the conversion of DRGs to MS-DRGs, looking at claims data from as far back as calendar year 2001. Using DRG data-mining software programs, the RACs are analyzing historic Medicare Provider Analysis and Review (MEDPAR) data and identifying accounts that possess the greatest potential for DRG overpayment error. Because the random account selection is not a part of the RAC demonstration program, a variety of DRGs were targeted for review.

A list of the top DRGs includes:

- Septicemia

- Wound débridement and skin graft

- Extensive operating room (OR) procedure unrelated to principal diagnosis

- Circulatory disorders except acute myocardial infarction (AMI), with cardiac catheterization and complex diagnosis

- Respiratory system diagnosis with ventilator support

- Other respiratory system OR procedures w/complication and comorbidity (CC)

- OR procedure for infectious and parasitic diseases

- Respiratory neoplasms

- Nonextensive OR procedure unrelated to principal diagnosis

- Coagulation disorders

- Major small and large bowel procedures w/CC

Identified Issues

Within this group of DRGs, the RAC has identified the three DRGs with the most changes:

- Septicemia

- Wound débridement and skin graft, except hand with débridement

- Coagulation disorders

Septicemia

Physician and clinical documentation regarding bacteremia and urosepsis continue to be inpatient coding challenges. The following scenarios are responsible for most RAC-designated changes.

- **790.7, Bacteremia**

  Target: Principal diagnosis assignment of bacteremia when other infectious diagnosis(es) has been documented and treated. Bacteremia is defined as the presence of bacteria in the blood. It is considered an abnormal laboratory finding for coding purposes. RAC findings indicate that coders should query physicians when bacteremia and other infectious disease processes such as pneumonia, infected ulcers, and urinary tract infections (UTIs) are documented and treated during the same admission.

- **599.0, Urinary tract infection**

  Target: Secondary diagnosis of UTI when the physician documents "urosepsis," but clinical and physician documentation do not support sepsis. RAC findings indicate that coders should query physicians when urosepsis is documented without conclusive evidence of clinical indicators for sepsis.

- **996.62, Line sepsis**

  Target: Secondary diagnosis of line sepsis. American Hospital Association's (AHA's) *Coding Clinic* states that documented cases of sepsis due to infected vascular access devices, catheters, or implants should have code 996.62 sequenced as principal diagnosis. Coders need to carefully review documentation and refer to AHA's *Coding Clinic* to confirm appropriate sequencing guidelines.

Wound Débridement and Skin Graft

Physician documentation regarding type of débridement (that is, sharp, excisional) as well as the depth and site of all excisional wound débridement procedures must be thoroughly reviewed by coding professionals in order to report the most appropriate ICD-9-CM procedure code. The following scenarios are responsible for most RAC-designated changes:

- **83.39, Débridement fascia/muscle**

  ICD-9-CM procedure code 86.22, Excisional débridement, is not appropriate for coding purposes when débridement of skin, subcutaneous tissue, and fascia are performed during the same surgical encounter. Coding professionals need access to complete documentation in order to properly assign débridement procedure codes.

- **81.5x, Joint replacements**

  ICD-9-CM procedure code 86.22, Excisional débridement, should not be assigned when a débridement is performed in conjunction with joint replacement and arthroplasty procedures. Débridement of joints and surrounding tissue is considered integral to joint replacement and arthroplasty procedures.

Coagulation Disorders

The 2004 third quarter AHA *Coding Clinic* provides explicit guidelines regarding the reporting of specific bleeding disorders resulting from Coumadin therapy. ICD-9-CM code 286.5, Hemorrhagic disorder secondary to circulating anticoagulants, should not be reported when the site or type of bleeding is documented by the physician. The following scenarios are responsible for most RAC-designated changes (Bryant 2007):

- 599.7, Hematuria

- 784.7, Epistaxis

- 578.x, GI bleeding

RAC Updates

Since RAC audits began nationwide, new topics and studies have been identified. Since this list is updated on a regular basis, it is important for the coding professional to keep updated on potential areas of risk. Table 8.1 is provided to show an example of RAC issues identified for the state of Tennessee.

The RAC Audit Process

This section, through the heading "Types of Audits," is adapted from AHIMA's Recovery Audit Contractor (RAC) Toolkit (AHIMA 2009b).

Who Is Eligible to Be Audited?

RACs are authorized to investigate claims submitted by all physicians, providers, facilities, and suppliers—essentially everyone who provides Medicare beneficiaries in the fee-for-service program with procedures, services, and treatments and submits claims to Medicare and/or their FIs, regional home health intermediaries (RHHIs), Part A and Part B Medicare administrative contractors (A/B/MACs), DME MACs, and/or carriers. More information on those eligible for RAC audits can be found within the "Preparation Checklist" in appendix A of the RAC toolkit (AHIMA 2009b).

Basis for the Audit

Now that the RACs have been assigned for a specific region of the country, they will receive a claim's file from CMS. The file contains the past claim's data from the National Claims History (NCH), compiling the claims that have been processed and paid after 10/01/07 in that assigned region. Monthly updates, including for the current fiscal year, will be sent thereafter. RACs employ their own custom-designed computer programs and processes, utilizing their uniquely developed criteria based on Medicare rules and regulations, accepted clinical standards of medical practice, and coding and billing policies to determine which specific sectors to review. They may also reference specific services included in the current year OIG's work plan as well as Government Accountability Office (GAO) and Comprehensive Error Rate Testing (CERT) findings. From this foundational information, the RAC will identify those situations

Table 8.1. RAC-approved issues for Tennessee

For inpatient hospital claims:
- Inpatient admissions without a physician's inpatient admit order

For non-medical necessity DRG validation reviews:
- Upper Limb and Toe Amputation for Circulatory System Disorders with MCC: MS-DRG 255
- Cirrhosis and Alcoholic Hepatitis with MCC: MS-DRG 432
- Septicemia without Mechanical Ventilation 96+ Hours without MCC: MS-DRG 872
- Nonextensive OR Procedure Unrelated to Principal Diagnosis without CC/MCC: MS-DRG 989
- Nonextensive OR Procedure Unrelated to Principal Diagnosis with MCC: MS-DRG 987
- Other Respiratory System OR Procedures without CC/MCC: MS-DRG 168
- Extensive OR Procedure Unrelated to Principal Diagnosis without CC/MCC: MS-DRG 983
- Other Respiratory System OR Procedures with CC: MS-DRG 167
- Other Digestive System Diagnoses with CC: MS-DRG 394
- Inflammatory Bowel Disease with CC: MS-DRG 386
- Major Gastrointestinal Disorders and Peritoneal Infections without CC/MCC: MS-DRG 372
- Other Respiratory System OR Procedures with MCC: MS-DRG 166
- Major Small and Large Bowel Procedures without CC/MCC: MS-DRG 331
- Major Small and Large Bowel Procedures with CC: MS-DRG 330
- Major Small and Large Bowel Procedures with MCC: MS-DRG 329
- Major Chest Procedures without CC/MCC: MS-DRG 165
- Major Chest Procedures with MCC: MS-DRG 163
- Major Chest Procedures with CC: MS-DRG 164
- Respiratory System Diagnosis with Ventilator Support 96+ Hours: MS-DRG 207
- Septicemia without Mechanical Ventilation 96+ Hours with MCC: MS-DRG 871
- Extensive OR Procedure Unrelated to Principal Diagnosis with MCC: MS-DRG 981
- Extensive OR Procedure Unrelated to Principal Diagnosis with CC: MS-DRG 982
- Nonextensive OR Procedure Unrelated to Principal Diagnosis with CC: MS-DRG 988
- Coagulation Disorders: MS-DRG 813
- Peritoneal Adhesiolysis with MCC: MS-DRG 335
- Nonextensive Burns: MS-DRG 935
- Other Kidney and Urinary Tract Procedures with CC: MS-DRG 674
- Full Thickness Burn with Skin Graft or Inhalation Injury with CC/MCC: MS-DRG 928
- OR Procedure with Principal Diagnoses of Mental Illness: MS-DRG 876
- Infectious and Parasitic Diseases with OR Procedure without CC/MCC: MS-DRG 855
- Infectious and Parasitic Diseases with OR Procedure with CC: MS-DRG 854
- Postoperative or Posttraumatic Infections with OR Procedure without CC/MCC: MS-DRG 858
- Infectious and Parasitic Diseases with OR Procedure with MCC: MS-DRG 853
- Postoperative or Posttraumatic Infections with OR Procedure with CC: MS-DRG 857
- Postoperative or Posttraumatic Infections with OR Procedure with MCC: MS-DRG 856
- Wound Debridements for Injuries with CC: MS-DRG 902
- Wound Debridements for Injuries with MCC: MS-DRG 901
- Wound Debridements for Injuries without CC/MCC: MS-DRG 903
- Other Kidney and Urinary Tract Procedures with MCC: MS-DRG 673
- Upper Limb and Toe Amputation for Circulatory System Disorders with CC: MS-DRG 256
- Cardiac Pacemaker Revision Except Device Replacement with MCC: MS-DRG 260
- Skin Grafts and Wound Debridement for Endocrine, Nutritional, and Metabolic Disorders without CC/MCC: MS-DRG 624
- Cardiac Pacemaker Revision Except Device Replacement without CC/MCC: MS-DRG 262
- Other Circulatory System OR Procedures: MS-DRG 264
- OR Procedure with Diagnoses of Other Contact with Health Services with MCC: MS-DRG 939
- OR Procedure with Diagnoses of Other Contact with Health Services with CC: MS-DRG 940
- Wound Debridement and Skin Graft Except Hand, for Musculo-Connective Tissue Disorders with MCC: MS-DRG 463
- Wound Debridement and Skin Graft Except Hand, for Musculo-Connective Tissue Disorders with CC: MS-DRG 464
- Skin Graft and/or Debridement for Skin Ulcer or Cellulitis without CC/MCC: MS-DRG 575
- Skin Graft and/or Debridement Except for Skin Ulcer or Cellulitis with MCC: MS-DRG 576
- Skin Graft and/or Debridement Except for Skin Ulcer or Cellulitis without CC/MCC: MS-DRG 578
- Other Hepatobiliary or Pancreas OR Procedures with MCC: MS-DRG 423

(continued on next page)

Table 8.1. RAC-approved issues for Tennessee *(continued)*

For non-medical necessity DRG validation reviews: *(continued)*

- Other Digestive System OR Procedures with CC: MS-DRG 357
- Skin Grafts and Wound Debridement for Endocrine, Nutritional, and Metabolic Disorders with MCC: MS-DRG 622
- Skin Grafts and Wound Debridement for Endocrine, Nutritional, and Metabolic Disorders with CC: MS-DRG 623
- Other Digestive System OR Procedures with MCC: MS-DRG 356
- Wound Debridement and Skin Graft Except Hand, for Musculo-Connective Tissue Disorders without CC/MCC: MS-DRG 465
- Skin Graft and/or Debridement for Skin Ulcer or Cellulitis with MCC: MS-DRG 573
- Skin Graft and/or Debridement for Skin Ulcer or Cellulitis with CC: MS-DRG 574
- Other Vascular Procedures with MCC: MS-DRG 252
- Respiratory system diagnosis with ventilator support < 96 hours: MS-DRG 208
- Extracranial procedures with CC: MS-DRG 038
- Cardiac defibrillator implant without cardiac catheterization without MCC: MS-DRG 227
- Amputation for circulatory system disorders except upper limb and toe with CC: MS-DRG 240
- Permanent cardiac pacemaker implant with MCC: MS-DRG 242
- Other OR procedures for multiple significant trauma with MCC: MS-DRG 957
- Minor small and large bowel procedures with MCC: MS-DRG 344
- Knee procedures without principal diagnosis of infection with CC/MCC: MS-DRG 488
- Fractures of femur with MCC: MS-DRG 533
- Cardiac valve and other major cardiothoracic procedures with cardiac catheterization with MCC: MS-DRG 216
- Spinal fusion except cervical without MCC: MS-DRG 460
- Percutaneous cardiovascular procedure with non-drug-eluting stent with MCC or 4+ vessels/stents: MS-DRG 248
- Cardiac defibrillator implant with cardiac catheterization with acute myocardial infarction/heart failure/ shock with MCC: MS-DRG 222
- Pneumothorax without CC/MCC: MS-DRG 201
- Rehabilitation with CC/MCC: MS-DRG 945
- Major joint replacement or reattachment of lower extremity without MCC: MS-DRG 470
- Psychoses: MS-DRG 885
- Heart failure and shock with MCC: MS-DRG 291
- Pulmonary edema and respiratory failure: MS-DRG 189
- Cardiac defibrillator implant without cardiac catheterization with MCC: MS-DRG 226
- Cholecystectomy except by laparoscope without C.D.E. with CC: MS-DRG 415
- Major cardiovascular procedures with MCC or thoracic aortic aneurysm repair: MS-DRG 237
- HIV with extensive OR procedure with MCC: MS-DRG 969
- Extensive burns or full thickness burns with mechanical ventilation 96+ hours without skin graft: MS-DRG 933
- Amputation for circulatory system disorders except upper limb and toe with MCC: MS-DRG 239
- Full thickness burn without skin graft or inhalation injury: MS-DRG 934
- Permanent cardiac pacemaker implant with CC: MS-DRG 243
- Percutaneous cardiovascular procedure with drug-eluting stent with MCC or 4+ vessels/stents: MS-DRG 246
- Other vascular procedures with CC: MS-DRG 253
- Other female reproductive system OR procedures with CC/MCC: MS-DRG 749
- Other OR procedures of the blood and blood-forming organs with CC: MS-DRG 803
- Lymphoma and nonacute leukemia with other OR procedure with MCC: MS-DRG 823
- Other circulatory system diagnoses with CC: MS-DRG 315
- Amputation of lower limb for endocrine, nutritional, and metabolic disorders with CC: MS-DRG 617
- Myeloproliferative disorders or poorly differentiated neoplasms with other OR procedure with CC/MCC: MS-DRG 829
- Knee procedures with principal diagnosis of infection with CC: MS-DRG 486
- OR procedure with diagnoses of other contact with health services without CC/MCC: MS-DRG 941
- Skin graft and/or debridement except for skin ulcer or cellulitis with CC: MS-DRG 577
- Other digestive system OR procedures without CC/MCC: MS-DRG 358
- Other ear, nose, mouth and throat OR procedures with CC/MCC: MS-DRG 133
- Other hepatobiliary or pancreas OR procedures with CC: MS-DRG 424
- Amputation of lower limb for endocrine, nutritional, and metabolic disorders with MCC: MS-DRG 616

(continued on next page)

Table 8.1.   RAC-approved issues for Tennessee   *(continued)*

- Other kidney and urinary tract procedures without CC/MCC: MS-DRG 675
- Other male reproductive system OR procedures except malignancy with CC/MCC: MS-DRG 717
- Peripheral/cranial nerve and other nervous system procedures with CC or peripheral neurostimulator: MS-DRG 041
- Major bladder procedures with CC: MS-DRG 654
- Stomach, esophageal, and duodenal procedures with CC: MS-DRG 327
- Rectal resection with CC: MS-DRG 333
- Cardiac valve and other major cardiothoracic procedures with cardiac catheterization with CC: MS-DRG 217
- ECMO or tracheotomy with mechanical ventilation 96+ hours or principal diagnosis except face, mouth, and neck with major OR: MS-DRG 003secondary diagnosis, and procedures affecting or potentially affecting the DRG
- Heart transplant or implant of heart assist system with MCC: MS-DRG 001
- Liver transplant with MCC or intestinal transplant: MS-DRG 005
- Rectal resection with MCC: MS-DRG 332
- Kidney transplant: MS-DRG 652
- Tracheotomy for face, mouth, and neck diagnoses with MCC: MS-DRG 011
- Tracheotomy for face, mouth, and neck diagnoses with CC: MS-DRG 012
- Intracranial vascular procedures with principal diagnosis of hemorrhage with MCC: MS-DRG 020
- Intracranial vascular procedures with principal diagnosis of hemorrhage with CC: MS-DRG 021
- Extensive burns or full thickness burns with mechanical ventilation 96+ hours with skin graft: MS-DRG 927
- Full thickness burn with skin graft or inhalation injury without CC/MCC: MS-DRG 929
- Craniotomy with major device implant/acute complex central nervous system principal diagnosis with MCC or chemo implant: MS-DRG 023
- Craniotomy with major device implant/acute complex central nervous system principal diagnosis without MCC: MS-DRG 024
- Lung transplant: MS-DRG 007
- Viral meningitis without CC/MCC: MS-DRG 076
- Bilateral or multiple major joint procedures of lower extremity with MCC: MS-DRG 461
- Splenectomy w MCC, w CC, w/o CC/MCC
- Respiratory infections & inflammations with MCC: MS-DRG 177
- Respiratory infections & inflammations with CC: MS-DRG 178
- Respiratory infections & inflammations without CC/MCC: MS-DRG 179
- Peripheral/cranial nerve and other nervous system procedures with MCC: MS-DRG 040
- Lymphoma and nonacute leukemia with CC: MS-DRG 841
- Cardiac pacemaker device replacement with MCC: MS-DRG 258
- Major bladder procedure with MCC: MS-DRG 653
- Kidney and ureter procedures for non-neoplasm with MCC: MS-DRG 659
- Stomach, esophageal, and duodenal procedures with MCC: MS-DRG 326
- Bone marrow transplant: MS-DRG 009
- Stomach, esophageal, and duodenal procedures without CC/MCC: MS-DRG 328
- Skin grafts and wound debridement for endocrine, nutritional, and metabolic disorders with CC: MS-DRG 623
- Other OR procedures of the blood and blood-forming organs with MCC: MS-DRG 802
- Osteomyelitis without CC/MCC: MS-DRG 541
- Cardiac procedures
- Lymphoma and nonacute leukemia with MCC: MS-DRG 840
- Zoledronic acid (Zometa)—dose vs. units billed—overpayment
- Percutaneous cardiovascular procedure with drug-eluting stent without MCC: MS-DRG 247

For outpatient hospital and physician claims:

- Medically unlikely edit list
- Nebulizer, demonstration and evaluation units billed
- Adenosine—dose vs. units billed
- Barium swallow studies—units billed
- Darbepoetin alfa (non-ESRD)—dose vs. units billed
- Bevacizumab—dose vs. units billed
- Carboplatin—dose vs. units billed
- Docetaxel—dose vs. units billed
- Irinotecan—dose vs. units billed
- Darbepoetin alfa (ESRD)—dose vs. units billed

Source: HCPro, Revenue Cycle Institute 2010.

in which claims have a high probability to be overpaid (and underpaid) in their region. These qualifiers are then entered into the RAC database for each claim to identify providers and begin the analysis and recoupment process.

RAC audits are based on proprietary methodologies developed by each contractor using CMS rules and regulations, national and local coverage determinations, and so on. This method is similar to those conducted by FIs when they are looking to identify improper payments and fraudulent claims. However, RACs are paid by contingency fees based on the amount of overpayments and underpayments they identify. Additionally, it is important to note the RAC will report potential fraud to CMS and potential quality issues to quality improvement organizations (QIOs). All RACs are required to employ professional clinicians, including a physician, medical director, nurses, therapists, and certified coders for their assessments.

Types of Audits

There are two types of audits: automated reviews and complex reviews. An *automated review* occurs when an RAC makes a claim determination at the system level without a human review of the medical record, such as data mining. Errors found must be clearly noncovered services or incorrect application of coding rules and must be supported by Medicare policy, approved article, or coding guidance.

A *complex review*, on the other hand, occurs when an RAC makes a claim determination utilizing human review of the medical record. Records requiring a complex review are those with high probability of noncovered service or where no definitive Medicare policy, Medicare article, or Medicare-sanctioned coding guideline exists.

Fraud and Abuse

Fraud and abuse consist of the acts of providers that are deemed to have defrauded the government or abused the right to bill for services rendered. Fraudulent activity means that the provider intentionally, or with reckless disregard for the truth, filed false healthcare claims. These findings can result in civil or criminal prosecution. Erroneous claims, or abuse, are innocent billing errors that result in the minimum of return of overpayments or funds received in error.

Federal Civil False Claims Act

The Federal Civil False Claims Act (FCA) (31 USC§3729–3733) is the legislation that provides the framework for federal fraud and abuse penalties and investigations. It defines liability for anyone who knowingly files a fraudulent claim with the intention of obtaining inappropriate funds from the government. The law specifies that a claim of fraud can be made up to 10 years from the date of violation.

The phrase "knew or should have known" is frequently used in conjunction with fraud and abuse. Professionals and facilities are required to adhere to all published rules and guidance. Whether they actually knew about a certain rule does not matter; if the rule was published, it should be followed.

Operation Restore Trust

Operation Restore Trust is a program set up by the OIG as a means of combating healthcare fraud and abuse. It uses an interdisciplinary project team of federal and state government and private-sector representatives to target Medicare abuse and misuse. The project consists of federal audits by the OIG, criminal investigations by CMS, and referrals by the OIG to appropriate law enforcement officials. Civil and administrative sanction and recovery actions by the OIG and other appropriate law enforcement officials are an integral part of this plan, with damages that can be triple the amount of the actual inappropriate payment, and with fines of more than $11,000 per occurrence.

Other OIG Guidance for Compliance Programs

The OIG also publishes studies and recommendations for program adjustments to prevent fraud and reduce waste and abuse. Additionally, it issues special fraud alerts to notify the public and healthcare community about schemes in the provision of healthcare services. The OIG Work Plan, published each fiscal year, is a projection of the various projects to be addressed by the Office of Audit Services, Office of Evaluation and Inspections, Office of Investigations, and Office of Counsel to the Inspector General. Current work plans are available online (OIG n.d.).

The government issued the first guidance for compliance programs for hospitals in 1998. The OIG (1998) stated:

> The adoption and implementation of voluntary compliance programs significantly advance the prevention of fraud, abuse, and waste in these health care plans while at the same time furthering the fundamental mission of all hospitals, which is to provide quality care to all patients.

Seven key elements were established as guidelines for an effective compliance program. A facility should:

- Establish written policies, procedures, and standards of conduct
- Designate a chief compliance officer and appropriate committee(s)
- Provide an effective training and education program
- Develop effective communication and a process for reporting compliance issues
- Enforce the program through well-publicized disciplinary guidelines
- Audit and monitor the program
- Respond promptly to allegations by taking corrective action

The OIG published the OIG Supplemental Compliance Program Guidance for Hospitals in 2005. This document (OIG 2005, 4858–4876) also is available online.

Policies and Procedures

Definitive policies and procedures should be established and maintained to ensure that all members of the organization are following the guidelines. Comprehensive policies and procedures should include accurate coding, documentation, retention, contracts, and outsourcing. Internal coding practices should be well written, clear, and indicative that the facility follows official coding guidelines. Written coding accuracy standards and commitment should be in place to provide adequate coding resources for all coding staff. If outsourced/contract coders are utilized in the facility, they must be educated on facility policies, and steps should be taken to ensure that they are following the same rules and regulations and are under the same quality measurements as hospital-employed coding professionals.

Moreover, the policies and procedures should be used to identify and target possible areas of risk. Some of the most common areas of risk include:

- Unbundling or fragmenting a service by reporting separate codes for services that are included in one procedure code

- Downcoding a service in order to assign an additional code. (This also can occur by inappropriately separating surgical approach from the major surgical service performed.)

Other areas of concern are as follows:

- Diagnosis or procedure misrepresentation

- Assignment of a code for a higher level of service than the service that was provided

- Diagnostic tests that are medically unnecessary

- DRG assignments including problematic areas such as pneumonia, sepsis, and respiratory failure

The policies and procedures should be communicated on a regular basis. A code of conduct should be developed that indicates a firm commitment to compliance as part of the daily routine and course of business.

Components of a Compliance Plan

The basic components of a compliance plan include designation of a compliance officer, training and education, communication strategies, auditing and monitoring activities, corrective action, and follow-up measures. In addition, mechanisms to ensure accurate and complete documentation in the health record must be in place to ensure coding and billing compliance.

Designation of Compliance Officer

In the compliance program guidance (CPG) for hospitals, the government recognized that facilities may have different needs in developing their compliance plan. The government recommends that hospitals appoint a chief compliance officer and establish a compliance committee to provide assistance and guidance, as needed.

Training and Education

Training and education are key components of all compliance plans. Annual training for new hires, professional staff, and physicians should be mandatory. Regular meetings should be held with coding staff to ensure compliance with any new rules and regulations. Focused training sessions should take place as problematic areas are identified, and compliance should be included in all performance evaluations. Facilities should establish job descriptions and qualification requirements for professional coders and billing staff.

Communication

Communication is an essential component in all compliance plans. A mechanism must be in place for reporting perceived compliance violations. If employees think that their complaints will be ignored or used against them in some way, they will not report problems, even though there are whistleblower laws to protect them. They need to know that compliance is not just a requirement from the government, but a part of the culture at the facility. No one member or group can be exempt from the system.

Auditing and Monitoring

Another key component of a thorough compliance program is auditing (which is discussed in greater detail in chapter 9). Auditing of the entire revenue cycle from patient service to payment should be completed on a regular basis. Some basic auditing steps include the following (OIG 2005, 4859):

- Use OIG target areas to ensure compliance with key efforts by the government to prevent fraud.

- Evaluate internal coding practices on a regular basis.

- Compare internal findings with external benchmarking practices. Frequency, scope, and size depend on the organization. There is no "one size fits all" compliance plan. Plans should be developed and reviewed on an ongoing basis to ensure that they are working properly and appropriately. "The OIG strongly encourages hospitals to identify and focus their compliance efforts on those areas of potential concern or risk that are most relevant to their individual organizations."

Corrective Action and Follow-up

With any compliance issues that are identified, corrective action and follow-up must occur in a timely manner. Although the definition of "timely" may vary depending on the scope of the problem, it is commonly recommended that corrective action and follow-up happen within 60 days of the date the complaint is reported. If employees think that their concerns are ignored, they are less likely to report possible violations in the future.

As hospitals work to maintain and promote compliance in their facilities, they should examine several areas. These include monitoring of case-mix index (CMI), comparison of coding and billing patterns, and monitoring and evaluation of denials and implementation of coding updates.

Monitor and Understand the CMI

The CMI is the average DRG weight for a set of patients for a given time period. A CMI close to 1.000 shows that the facility's patients are using approximately the same amount of resources as the average Medicare patient. A higher CMI indicates patients who are more acutely ill than the average Medicare patient. As the government monitors submitted data in the MEDPAR database, a hospital with a CMI that is statistically higher than that of hospitals in surrounding areas may raise concern. In the early days of fraud and abuse investigations, several hospitals with unusually high CMIs were found to have improper coding and billing practices. (See table 8.2 for a typical CMI.)

Table 8.2. Example of CMI

Patient	MS-DRG	MS-DRG Weight
1	89	0.9298
2	434	0.6489
3	55	1.0613
4	478	2.1321

Total MS-DRG Weight = 4.7721/4 = 1.193025 CMI.

The CMI should be calculated and tracked over time to allow the facility to monitor for unusual events that have an impact on the overall CMI. For example, one or two highly weighted DRGs (such as MS-DRG 002 with a relative weight of 11.754) will create an abnormally high CMI. If the facility in this example had one additional patient in MS-DRG 927 with a relative weight of 13.7351, the CMI would jump to 3.70144. This high CMI does not accurately reflect the amount of resources used by the average patient in the facility.

Compare Utilization and Billing Patterns with National, State, and Regional Norms

A common practice is to benchmark with other facilities with similar traits, such as bed size and patient mix. This allows the hospital to evaluate its performance statistics in comparison with like hospitals and review any unusual findings.

Compare Coding and Billing Patterns Over Time

Facilities also can benchmark internally. The facility might use a simple graph to chart patterns over different time periods to determine problem areas. It also should look for areas of concern, such as an unusually high CMI or a drop in reimbursement.

Monitor Claims Denials and Error Reports

As much as possible, facilities should have staff dedicated to monitoring all denials and claims that are returned to provider (RTP). A simple spreadsheet, as shown in table 8.3, can be developed to monitor denials to evaluate areas for education and improvement in coding and billing practices.

Monitor Coding and MS-DRG Changes

Facilities should monitor claims carefully in the first few months after coding changes take effect. These changes affect coding, billing, and documentation practices and should be reviewed to ensure that correct and complete claims are submitted. Some insurance companies may not have uploaded coding changes into their computer systems and may erroneously deny claims that make use of new codes.

Appeal Inappropriate Denials

As denials are being monitored, it is imperative that incorrect or inappropriate denials be appealed.

Table 8.3. Example of denial spreadsheet

Reason for Denial	No. of Patients	Amount
Medical necessity	15	$4,345
Noncovered services	3	$2,356
Bundling edits	5	$6,742

Documentation Requirements

As discussed in other chapters, documentation in the health record is key to ensuring coding and billing compliance. According to Medicare, documentation should be available to the coder at the time of coding and sufficient to support the claim. It should be timely, with dictation and transcription completed as soon as possible after discharge. An established mechanism must be in place for obtaining physician clarification when the documentation is incomplete, illegible, or ambiguous so that billing accurately reflects the services provided.

Quality Improvement Organizations

To ensure that the federal government pays only for medically necessary, appropriate, and high-quality healthcare services, CMS contracts with medical review organizations called quality improvement organizations (QIOs). These organizations were formerly known as peer review organizations (PROs). QIOs work with hospitals and other healthcare organizations in their area to conduct studies designed to help improve quality of care for Medicare beneficiaries. The QIO's contract with CMS is known as the Scope of Work (SOW), a document that specifies the goals and topics for review. According to Qsource (2005), for the state of Tennessee, the QIO's "approach to quality improvement focuses on patterns of care, with the primary goal of studying and improving the mainstream of care."

Hospital Payment Monitoring Program

Through the SOW, CMS has reviewed problematic DRGs over the past several years. Originally, in 1999, this program was known as the Payment Error Prevention Program (PEPP). The QIOs worked with hospitals to monitor their documentation and coding practices to ensure compliance with Medicare initiatives to prevent fraud and abuse.

Medicare Quality Initiative

Section 501(b) of the Medicare Modernization Act (MMA) requires that certain inpatient hospitals submit quality data to the HHS Secretary on a set of indicators, as established by the Secretary as of November 1, 2003, in order to receive a full-payment update. Hospitals that do not submit data in the form and manner specified will have their payment update reduced by two percentage points. The requirements for the Hospital Inpatient Quality Reporting Program are available online from Quality-Net (n.d.).

Specific Coding Problem Areas

Based on studies of coding patterns, the OIG is able to target specific problem areas that result in inaccurate coding and payment. Pneumonias constitute one such problem area; septicemia and related conditions are another.

Pneumonias

The OIG has performed several studies related to the issues of pneumonia coding because of patterns indicating inaccurate coding and payment for bacterial cases of pneumonia. Clinically, there are many different types of pneumonia. Code 486, Pneumonia, organism unspecified, should be used only when the health record does not identify the causative organism. Therefore, it is important that the coder review the entire medical record and possibly query the physician to determine whether a more specific code can be used. Even when the coder finds a positive culture in the laboratory findings, such as for *Klebsiella pneumoniae,* this cannot be coded as Pneumonia due to Klebsiella pneumoniae without confirmation from the physician of a cause-and-effect relationship.

Viral pneumonia is highly contagious and typically affects the trachea and bronchi of the lungs. Pneumococcal pneumonia is caused by pneumococcal/streptococcus pneumoniae bacteria. Clinical indicators include documentation of pleural friction and chest x-ray showing consolidation from pus. Other bacterial pneumonias caused by agents such as *Klebsiella, Pseudomonas,* and *Streptococcus* are common in the adult population and are usually identified through Gram staining of sputum. Because of differences in the quality of a sputum culture and the possibility of contamination as the sputum travels through the airway, *Coding Clinic for ICD-9-CM* states that a gram-positive cocci finding should not be coded as the cause of bacterial pneumonia without further clinical findings and documentation by the physician.

Coding Clinic guidelines for coding gram-negative pneumonia include findings such as worsening of cough, dyspnea, reduction of oxygen level, fever, purulent sputum, and patchy infiltration on chest x-ray. It may appear as a complication of surgery, trauma, or chronic illnesses, or in patients with chronic obstructive pulmonary disease (COPD) and those receiving immunosuppressive drug therapy.

Septicemia

Another problem identified by the OIG is that of incorrect coding of sepsis. Clinically, sepsis may have characteristics similar to a urinary tract infection, which is often documented as urosepsis, and there is a large difference in DRG payment. It is very important that the coder understand findings in the health record in order to code the diagnoses appropriately.

In the past, sepsis and septicemia were coded the same, but over the past several years, the "systemic inflammatory response syndrome-sepsis-severe sepsis-septic shock continuum" has been established. The patient first may exhibit signs of bacteremia. Bacteremia is the presence of bacteria in the blood and is coded to 790.7. It can lead to sepsis but is not necessarily the same thing. The coder should query the physician, especially when bacteremia is found with two or fewer signs of sepsis. Transient bacteremia may occur in other diseases such as pneumonia, but if it lasts over several days, it may mean that there is an infected vessel or heart valve.

Septicemia, code 038.X, is defined as "an infectious disease due to the accumulation and persistence of bacteria and/or their toxins in the blood and marked by high fever, shaking chills, prostration, and if untreated, hypotension, shock and death" (Channel 2009, 446). It is a systemic disease.

Systemic Inflammatory Response Syndrome (995.9x)

Systemic inflammatory response syndrome (SIRS) is considered a major complication consisting of the body's reaction to infection or trauma. It includes systemic inflammation, rapid heart rate and respiration, and an elevated white blood cell (WBC) count that may develop into multiorgan dysfunction (MOD) or failure (Channel 2009, 1053). Sepsis codes are sequenced after the code for the underlying infection, such as septicemia.

Sepsis (995.91)

The definition of sepsis is a SIRS reaction plus documented infection. Common symptoms include mental status changes, especially in the elderly patient; oliguria; and sustained hypotension.

Severe Sepsis (995.92)

Severe sepsis consists of sepsis plus end-organ dysfunction. It may include multiple organ failure, including kidney and respiratory failure, encephalopathy, or critical illness myopathy or polyneuropathy. Each organ dysfunction should be coded along with the severe sepsis code. If there is question in the documentation whether the organ dysfunction is or is not from the sepsis, then query the physician. This patient typically requires extensive treatment with high-cost medications such as Xigris.

Septic Shock (785.52)

The last phase of the continuum is septic shock, which is defined as "sepsis with sepsis-induced hypotension despite fluid resuscitation and inadequate tissue perfusion (failure of peripheral circulation)" (Channel 2009, 968). Many patients do not recover when they reach this point in the continuum.

Coding Guidance for Septicemia

According to *Coding Clinic for ICD-9-CM*, a negative blood culture does not mean the patient does not have septicemia. If clinical signs substantiate the diagnosis, however, the physician must show a clear link between the culture findings and the diagnosis.

Treatment for sepsis usually includes high dosages of intravenous antibiotics; thus, if a patient has been on antibiotics prior to the blood culture, this may account for a negative-appearing (normal) result. Clinical indicators include positive blood cultures, WBC count greater than 14,000/mm, fever, and oliguria. When the term *urosepsis* is used, the physician should be queried to determine the proper diagnosis. The main problem identified in government DRG validation studies included "clinical findings in the chart not specified/verified by physician"; thus, it is very important that coders review the chart carefully and query the physician to ensure correct coding. Facilities should continue to review cases in MS-DRGs for sepsis and septicemia, especially those with a short length of stay, and to continue to educate physicians on updated terminology to assist with proper coding. The coding professional should also carefully review the chart for mechanical ventilation, as patients with 96 or more hours of mechanical ventilation tend to stay in the hospital longer and utilize more resources. *Coding Clinic for ICD-9-CM* and *ICD-9-CM Official Guidelines for Coding and*

Reporting should be reviewed for more detailed information as noted below in the chapter-specific guidelines:

The coding of SIRS, sepsis, and severe sepsis requires a minimum of two codes: a code for the underlying cause (such as infection or trauma) and a code from subcategory 995.9 Systemic inflammatory response syndrome (SIRS). These codes are detailed below.

(i) The code for the underlying cause (such as infection or trauma) must be sequenced before the code from subcategory 995.9 Systemic inflammatory response syndrome (SIRS).

(ii) Sepsis and severe sepsis require a code for the systemic infection (038.xx, 112.5, etc.) and either code 995.91, Sepsis, or 995.92, Severe sepsis. If the causal organism is not documented, assign code 038.9, Unspecified septicemia.

(iii) Severe sepsis requires additional code(s) for the associated acute organ dysfunction(s).

(iv) If a patient has sepsis with multiple organ dysfunctions, follow the instructions for coding severe sepsis.

(v) Either the term sepsis or SIRS must be documented to assign a code from subcategory 995.9.

(vi) See Section I.C.17.g, Injury and poisoning, for information regarding systemic inflammatory response syndrome (SIRS) due to trauma/burns and other noninfectious processes.

Due to the complex nature of sepsis and severe sepsis, some cases may require that the provider be queried prior to assignment of the codes (NCHS 2009, 17).

According to Official Coding Guidelines, the codes should be sequenced based on whether the patient had evidence of sepsis on admission and should follow the definition of principal diagnosis. The instructional note under subcategory 995.9 instructs to assign the underlying condition first.

- Note: The term *urosepsis* is nonspecific. If it is the only term documented, only code 599.0 should be assigned based on the default for the term in the ICD-9-CM index, in addition to the code for the causal organism, if known.

- For patients with severe sepsis, the code for the systemic infection (038.xx, 112.5, and so forth) or trauma should be sequenced first, followed by either code 995.92, Systemic inflammatory response syndrome due to infectious process with organ dysfunction, or code 995.94, Systemic inflammatory response syndrome due to noninfectious process with organ dysfunction. Codes for the specific organ dysfunction also should be assigned.

- If septic shock is documented, it is necessary to code first the initiating systemic infection or trauma and then either code 995.92 or 995.94, followed by code 785.52, Septic shock.

ICD-10 Impact on Fraud and Abuse Prevention

The use of ICD-10-CM and ICD-10-PCS may help reduce the opportunities for fraud and improve fraud detection capabilities. Field testing has shown that ICD-10's greater specificity results in improved data accuracy and coding due to the level of detail in the code descriptors

(AHIMA 2009a). The improved logic and increased specificity in ICD-10 will facilitate the development of sophisticated edit tools for detection of questionable patterns and suspected fraud, whereas continued use of ICD-9-CM inhibits the development of computer-assisted coding systems that can reduce fraud. The report of the antifraud study conducted by the Office of the National Coordinator for Health Information Technology (ONC) is available at http://www. hhs.gov/healthit/documents/ReportOnTheUse.pdf.

Applying the Guidelines

The following case examples are designed to increase the reader's understanding of and ability to select appropriate principal and secondary diagnoses. The correct answers are found at the end of the chapter.

Case 8.1

History of Present Illness: The patient is a 54-year-old man with a 5-day history of feeling ill. When his daughter went to his house today to check on him, she found him clammy with a fever and very disoriented. Laboratory results in the emergency department showed UTI, probable sepsis, renal insufficiency. Blood urea nitrogen, creatinine elevated. WBC count was 23,000. The patient was admitted for treatment of probable urinary sepsis.

Findings While in the Hospital: WBCs fell during hospitalization to 9,000. Urine culture grew *Escherichia coli;* blood cultures also grew *E. coli.* No other abnormalities noted.

Hospital Course: The patient was started on IV fluid rehydration; electrolytes improved throughout stay. He was started on IV antibiotics and switched to oral antibiotics the day of discharge. The patient was discharged to his daughter's care at her home until he gets back on his feet.

Answer:

Principal Diagnosis: _____

Secondary Diagnoses: _____

Questions for Physician: _____

Case 8.2

Discharge Diagnoses: UTI, Urosepsis, Pneumonia

History: The patient is a 74-year-old man who complains of fever, chills, and not feeling well generally. Urine culture had been done the day prior to admission due to frequent UTI problems and was positive for *E. coli,* so he was started on Cipro. Admission urinalysis showed a large number of WBCs and nitrate. WBC count was 14,000. Sputum cultures were positive for *Klebsiella pneumoniae.*

Hospital Course: The patient was started on IV fluids to rehydrate him and Ancef added to his Cipro meds. Urine cultures continued to have increased white cells. Blood cultures taken on the second day were normal. Chest cleared to normal by discharge.

Answer:

Principal Diagnosis: _____

Secondary Diagnoses: _____

Questions for Physician: _____

Summary

Because hospitals are paid for inpatient care based primarily on codes, it is vital that coders have a clear understanding of appropriate and compliant coding. Facilities throughout the country have had to make repayments to the government because of improper coding, sequencing, and billing of diagnosis and procedure codes. Most facilities have not set out to defraud the government purposely but, rather, have made mistakes because of a lack of policies, procedures, and appropriate compliance training. Compliance should not be another buzzword; rather, it should be part of a culture in which all members of the healthcare team work together to ensure that complete and accurate documentation leads to correct and adequate payment for services.

References

American Health Information Management Association. 2009a. About ICD-10 Codes. http://www.ahima.org/icd10/about.aspx.

American Health Information Management Association. 2009b. Recovery Audit Contractor (RAC) Toolkit. http://library.ahima.org/xpedio/groups/public/documents/ahima/bok1_044065.pdf.

Bryant, Gloryanne. 2007 (Mar.). *CodeWrite Community News.* Chicago: AHIMA.

Centers for Medicare and Medicaid Services. 2010. Recovery Audit Contractor Overview. http://www.cms.hhs.gov/RAC/.

Channel. 2009. *Educational Annotation of ICD-9-CM.* Reno, NV: Channel Publishing.

HCPro, Revenue Cycle Institute. 2010. CMS-Approved RAC Audit Issues: CMS-Approved RAC Issues by Region, Updated 7-6-10. http://blogs.hcpro.com/revenuecycleinstitute/tools/.

Office of the Inspector General. n.d. Work Plan. http://oig.hhs.gov/publications/workplan.asp.

Office of the Inspector General. 1998 (Feb. 23). Publication of the OIG Compliance Program Guidance for Hospitals. *Federal Register* 63(35):8987–8998. http://oig.hhs.gov/authorities/docs/cpghosp.pdf.

Office of the Inspector General. 2005 (Jan. 31). OIG Supplemental Compliance Program Guidance for Hospitals. *Federal Register* 70(19):4858–4876. http://oig.hhs.gov/fraud/docs/complianceguidance/012705HospSupplementalGuidance.pdf.

QSource. 2005. Hospital Payment Monitoring Program Resources. http://www.qsource.org/workbook.htm.

QualityNet. n.d. Hospital Inpatient Quality Reporting (IQR) Program Overview. http://www.qualitynet.org/dcs/ContentServer?cid=1138115987129&pagename=QnetPublic%2FPage%2FQnetTier2&c=Page.

Answers to Case Studies

Case 8.1

Principal Diagnosis: The physician states "probable sepsis" and all clinical evidence (blood cultures, mental status changes) points to that as the main reason for admission. Underlying cause (such as *E. coli* septicemia) would need to be verified. Because the patient has renal insufficiency, the coder needs to query the physician to see if this is more appropriately coded to severe sepsis. Because official coding guidelines do allow for coding "probable" at present, it is technically correct to code sepsis; however, a query to the physician would be indicated to obtain the most appropriate information. Urinary sepsis codes to 599.0; however, it appears the physician may mean sepsis, which would be coded to 038.9, 995.91. The coder should query for cause-and-effect relationship of positive blood culture *E. coli* to sepsis for 038.42 and would need more information from the chart to determine if the patient had acute renal failure and the 995.92 severe sepsis with organ dysfunction for acute renal failure (584.9).

Secondary Diagnoses: UTI 599.0

E. coli 041.4

Patient was started on IV fluid rehydration. Clarify with the physician: Is dehydration a codeable diagnosis?

MS-DRG Grouping Issues: If this case is grouped with the UTI as the principal diagnosis, it falls into MS-DRG 690, Kidney and Urinary Tract Infection without MCC, which is weighted 0.7708 and has an approximate payment of $4,378.35. If the physician query justifies the septicemia as the principal diagnosis, it groups to MS-DRG 872, Septicemia without Mechanical Ventilation Greater than 96 hours, without MCC. The weight is 1.1155 with approximate payment at $6,336.35. Severe sepsis with acute renal failure would group to MS-DRG 871 with a weight of 1.8437 and approximate payment rate of $10,472.70.

Case 8.2

Principal Diagnosis: The coder needs to verify in the record and query the physician as to the main reason for admission. Nonspecific diagnosis of urosepsis needs to be clarified; it could mean urinary sepsis (coded as UTI, 599.0) or sepsis. Blood cultures were negative, but this does not preclude a diagnosis of sepsis according to *Coding Clinic*. Also, sputum culture grew out *Klebsiella*. The coder should verify that documentation supports that as the cause for the pneumonia (482.0) by querying the physician. This case could be "multiple conditions present on admission" because it appears that either the pneumonia or UTI/sepsis could be the chief reason for admission.

Secondary Diagnoses: UTI 599.0

E. Coli 041.4

MS-DRG Grouping Issues: The order of the diagnoses and level of specificity provided through the query process can have a tremendous impact on correct reimbursement in this case. After querying the physician, if the UTI is found to meet the definition of principal diagnosis, with the pneumonia due to *Klebsiella* as secondary (counting as an MCC), it groups to MS-DRG 689 with a weight of 1.2122 and an approximate payment of $6,885.62.

If septicemia is determined to be the principal diagnosis, MS-DRG 871 is weighted at 1.8437 with an approximate payment of $10,472.70.

If the *Klebsiella pneumoniae* is the principal diagnosis with a secondary diagnosis of UTI instead of septicemia, the correct MS-DRG is 178 with a weight of 1.486 and an approximate payment of $8,440.88. If *Klebsiella pneumoniae* is the principal diagnosis with both UTI and sepsis/septicemia coded as secondary diagnoses, the MS-DRG 177 would be assigned, which has a weight of 2.0483 and approximate payment of $11,634.89.

MS-DRG	Relative Weight	Approximate Payment
689	1.2122	$6,885.62
871	1.8437	$10,472.70
178	1.486	$8,440.88
177	2.0483	$11,634.89

Chapter 9

The Health Record Auditing Process

In simplest terms, an inpatient health record audit is a methodical examination and review of a hospital's coding and billing processes. This chapter discusses the types of code audits, the different methods for reviewing them, and how to design and implement a code audit.

Plan of Action for Setting Up or Updating a Health Record Auditing Process

When establishing or updating an auditing process, the healthcare facility should develop a plan of action based on consideration of the following issues:

- What does the facility want to accomplish with the auditing program? What are its goals and objectives?

- What resources are needed in terms of personnel, time, finances, and so forth?

- What should the time frame be? One big audit per quarter? Several ongoing audit and monitoring projects?

- What forms are needed? Several companies and textbooks provide audit samples, or the facility can create its own forms.

- How can the facility achieve buy-in from staff, physicians, and administration? The more people feel ownership of a program, the more likely they are to participate willingly.

During the audit, the reviewers should look for patterns and trends, strengths and weaknesses, and problems that might be uncovered during the auditing process. They also should have access to all documents and be able to work independently so that they can remain objective in all areas. With strong commitment from the facility's administration, the reviewers should be able to obtain a true picture of its compliance program without worrying about "stepping on toes" or feeling that a particular group of people is off-limits or exempt from compliance activities.

Compliance Program Guidance

The Hospital Payment Monitoring Program (HPMP) and its precursor, the Payment Error Protection Program (PEPP), have resulted in a number of excellent methods and structures for coding and reimbursement evaluation. Health information management (HIM) professionals can look to resources provided by quality improvement organizations (QIOs) (and the earlier peer review organizations), under contract with government agencies for reliable means to improve processes and minimize the risk of noncompliance.

An effective auditing and monitoring program shows that standards and procedures are current and accurate and that the compliance program is being carried out effectively. In its 2005 OIG Supplemental Compliance Program Guidance for Hospitals, the Office of the Inspector General (OIG) identified the following areas of potential risk for hospitals that should be incorporated into the auditing portion of their compliance programs (OIG 2005):

- *Submission of accurate claims and information:* Ensuring that claims are accurate and complete remains the largest area of risk for hospitals. Documentation must support all services provided and billed and show that the service is "reasonable and necessary" for treatment of the patient's condition.

- *Referral statutes:* The physician self-referral law (Stark) prohibits hospitals from submitting claims for services provided as part of a "prohibited financial relationship." This includes certain joint ventures and compensation relationships with physicians, such as recruitment or discounts.

- *Payments to reduce or limit services:* This includes inappropriate gain-sharing or cost-sharing procedures whereby the physician may have an incentive to reduce or limit services to a beneficiary.

- *The Emergency Medical Treatment and Labor Act (EMTALA):* EMTALA was established to prevent hospitals from inappropriately transferring patients who are unstable or in active labor. Documentation must substantiate that appropriate screening and approval was done prior to any transfer or referral to other healthcare facilities.

- *Quality of care:* Providing substandard care can be viewed as a form of fraudulent activity even when services are billed correctly. Hospitals are obligated to review the quality of services provided by their medical staff and employees for all patients, not just Medicare or Medicaid patients.

- *Relationships with federal health beneficiaries:* Hospitals must take care to avoid inappropriate incentives to patients by refraining from providing any prohibited services such as gifts or free transportation.

- *Health Insurance Portability and Accountability Act (HIPAA) Privacy and Security Rules:* The facility must ensure strict compliance with the rules governing the privacy and security of patient information established by HIPAA of 1996.

- *Medicare or Medicaid billing:* The facility must ensure that it is not billing Medicare or Medicaid in excess of usual charges.

Types of Audits

The main types of audits are coding audits, claims audits, and audits of policies and procedures. Some organizations choose to review coding accuracy and conduct claims review separately. Coding accuracy requires individual record assessment whereas some aspects of claims review are based on aggregate data analysis.

Coding Audits

All facilities should perform coding audits on at least a quarterly basis with the understanding that compliance must be an ongoing process. A comprehensive review should include a sample of all physicians, types of patients, and common diagnoses and procedures. The internal auditor should act as an external auditor by avoiding assumptions, and the record should reflect enough documentation to substantiate any diagnosis or procedure performed. A summary of the results should be prepared and shared with coders, physicians, and administration as needed. Any coding assessment should include verification that the codes selected for cases are the same codes reported for any external purpose, such as reimbursement from a third party.

Claims Audits

Claims audits are performed on a regular basis to ensure that claims are processed in accordance with required healthcare program and billing regulations. In addition, they are done to determine the completeness of medical record documentation in supporting the services billed. Audits or chart reviews also help to verify that the codes selected are exactly the same as those submitted to the insurance company.

Audits of Policies and Procedures

The organization's compliance plan, coding policy, and other policies and procedures should be reviewed at least annually. Adherence to the hospital's compliance plan should be audited and monitored periodically to ensure its effectiveness. The procedure manual should be a fluid, current document that is frequently used by staff as a reference tool.

Methods for Review

The method used to review code audits may vary depending on whether an initial diagnostic audit or a focused review based on a specific problem area is being performed. One common approach is to use published statistical reports for comparison. For example, *The Medicare DRG Handbook*, published by Solucient, could be used for this purpose. This manual is compiled from the Medicare Provider Analysis and Review (MEDPAR) file and summarizes key findings by the top 50 highest-volume diagnosis-related groups (DRGs), which constitute a large percentage of the total discharges of more than 500 total DRGs. Any organization's data can be compared and contrasted with the key findings in this manual. Although this book and others like it are still available, with the implementation of the MS-DRG system in fiscal year (FY) 2008, facilities should monitor data carefully. As data are compiled using the

MS-DRG groupings, updated publications will be available. The American Health Information Management Association's (AHIMA's) book *Analyzing the Impact of MS-DRGs* (Hyde and Spencer 2008) is designed to assist facilities in converting their top 10 high-risk, high-volume DRG data into MS-DRG data and performing audits based on that facility-specific information.

Inpatient coding quality measures include (Wilson 2008):

- Accurate ICD-9-CM code assignment to the principal and secondary (additional) diagnoses.

- Accurate ICD-9-CM code assignment to the principal and other procedures.

- Accurate DRG assignment for inpatient reimbursement.

- Accurate present on admission (POA) indicator for all ICD-9-CM diagnosis codes, excluding codes published on the exempt list.

- Accurate patient status (discharge disposition) assignment.

Two types of record review methods are used in inpatient settings: the record method and the code method.

Record Method

The record method considers each incorrectly coded record to be one error. There are several advantages to this method, including:

- It is commonly used in hospitals, which allows for benchmarking.

- It permits the reviewer to track errors by case type.

- It enables the reviewer to relate productivity to quality errors on a case basis.

The disadvantages to the record method include the following:

- It oversimplifies the type of records coded because it does not recognize the coder's identification of codes that should be reported.

- It identifies neither the number of secondary diagnoses nor procedures missed by the coder.

Code Method

The code method compares the total number of codes identified by the coder to the total number of possible codes that should have been reported. The advantages to the code method include the following:

- It recognizes the coder's ability to identify all codes.

- It weighs the more resource-intensive cases by code.

- It better identifies the kinds of errors the coder is making (for example, omission of secondary diagnoses or missed sequencing).

The disadvantages to the code method include the following:

- It is difficult to compare results with benchmarking activities of other organizations.

- It does not assist with the diagnosis of case-type coder educational needs.

Benchmarking best practices shows that the code-on-code methodology is a more accurate way to calculate error rate. "A coding error is any code that is revised, added, or deleted" (Wilson 2008). These are defined as:

- **Revised code:** Revised codes are counted as *one error* or *one revision* when the *condition* or *procedure* being validated requires any of the following types of code changes: resequencing such as moving a secondary diagnosis or procedure to principal diagnosis or principal procedure; deleting one code and revising the second code to report the combination code for the condition or procedure (300.00 and 311 being validated, auditor deletes one code and revises second code to 300.4); revising one code to more accurately reflect the condition (496 being validated, auditor revises to 491.21) or procedure (45.13 being validated, auditor revises to 45.16); or other similar revision or resequencing to the code(s) being validated.

- **Added code:** Code not reported by coder but meets secondary diagnosis or procedure reporting guidelines. Auditor counts one error for each code added; for example, adding a diagnosis or procedure code to more completely reflect a condition or procedure (for example, the auditor adds 995.91 to sepsis; adds a manifestation code; or adds a "code also" procedure code as in the case of a type of bearing surface 00.74–00.77).

- **Deleted code:** Code reported by coder but does not meet secondary diagnosis or procedure reporting guidelines. Auditor counts one error for each code deleted.

- **Correct code:** A correct code is any code that is not revised, added, or deleted.

- **Reviewed code:** Reviewed codes are the total number of codes reviewed (after auditing): correct codes + coding errors (+ revised codes + added codes – deleted codes).

NOTE: Do *NOT* count the number of codes coded by the coder for the denominator. Count the number of codes validated by the auditor as "reviewed codes" for the denominator.

Design and Implementation of a Coding Audit

The design and implementation of a coding audit begins with goal setting, which includes establishing an ongoing monitor for identifying problems or opportunities to improve the quality of coded data for inpatient and outpatient cases. The plan should clarify monitoring and evaluation methods. The appropriate supervisor will be responsible for identifying problems that relate to coding issues based on analysis of the review results.

Audit Team

Facilities should consider having an audit team made up of members from several key departments, including HIM/coding, billing, finance, compliance, and case management. The team should be educated on aspects of auditing and the billing cycle to ensure that all members are aware of the important role each department plays in revenue cycle management. Training should include an overview of the coding process, as well as discussion of payment systems, *ICD-9-CM Official Guidelines for Coding and Reporting,* and facility-specific policies and procedures.

Sample Review Size

The type of review being planned determines the sample size. A 200-case review is usually adequate for an initial diagnostic review. Focused MS-DRG reviews may be limited to only 10 to 15 percent of the cases, or 100 percent of the cases may be pulled. Of course, the larger the sample size, the greater the confidence in the results. The number of cases to pull for a coder-specific review depends on the number of cases the individual codes. For an annual review of coding quality for a specific coder, 50 cases should be pulled for full-time staff and 25 for part-time staff.

Although there is no absolute correct number of charts to audit, the industry standard is approximately 10 to 25 charts per provider. For many years, the Joint Commission recommended that studies include 5 percent or 30 charts, whichever is greater. The hardest part of auditing is selecting a good sample that is reflective of the entire population. Several software packages and auditing books are available to help establish a good (fair) sample. One way to establish an appropriate sample is to pick every "nth" chart, such as every 10th chart coded, every 5th surgical case, and so forth. Additionally, the facility might select an occurrence to study and have coders, transcriptionists, and/or chart-processing staff maintain a log to record whenever an event occurs. For example, in the past, sepsis stays of less than 3 days were referred to as occurrence screening.

Recommendations from the AHIMA e-HIM workgroup are illustrated in figure 9.1.

Recommended Topics for Auditing

Although facilities vary according to patient mix, problems identified, and so forth, certain topics lend themselves to auditing. Some recommended topics for auditing include:

- OIG Work Plan
- Fraud alerts
- Top 10 surgeries
- Top 10 MS-DRGs
- High-volume, high-risk procedures
- Top 10 denials
- Top 10 services provided
- Use of most specific code available
- Data-entry errors
- All orders written and signed by physician
- Review of assignment codes and modifier usage
- All tests ordered were actually performed
- MS-DRG payments
- Inpatient outliers

Figure 9.1. Inpatient coding quality audits

Type of Review:

Established coder: Quarterly or biannual.

New-hire coder: Baseline or 100 percent of reviews during Orientation and Training until passing to an established coder.

- Type of review may be further refined by prebill and postbill.
  Note: Coding accuracy is calculated the same for prebill or postbill reviews regardless of the DRG billed.

- Type of review may be further refined by representative sample or focused sample.
  —A *representative sample* is a selection of records at random with no preidentified DRG, documentation, coding, or coder issue.
  —A *focused sample* is a selection of records with a preidentified DRG, documentation, coding, or coder issue.

Record Sampling Methodology:

- **Time Frame**

  —*For quarterly,* the 3-month time frame not previously reviewed.

  —*For biannual,* the 6-month time frame not previously reviewed.

Note: The records selected should occur after the coder education date of the last audit. In addition, the most recent discharges should be selected.

Number of Records

Representative sample: Random selection of 2 percent of the required productivity standards per patient type coded (including maternity and newborn if applicable) by the coder for the time frame selected for the review (quarterly or biannual).

Note: This random selection may be selected by first picking a number 0 through 9. For example, if 5 is selected, then consecutively select every account number ending in 5 per patient type as part of your sample until you have the total records selected for your sample size.

Focused sample: Selection of 30 records or all records in the time frame if fewer than 30 are available.

Source: Wilson 2008, 5–6.

- Consecutive inpatient stays
- Medical necessity
- Restraint-related deaths
- Coronary artery stents

Focused Coding Reviews

When the initial diagnostic review has been completed, focused reviews based on specific problem areas should be planned. Topics identified for the focused reviews also may be based on controversial issues identified through *Coding Clinic for ICD-9-CM*. Some potential topics for the focused reviews include:

- Surgical complications
- Obstetric complications
- Error MS-DRGs

- Diabetes mellitus

- Dehydration as principal diagnosis

- Gastrointestinal bleeding

- OIG-identified paired/families of MS-DRGs

- Recent issues identified by external review agencies and/or professional journals

In *Benchmarking to Improve Coding Accuracy and Productivity*, Wilson discusses common target areas for inpatient coding audits (2008):

1. Review and compare patients with sepsis and urinary tract infections to assure correct coding.

2. Review Complex Pneumonia patients in comparison with Community Acquired Pneumonia patients. For example, some organizations were placed under focused review by the OIG for upcoding complex pneumonia based on clinical indications such as: an elderly patient who lives in a nursing home and who has a gastrostomy/percutaneous endoscopic gastrostomy (PEG) tube and a fever.

3. Review patient status (discharge disposition) code assignments on all records selected for a coding review. The patient status (discharge disposition) code is the code assignment for the destination of the patient at discharge. It will save the coding quality manager time if, while the manager is performing coding reviews, the discharge disposition code is also verified.

An MS-DRG example audit would be to analyze specific documentation of congestive heart failure (CHF). A report detailing principal and secondary ICD-9-CM codes 428.0 (CHF) by physician will enable the coding manager to determine which physicians need education regarding the appropriate documentation of heart failure.

The Review Process

For a coding audit, the coder first reviews the medical record to ensure that the diagnosis billed as principal meets the official Uniform Hospital Discharge Data Set (UHDDS) definition. The principal diagnosis is defined as the reason determined after study to have occasioned the admission of the patient to the hospital for care. It must have been present on admission, been a principal reason for admission, and treated or evaluated during the stay. When several diagnoses meet all these requirements, any of them may be selected as the principal diagnosis. If the principal diagnosis was chosen incorrectly, the correct diagnosis must be determined. If this can be done using coding conventions and guidelines, the attending physician does not need to be consulted. However, if the documentation in the medical record is unclear, the attending physician should be asked to clarify. If any changes affect the MS-DRG, the case will need to be rebilled. Physician clarification should be included as an addendum to the medical record that supports the code selection. The problem and its source should be identified and corrective action implemented to prevent a recurrence.

Identifying Data Quality Evaluation Indicators for Inpatient Cases

The error types identified during review will fall into the categories listed below:

- Incorrect selection of principal diagnosis

- Principal diagnosis not supported by documentation in the health record

- Substitution of a secondary diagnosis for the correct principal diagnosis

- Miscoding

- Incomplete identification of all secondary diagnoses

- Principal procedure not selected or coded correctly

- Other procedures not coded correctly

See AHIMA's *Benchmarking to Improve Coding Accuracy and Productivity* for the survey and analysis (Wilson 2008).

Reporting the Review Results

A summary of the results should be prepared and shared with coders, physicians, and other healthcare providers, including nursing staff, physical and occupational therapists, respiratory therapists, others whose documentation may have been reviewed, and administration, as needed. Often one of the hardest aspects of auditing and monitoring is that of presenting the findings to the team, but this is an essential part of the compliance program. Most physicians and staff want to know the results of audits and recommendations on how to improve their processes.

Findings should be presented as a pictorial display, using bar graphs or pie charts as appropriate. When poor or inadequate documentation is found to be a key factor causing the coding error or when physicians consistently do not respond to query requests, it is important to share these findings with the physician. If education does not help to alleviate the problem, it may be necessary to report these findings to the chief of the department/chief of the medical staff, and/or administration of the facility.

If the coding staff includes a large number of clinical coding specialists, a rotating schedule should be established to include all coders on an annual basis. The review schedule depends on the number of coders and the identified problems. Initially, a large study including all coding staff and representative common diagnoses and procedures should be conducted.

Taking Action

When a problem is identified, it is important to take appropriate action in a timely manner. It is likewise important to remember that the auditing process is a learning process, not a police action. A compliant culture is one in which the information discovered during the review is used to train employees and educate physicians and to identify resources and training needs for the future, with the ultimate goal of making the billing process more accurate and effective.

Appendix F provides further details on how to develop an effective compliance audit process. Sample audit forms and tools can be found in appendix G.

Summary

The health record audit process allows a facility to systematically examine and review its coding and billing processes with the goal of identifying and correcting problem areas. Regular health record audits provide the foundation for coding and corporate compliance.

References

Hyde, L.A., and C. Spencer. 2008. *Analyzing the Financial Impact of MS-DRGs.* Chicago: AHIMA.

Office of the Inspector General. 2005 (Jan. 31). Supplemental Compliance Program Guidance for Hospitals. *Federal Register* 70(19):4858–4876. http://oig.hhs.gov/fraud/docs/complianceguidance/012705HospSupplementalGuidance.pdf.

Wilson, D.D. 2008. *Benchmarking to Improve Coding Accuracy and Productivity.* Edited by Dunn, R. Chicago: AHIMA.

Exercises

Under the inpatient prospective payment system (IPPS), health record documentation must support the principal diagnosis (PDX) and principal procedure designations, as well as all other diagnoses and procedures submitted on the claim. Documentation should also support present on admission (POA) indicator assignment when required.

For each coding problem in this section, the documentation should be reviewed to identify:

1. The principal diagnosis as defined as the reason, after study, that caused the patient to be admitted to the hospital. The coding professional must remember that this may not be the diagnosis listed first by the physician.

2. Other diagnoses and procedures that meet secondary reporting requirements

3. The principal procedure

4. Information to be clarified with the attending physician in a query

In selecting diagnoses or procedures for coding, the coder should assume that the documentation provided is the only documentation available. If no documentation is available to indicate a condition affecting treatment or length of stay, do not report this condition.

On the job, the coder may review other sections of the health record and consult the attending physician, if necessary, for assistance in sequencing and code selection. In the following exercises, however, the discharge summary is the only documentation available to the coder. Answers for each sequencing or coding problem must be based solely on *ICD-9-CM Official Guidelines for Coding and Reporting,* including sequencing guidelines, ICD-9-CM coding conventions and principles, and the American Hospital Association's ICD-9-CM *Coding Clinic* advice. The attending physician has approved the diagnoses as listed in the discharge summary.

Exercise 1

History of Present Illness: This 72-year-old female presented to the ENT clinic complaining of her current epistaxis for 7 days prior to admission. The bleeding usually occurred from the right nostril. She had no prior history of epistaxis and denied any rhinorrhea, congestion, or anosmia. On admission she also complained of weakness. Four days prior to admission, her hematocrit level was 35, and the night before her admission, her hematocrit level was 29 when measured at an outside hospital. Her past medical history was significant for rheumatoid arthritis. Her past surgical history included status post bilateral knee replacement and right hip replacement. Medications at the time of admission included prednisone 2 mg PO b.i.d.. and aspirin, six to eight per day for the past several months. Allergies: none.

Physical Examination: On physical examination at the time of her admission, she was afebrile. Her blood pressure was 114/70 and her pulse was 92. Examination of the head and neck was significant for nasal cavities, which were without lesions and without physical bleeding sites. The remainder of the head and neck examination was within normal limits. Her neck was normal with no jugular venous distention. The lungs were clear. The heart rate was regular, and heart rhythm was without murmurs. The abdomen was soft without masses, and the extremities had no bruises, cyanosis, or edema.

Laboratory Data and Hospital Course: The patient was admitted, and a right anterior nasal pack was placed. Serial hematocrit levels were also obtained. The night of her first day of admission, she required replacement of an anterior pack because of refractory bleeding. The day following her admission, she underwent transfusion with two units of packed red blood cells for a hemoglobin level of 8.

On the second day of her admission, bleeding was noted around the anterior pack. For this reason, she was taken to the treatment room, where a posterior nasopharyngeal pack and a new anterior pack were placed. She was then transferred to the special care unit and monitored on the cardiac monitor and with pulse oximetry. The posterior pack was left in place for 2 days. At this time, a repeat episode of bleeding showed that her bleeding time had normalized from its previous elevated level. She was observed overnight for 1 day without a pack in place. The patient did well during this observation period without any further bleeding.

When it was confirmed that the patient had no further bleeding for 48 hours after pack removal and the hematocrit level was stable, she was discharged to home. She was instructed to follow up with her private physician. She was also instructed to refrain from taking aspirin and to use Disalcid 750 mg t.i.d., instead, for her arthritic pain. She was also placed on iron supplements 300 mg three times a day and told to continue using saline and Prenaris nasal drops.

Final Diagnosis: Epistaxis

Additional Diagnosis: Rheumatoid arthritis

1.   PDX:

2.   Other diagnoses:

3.   Principal procedure:

4.   Other procedures:

5.   Conditions to clarify with physician:

Exercise 2

History of Present Illness: The patient is an 80-year-old white female with a known history of advanced, widely metastatic carcinoma of the breast. The patient was admitted because of increasing shortness of breath and severe pain. The pain, which was worse in her left chest, was associated with increasing shortness of breath. At the time of admission, the patient was in so much pain she was unable to remember her history. The patient initially presented for congestive heart failure over a year ago. This condition was subsequently found to be secondary to metastatic breast cancer, post left mastectomy, 3 years ago. The patient previously received chemotherapy.

Laboratory Data and Hospital Course: The patient was initially treated with intravenous pain medication to control her pain. Subsequently, her condition stabilized with oral medication. By the time of discharge, the patient's condition was stablized with oral Vicodin and she was able to eat. Blood sugar levels were improved and her Tolinase was able to be held. Laboratory values at time of discharge included BUN 17, creatinine 1, sodium 141, potassium 4.5, chloride 105, CO_2 25, alkaline phosphatase elevated at 170 with GGT 267, SGOT 68. Admission BUN was up to 38 with creatinine 1.3 secondary to dehydration. By the time of discharge, these had improved. Admission glucose 225, down to 110 at discharge.

Medications at Discharge: Aldactone, 25 mg twice a day; Tamoxifen, 10 mg b.i.d. with meals; Lanoxin, 0.125 mg daily; Metamucil, 5 cc in four ounces of juice twice a day; Tolinase, 250 mg half tablet b.i.d. (but hold if preceding AccuCheck is less than 125); Reglan, 10 mg PO ac; Timoptic 0.5% eye drops, one to each eye twice a day; Pepcid, 20 mg b.i.d.; Lasix, 40 mg daily (only if pedal edema is present); Vicodin tablets, one every 3 hours prn for pain.

Discharge Diagnosis: Uncontrolled pain, secondary to widely metastatic breast carcinoma. Dehydration. Type II diabetes mellitus, uncontrolled. Congestive heart failure.

1. PDX:

2. Other diagnoses:

3. Principal procedure:

4. Other procedures:

5. Conditions to clarify with physician:

Exercise 3

History of Present Illness: This 70-year-old female with a past history of endometrial carcinoma was admitted to medical oncology for blood transfusion. The patient complains of GI bleeding on and off for the past 2 months. She has no changes in bowel movements, no diarrhea or constipation, and no nausea or vomiting. There is mild abdominal pain in the lower part of the abdomen, no radiation, relieved by analgesics. Endometrial carcinoma, stage 2, was diagnosed in November of last year. Status post radiation therapy externally and internally in January. CT scan of the abdomen in March showed a decrease in the size of the mass, and the patient had total abdominal hysterectomy and bilateral salpingo-oophorectomy at that time. The patient presented 1 month ago with GI bleeding, which was thought to be secondary to radiation colitis, but proctoscopy revealed a necrotic mass in the anterior wall. Biopsy was negative times two. There is a 6-year history of hypertension, and a 10-year history of type II diabetes mellitus. Medication: Nifedipine, 90 XL once a day; Tolbutamide, 500 mg once a day. No alcohol. Patient smokes one pack of cigarettes per day.

Physical Examination: Alert and oriented in no active distress. Blood pressure 110/60. HEENT: pale conjunctiva. Neck supple, no lymphadenopathy. The lungs were clear to auscultation, resonant to percussion. Heart regular rate and rhythm, no murmurs, no S3. Abdomen soft; there is tenderness in the lower parts; no hepatosplenomegaly. The bowel sounds are positive. Rectal positive for heme. Extremities plus two edema in the left more than the right.

Laboratory Data: Hemoglobin 6.7, hematocrit 20.8, white blood cells 9.7, neutrophils 81, lymphocytes 14 and monocytes 4, eosinophils 1. Platelet count 448,000. Sodium 142, potassium 4.8, chloride 108, CO_2 21, BUN 40, calcium 8.2, phosphorus 3, magnesium 1.4 and glucose 123, SGOT 50, alkaline phosphatase 137, SGPT 42, albumin 2.0; total bilirubin 0.3, direct bilirubin 0. PT 11.7, PTT 27.6.

Hospital Course: Problem #1: Lower GI bleed and melena. The patient presented 2 months ago with lower GI bleed, which was most likely secondary to radiation therapy. At that time, proctoscopy was done and showed necrotic mass in the anterior wall of the rectum. Biopsy was also done and was negative. Proctoscopy was repeated and was negative the second time. For current admission, the patient presented with the same complaint. Hemoglobin level was 6.7; hematocrit level was 20. The patient was transfused with four units of packed red blood. Hemoglobin level rose to 14.2, hematocrit level to 41.8, and the patient was stabilized. GI staff were contacted regarding repeating proctoscopy. Their suggestion was to discharge and follow her in GI clinic.

Problem #2: Endometrial carcinoma, status post radiation therapy, status post resection. No further therapy now.

Problem #3: Anemia, secondary to lower GI bleed.

Problem #4: Type II diabetes mellitus, which is stable on Tolbutamide, 500 mg once a day.

Problem #5: Hypertension, which is stable on Nifedipine, 90 XL once a day.

Problem #6: Increased creatinine and BUN, which was not corrected after the hydration. On discharge, creatinine was 3.2 and BUN was 39. Testing will be repeated as an outpatient. The patient is known to have increased creatinine and BUN, most likely secondary to hypertension. The patient was discharged home in stable condition to be followed up in Oncology. Discharge medications: Nifedipine, 90 XL once a day; Tolbutamide, 500 mg once a day.

Final Diagnosis: Lower gastrointestinal bleeding secondary to radiation colitis.

1. PDX:

2. Other diagnoses:

3. Principal procedure:

4. Other procedures:

5. Conditions to clarify with physician:

Exercise 4

History of Present Illness: The patient is a 72-year-old male who was involved in an interpersonal altercation at approximately 1:30 a.m. He presented to the emergency department with complaints of pain and swelling to the right side of the face. The patient had been struck multiple times with the butt end of a handgun. He denied loss of consciousness. The attack was witnessed, and the witnesses also claim there was no loss of consciousness. He presented with pain and swelling on the right side of his face in the temporal region and in the right eye region. He had a small abrasion on the top of his head and on the right forehead. No lacerations were noted. He had no diplopia. The past medical and surgical histories were noncontributory. The patient was taking no medications and had no allergies.

Laboratory Data: Admission x-rays and CT scan revealed a nondisplaced right zygoma fracture and an orbital floor fracture with slight limitation of his upward gaze on physical examination.

Hospital Course: He was taken to the operating room for open reduction of the facial fracture and placement of Silastic implant to right orbital floor fracture, which was accomplished without difficulty or complication. The patient tolerated the procedure well. Postoperative course was uncomplicated. He received intravenous antibiotics throughout his hospital stay. Currently, he is tolerating a general diet without problems. He was up and about, ambulating without difficulty. He will be seen here at the hospital on Saturday for suture removal. Discharge medications: Keflex, 500 mg to be taken q.i.d. for 1 week.

Final Diagnoses: Right orbital fracture

Right zygoma fracture

Abrasions of head

Operations: Exploration and placement of Silastic implant to right orbital floor fracture

1. PDX:

2. Other diagnoses:

3. Principal procedure:

4. Other procedures:

5. Conditions to clarify with physician:

Exercise 5

History of Present Illness: This 66-year-old female was initially admitted on September 1, following a 7-month history of left upper quadrant and left flank abdominal pain. This pain was severe, constant, and not related to food intake. The patient had undergone further workup at her home in Michigan. At that time, only gastritis was found with esophagogastroduodenoscopy and upper gastrointestinal swallow. Thus, the patient chose to come here for further evaluation.

She was admitted on September 1, discharged on September 6, and underwent several diagnostic studies. An ultrasound of the abdomen did not show any evidence of retained gallstones or common duct stones, as she had undergone a cholecystectomy in the past. The patient underwent CT scan of her abdomen, which demonstrated a mass in the tail and the body of her pancreas that involved the left kidney and the spleen. The presence of enlarged periaortic nodes and also an enlarged left adrenal gland was questioned. The patient also underwent an intravenous pyelogram, which demonstrated splaying of the left kidney. Renal scan demonstrated good renal perfusion to both kidneys. Upper and lower GI endoscopies in this initial hospitalization demonstrated no involvement of the stomach, esophagus, or duodenum, or of the colon.

Because of the severity of the pain, the assessment was that the patient probably had pancreatic carcinoma. Consultations were made with the radiology department and the urology service. The final consensus was that this was most likely a pancreatic tumor. The patient had severe, unrelenting pain that was only controlled with narcotics at this time. After a thorough discussion with the patient of the possible treatments, the patient chose to pursue a possible surgical resection. The patient stated that the pain appeared to be getting worse and she also was experiencing weight loss. Therefore, the patient was admitted to the hospital.

Hospital Course: The indications for surgery in this patient were a possible resection of this tumor for palliation and control of her pain. Based on her CT scan, it did not appear that this tumor was involved with any other vascular structures that would preclude resection.

On September 12, the patient was taken to the operating room for left nephrectomy. At this time, she underwent resection of her distal pancreas and spleen after a left kidney en bloc. However, this tumor involved her celiac access. A surgical injury to the superior mesenteric artery was repaired at the time of the operation with a reversed interposition vein graft. Her surgical course was complicated by diffuse intravascular coagulation, persistent bleeding, and hypothermia following anesthesia, requiring massive blood transfusions. Following revascularization of her small bowel, the patient's wound needed to be packed and she was returned to the surgical intensive care unit in critical condition.

The patient had a rocky postoperative course and went into cardiac arrest several times in the first 4 hours following return to the intensive care unit. Four hours following her return to the intensive care unit, the patient went into cardiac arrest and could not be resuscitated. The final cause of death was carcinoma of the pancreas and was related to resection of this cancer.

Final Diagnosis: Carcinoma of the tail of the pancreas with extension to spleen and left kidney

1. PDX:

2. Other diagnoses:

3. Principal procedure:

4. Other procedures:

5. Conditions to clarify with physician:

Exercise 6

History of Present Illness: This 87-year-old woman with type II diabetes underwent an amputation of her fourth digit of the right foot approximately 5 weeks ago. She was referred elsewhere for angioplasty. At that time, insulin therapy was discontinued and she is currently following a 1,500-calorie diet. She was sent back to the nursing home and has since developed an increasing amount of pain and cellulitis of her right foot. The patient is a poor historian. She is alert, but her orientation seems to be off. Information is obtained from her old records and from the transfer sheet sent from the nursing home. February 2004: pacemaker implantation secondary to sick sinus syndrome with congestive heart failure (stable with Lasix, 40 mg PO) and bradyarrhythmia, as well as pleural effusion. October 2006: acute MI.

Physical Examination: General: Reveals an 87-year-old white female in no acute distress. BP 152/70, temperature 99.8 orally, pulse 66, respirations 24. Skin: Warm and dry. HEENT: Head is normocephalic, atraumatic. Pupils are equal, round, and reactive to light and accommodation. Extraocular muscles are intact. Fundi are not seen. No conjunctivitis or icterus noted. Canals are clear with good cone of light reflex on TMs. Gross hearing is within normal limits. Septum is midline. No discharge. No erythema or exudate of throat. Uvula raises midline. Neck: Supple with full range of motion. No lymphadenopathy or thyromegaly. No carotid bruits or JVD. Breasts: No masses or nipple discharge. Lungs: Clear on the left with rales in right lower lobe. Heart: Grade II/VI systolic ejection murmur elicited with a paced beat. Abdomen: Distended. Positive bowel sounds X4. No hepatosplenomegaly. No masses upon palpation. GU: Rectal: Deferred at this time. Musculoskeletal: Right foot is status post fourth toe amputation with open incision with exudate, as well as surrounding erythema of approximately 3 cm. Skin is warm to touch and tender. Right arm paralysis with slight weakness of the right leg. Neurologic: Cranial nerves II through XII grossly intact. No major deficits noted.

Impression: Cellulitis of right foot, status post amputation; noninsulin-dependent diabetes mellitus; arteriosclerotic heart disease with history of sick sinus syndrome and pacemaker implantation; and residual right hemiparesis from cerebral thrombosis.

Plan: Admit for intravenous antibiotics.

Hospital Course: Following angioplasty, it was thought the circulation was good in her foot at the time of her discharge from St. Mary's Hospital. However, soon after returning to the nursing home, her cellulitis began to increase, which led to her being brought here. Culture revealed a *Staphylococcus aureus* infection. White blood cell count on admission was essentially normal with 7,800 white blood cells, 80 segs. Glucose level was 149 with normal follow-up. Urinalysis was normal. Creatinine level was 1.5; BUN was 18; platelet count was normal. Digoxin level was high normal. The patient was treated with bed rest, elevation of the foot, Betadine soaks, intravenous Garamycin, and Cleocin. With the treatment here, the patient's pain subsided. Doppler pressures in her ankle were adequate. The wound drainage decreased. At the time of her discharge to a skilled care facility, there was no real evidence of cellulitis. However, I think she will benefit from continued intravenous antibiotic therapy and local care. She was discharged to a skilled care facility to continue the intravenous administration of Garamycin and Cleocin.

Diagnoses: Cellulitis, right foot, postamputation

Diabetes mellitus

Diabetic peripheral vascular disease with recent angioplasty

1.   PDX:

2.   Other diagnoses:

3.   Principal procedure:

4.   Other procedures:

5.   Conditions to clarify with physician:

Exercise 7

History of Present Illness: This is a 69-year-old female with previous myocardial infarction, known hypertension, who started complaining of cough, chills, and fever about 4 days prior to admission. One day prior to admission, she started to complain of progressive dyspnea associated with hemoptysis. She went to the emergency department and was noted to be extremely dyspneic and wheezing. She was given an aerosol treatment with good response. However, chest x-ray showed evidence of bilateral lower pneumonia with a PO$_2$ of 66 and white blood cell count of 12,400, for which admission was advised. The patient had been taking Methyldopa 500 mg b.i.d., Ascriptin one tablet daily, Transderm Nitro 5 once daily, Capoten 30 mg b.i.d., and Lanoxin 0.725 mg daily. The patient had an inferior wall myocardial infarction 10 months ago. She is known to have chronic anxiety problems and had been under the care of the mental hygiene clinic.

Physical Examination: Revealed a well-developed, well-nourished female whose respirations had improved since the aerosol therapy was given. Blood pressure is somewhat elevated. Respirations 24. Pulse 110/minute. HEENT: Unremarkable. No carotid bruits. No distended neck veins. Chest: No deformity. Equal expansion. Lungs: Crepitant rales over the lower half of end hemithorax. No wheezing. No pericardial or pleural rub noted. Heart: Regular rhythm. No murmurs. Abdomen: Soft. Liver, spleen, and kidneys not enlarged. No tenderness. Extremities: No clubbing. No cyanosis. Peripheral pulses strong and equal. Rectal: Deferred.

Impression: Lobar pneumonia associated with hemoptysis. Previous inferior wall myocardial infarction. Hypertension. Chronic anxiety.

Plan: After appropriate cultures are obtained, the patient will be empirically started on Kefzol. Nasal oxygen will be administered. Patient will be hydrated and aerosol therapy will be continued.

Laboratory Data and Hospital Course: Sputum smear showed moderate white blood cells, many epithelial cells, and many mixed respiratory microflora. Sputum culture showed normal growth. Blood cultures after 10 days showed no growth. Chest x-ray report revealed mild congestive cardiac failure pattern. Significant improvement in congestive heart failure noted on second x-ray but not complete resolution, although the pneumonia has resolved. EKG showed right bundle branch block with old inferior myocardial infarction, left ventricular strain; no change when repeated prior to discharge. The patient's previous medications were continued.

After cultures were obtained, she was empirically started on intravenous Kefzol. Because of initial bronchospasm, she was also started on aerosolized bronchodilator therapy consisting of Alupent. She remained afebrile during her stay in the hospital. She had no further wheezing after 24 hours, but continued to have mild hemoptysis and crepitant rales in both bases. Hemoptysis disappeared after 48 hours. She had one episode of mild angina pains relieved by nitroglycerin during her stay. With improvement in her respirations and x-ray findings, she was discharged. Her BP was 154/110 on discharge, but this is not considered unusual because her BP is quite unstable as an outpatient, with variable high and low readings. This will, however, be followed up in the office.

Final Diagnoses: Bilateral lobar pneumonia and hemoptysis

Old myocardial infarction with angina

Hypertension

Chronic anxiety

Congestive heart failure

1. PDX:

2. Other diagnoses:

3. Principal procedure:

4. Other procedures:

5. Conditions to clarify with physician:

Exercise 8

History of Present Illness: The patient is a 72-year-old male with a history of abdominal perineal resection for colon cancer in 1994 and left hemicolectomy in 1995 for splenic flexure recurrence of cancer. Subsequent right nephrectomy, right adrenalectomy, right posterior hepatic wedge resection in February for metastatic colon carcinoma. The patient is admitted with complaints of lower back pain and bilateral thigh pain times 2 months' duration, increasing in intensity.

Physical Examination: Examination on admission: temperature 99, pulse 72, respirations 24, blood pressure 150/90. The examination was remarkable for left lower quadrant colostomy from previous surgery, mildly tender lumbar spine, and the patient was barely able to stand. It was also noted that the patient had decreased sharp, dull discrimination on the neural examination of the lateral thighs.

Laboratory Data: On admission the laboratory values were: Urinalysis: Specific gravity 1.021, pH 5; Chem tests were negative; Nitrite negative; Blood negative, 12 white blood cells, moderate bacteria. The clinical chemistry results were: serum sodium 141, BUN 42, potassium 4.9, chloride 104, CO_2 28, glucose 99, creatinine 1.8, SGOT 12, SGPT 16, alkaline phosphatase 68, total protein 6.6, albumin 3.8, total bilirubin 0.7, direct bilirubin 0.0, GGT 87, calcium 10.3, magnesium 2.0, phosphorus 3.2, uric acid 5.7, PT 12.9, PTT 28.4, white blood cell count 8.0, hemoglobin 15.0, hematocrit 43.8, platelets 223,000. The CEA level was noted to be 508 ng/mL on admission. Metastatic workup for the colon carcinoma revealed no evidence of metastatic disease to the head or the thoracic and cervical spine.

Radiologic Studies: CT and MRI revealed left celiac ganglion node plexus enlarged, suspicious for metastasis. Multiple small lung nodules bilaterally suspicious for metastasis. Pathologic fracture of L2, with compression of L2, effacement of the spinal canal space and apparent cord compression at the L2 level. Subsequent urine culture grew out greater than 10^5 *Pseudomonas aeruginosa,* which was sensitive to Ciprofloxacin. The patient was treated with Ciprofloxacin 500 mg PO q 8 hours and subsequent urine culture showed no growth.

Hospital Course: The patient was taken to the operating room for L2 laminectomy with decompression and anterior allograft bone fusion. The postoperative course was marked by slow recovery with nausea and difficulty with pain control. The patient slowly improved and began ambulating 8 days later. The patient fell 3 days later while ambulating but had no significant injuries. Further physical therapy was marked by continued improvement in ambulation with walker and no further setbacks. Clinically, the patient is afebrile without signs and symptoms of infection, no CVA tenderness, no dysuria. The patient will be discharged home today. Condition on discharge fairly good.

Treatment: The patient will go home on Vicodin (PO q 4 to 6 hours for pain) and Capoten. He will resume Capoten b.i.d. dosing per his internist's recommendations, 25 PO b.i.d. Prognosis: The long-term prognosis is poor because the patient has metastatic colon CA; short-term prognosis is fairly good with improvement in ambulation. Ambulation with assistance with walker. Follow-up: The patient will return to see me next Wednesday.

Final Diagnoses: Metastatic colon cancer to lung and bone

Pathologic compression fracture of L2 vertebra with cord compression at L2 level

UTI due to *Pseudomonas*

1.   PDX:

2.   Other diagnoses:

3.   Principal procedure:

4.   Other procedures:

5.   Conditions to clarify with physician:

Exercise 9

History of Present Illness: This 71-year-old male was the pedestrian who was struck by a motor vehicle. He had no loss of consciousness at the scene but was confused at the time of admission. He had vital signs that were stable in the field. He sustained head lacerations.

Physical Examination: The patient was alert, but confused. He was in a cervical collar and had a laceration of the scalp posteriorly and a small laceration under the chin. Chest: Clear to auscultation. Heart: Regular. Abdomen: Soft and nontender with positive bowel sounds. He had a palpable right inguinal hernia, which was large. Extremities: His pedal pulses were intact bilaterally. He was able to move all extremities well. Head and neck examination: Revealed eyes intact. Neck was nontender to palpation, but the patient remained in the C-collar.

Laboratory Data and Hospital Course: Chest x-ray and EKG revealed no gross lesions. The EKG revealed atrial fibrillation. Laboratory examination was unremarkable. Chest x-ray revealed cardiomegaly. Odontoid tomograms did not show a fracture. He had a right small subarachnoid hemorrhage on CT scan of the head. The patient was admitted to the intensive care unit for observation. He was stable in the intensive care unit and was transferred to the ward, where he was monitored on telemetry. Social Work was immediately contacted for discharge planning. Neurosurgery was consulted. They thought the patient had a traumatic subarachnoid hemorrhage, which was small, and they would follow it clinically. They stated that he had a history of syncope and suggested an MRI of his head.

On February 7, the patient was attempting to ambulate when the Trauma Service noted he had left knee pain. X-rays revealed a Schatzker IV tibial plateau fracture. The patient was then evaluated preoperatively for open reduction and internal fixation of his left lower extremity. Preoperative laboratories were unremarkable. Both the patient and his wife then refused surgery. The decision was made to treat the tibial plateau fracture in a long-leg plaster cast. X-rays following placement of the plaster showed adequate reduction of the fracture. It was discussed with the patient and his wife that arthroplasty of the knee may be required in the future, but the tibial fracture would be well treated in the plaster. It was the preference of the surgical team to perform open reduction and internal fixation, but the patient and his wife were against a surgical procedure at that time. Psychiatry was also consulted to evaluate the competency of the patient. They thought that the patient was somewhat demented, but that he did understand the benefits and risks of surgery and was competent to make decisions.

On February 9, the patient was noted to be quite lethargic and had apnea as well. Neurosurgery evaluated the patient and administered intravenous fluids. They checked laboratory values and found the patient was hypovolemic. The patient improved following administration of intravenous fluids. By February 10, the patient was oriented and much improved. He was discharged to home on February 15. At the time of discharge, vital signs were stable and he was afebrile. Circulation, motor skills, and sensory functions of the left lower extremity were intact. The plaster was intact.

Final Diagnoses: Closed head trauma with subarachnoid hemorrhage

Closed left tibial plateau fracture

Dementia senile

Hypovolemia

1. PDX:

2. Other diagnoses:

3. Principal procedure:

4. Other procedures:

5. Conditions to clarify with physician:

Exercise 10

History of Present Illness: The patient is a 75-year-old female with coronary arteriosclerosis status post coronary artery bypass graft. The patient complains of shortness of breath that began 3 to 4 days prior to admission and became worse on the day of admission. She complains of wheezing and cough productive of whitish sputum. No fever, chills, nausea, or vomiting. Paroxysmal nocturnal dyspnea, orthopnea is unchanged. Past medical history, as above.

Physical Examination: On physical examination, the patient is alert and oriented, in mild distress. Her blood pressure is 150/70, heart rate 70, respiratory rate 16. The temperature is afebrile. The head and neck examinations are within normal limits. Patient wheezes. Abdomen soft, nontender. The extremities are 2+ edema bilaterally. Neurological: Left upper extremity and left lower extremities were weak and the patient is unable to ambulate.

Laboratory Data: The WBC is 7.5, hemoglobin 11.0, hematocrit 34.2. The platelets are 292,000. The digoxin level is 0.5. The chest x-ray revealed cardiomegaly and congestive heart failure. Pulmonary vascularity within normal limits. The sodium is 143, potassium 4.5, chloride 111, bicarbonate 21. The BUN is 23, creatinine 1.2, glucose 207.

Hospital Course: The patient was admitted with chronic obstructive pulmonary disease exacerbation. She responded well to nebulized breathing treatments and intravenous Solu-Medrol. She was then switched to oral steroids. The patient was discharged home in stable condition on the following medications: Prednisone 40 mg on an untapering dose; aspirin, enteric-coated, one PO q a.m.; Atrovent and albuterol inhaler; Persantine 75 mg t.i.d.; Captopril 12.5 mg t.i.d.; Theophylline 300 mg b.i.d.; Diltiazem 90 mg t.i.d.; Nitropaste 7.5 mg q a.m.; Lasix 40 mg q a.m.; and digoxin 0.25 mg q a.m.. She is to follow up in 2 weeks in the pulmonary clinic. The patient also has follow-up in the cardiology clinic.

Final Diagnosis: Acute exacerbation of chronic obstructive pulmonary disease

Secondary Diagnoses: Congestive heart failure, acute diastolic

Type II diabetes mellitus controlled by diet

Hypertension

1. PDX:

2. Other diagnoses:

3. Principal procedure:

4. Other procedures:

5. Conditions to clarify with physician:

Case Studies

Directions

Under the inpatient prospective payment system (IPPS), health record documentation must support the principal diagnosis and principal procedure, as well as all other diagnoses and procedures submitted on the claim.

The coder should review the documentation to identify:

1. The principal diagnosis, which may not be the diagnosis listed first by the physician

2. The principal procedure

3. Other diagnoses and procedures to be included on the claim

4. Any other diagnoses or procedures that require coding for the healthcare facility to have appropriate databases

In selecting diagnoses/procedures for coding, the coder should assume that the documentation provided is the only documentation available. If no documentation is available to indicate that a condition affected treatment or length of stay, do not code this condition. Identify these types of conditions on the answer sheet in the space titled "Issues to clarify with physician."

On the job, the coder may review other sections of the health record and consult with the attending physician, if necessary, for assistance in sequencing and code selection. In the following cases, however, the information available to the coder is limited. Answers for each sequencing/coding scenario must be based solely on sequencing guidelines, ICD-9-CM coding conventions and principles, the prospective payment system (PPS) regulations, and the information provided in the case.

Case 1

History

Chief Complaint: Feeling weak and passing bright red blood

History of Present Illness: The patient says for the past 3 days he has had huge amounts of bright red blood going through his rectum. Yesterday, this seemed to slow down; he just had a little black color on top of the stool, but there was no bright red blood. He denies any abdominal pain, fever, chills, or back pain. No nausea or vomiting. No runny nose or cough. He says most of the blood was in the toilet bowl and some was on the tissue paper. This a.m., he had a little bit of nausea while eating lunch. He also is complaining of some chest pain, which was dull and lasted for about $1^{1}/_{2}$ hours after he ate lunch. This was not like his previous MI pain. He denies any diaphoresis.

I saw him in the office on Feb. 11, with all his symptoms. I did an EKG in the office and it did not show any change. He looked a little bit pale. I scheduled him for a flexible sigmoidoscopy and did a CBC. The CBC came back later on the same day saying the hematocrit was about 22. I did a flexible sigmoidoscopy on him after admission this morning. The bowel prep was inadequate. Almost all the sigmoid colon was covered with loose, slightly greenish stool, but a whole lot of diverticula was all over the sigmoid colon. I could go up to 45 cm, but there was a lot more stool and I could not get past it. The patient was also complaining of pain, so I stopped the sigmoidoscopy at that time. The patient also states he has been feeling pretty weak. He denies any shortness of breath, paroxysmal nocturnal dyspnea, or swelling of the feet.

Past Medical History: Significant for: (1) Chronic back pain. He is status post laminectomy of L5-S1 5 years ago. He recently had some surgery in the lower back and also some surgery in the cervical spine with stenosis. (2) He had degenerative joint disease. (3) He says he had an MI about 20 or 25 years ago. (4) History of hypercholesterolemia. (5) Status post carotid endarterectomy about 5 or 8 years ago. (6) History of CVA with right hemiparesis, more than 5 years ago; complete recovery. (7) Extreme anxiety. (8) He does exhibit some sleeping pill addictive behavior. He has been weaned off a lot of sleeping pills. He used to take Valium (up to 50 mg) in the past. He was also taking a lot of Percocet for his back pain. He is off all those medications. The only medication he takes is Restoril, 15 to 20 mg at bedtime.

Family History: Mother died from stomach cancer. Father had angina, no MI.

Social History: He used to be in the dry-cleaning business. He does not smoke now and quit smoking 20 years ago. No alcohol. He lives with his wife at home.

Review of Systems: As per HPI and PMH.

Physical Examination

The patient is alert and in no distress, somewhat pale.

Neck: Supple. No JVD. Good carotid upstrokes.

Lungs: Clear.

Heart: S1 and S2. Grade I over VI systolic murmur.

Abdomen: Soft, nontender. No masses are felt. No hepatosplenomegaly. Bowel sounds are normal. There is no pedal edema.

Rectal: Definitely heme positive.

Impression: Patient is a 74-year-old white male with lower GI bleed and anemia, probably secondary to the lower GI bleed. He is symptomatic with anemia. Will admit him to the hospital and give him blood. Will get a barium enema tomorrow to see if there is any etiology of his lower GI bleed other than diverticula, which are probably bleeding. He has had one such episode in the past. We want to make sure he has no evidence of any carcinoma or any other etiology for cancer while he is here in the hospital.

Progress Notes

2/13   Doing fine. Hemoccult neg. Lungs clear. Hct about 27 today.

2/14   Hemoccult neg. No major complaints. Says he is feeling much stronger.

Exam: WNL

Hgb/Hct: 9.2/28.4

B.E shows extensive diverticula

Discharge Dx: Blood loss anemia secondary to bleeding diverticula, anxiety

D/C home on FeSO4 and lots of fiber

F/U in 3 to 5 days

Radiology Consultation

Barium Enema: Examination of the colon with barium shows no constant filling defect or mucosal ulceration. There are multiple, somewhat large diverticula involving the left colon. No extrinsic pressure deformity is noted. Scattered loops of small bowel are noted without evidence of reflux into the terminal ileum.

Impression: Rather marked diverticulosis of the left colon without evidence of diverticulitis. Suggestion of some small bowel ileus.

Laboratory Tests

Test	2/12	2/13	2/14	Reference	Units
WBC	6.2		5.7	4.8–10.8	x10-3
RBC	3.06 L		3.93 L	4.70–6.10	x10-6
Hemoglobin	6.4 C (1)	8.9 C	(*) 9.2 L	14.0–18.0	9
Hematocrit	20.8 C (1)	27.8 L	(*) 28.4	42.0–52.0	%
MCV	67.9 L		72.3 L	80.0–94.0	u3
MCH	20.9 L		23.4 L	27.0–31.0	uug
MCHC	30.8 L		32.4	32.0–36.0	%
RDW	17.6 H		20.3 H	11.8–14.1	%
Platelet Estimate	Adequate		Adequate	Adequate	
SEGS	67		71 H	40–70	%
Bands	0		0	0–4	%
Eosinophils	0		1	0–3	%
Basophils	1		0	0–1	%
Lymphocytes	30		25	20–45	%
Monocytes	2		3	0–4	%
Metamyelocytes	0		0	0–0	%
Myelocytes	0		0	0–0	%
Anisocytosis	2+ A		3+ A		
Poikilocytosis	1+ A		1+ A		
Microcytic			1+ A		
Hypochromia	3+ A		1+ A		
Polychromia			1+ A		
Test Result Comments					
*1 Result verified by repeat analysis					

Case 1: Solution

1. Principal diagnosis: _____

   _____

2. Other diagnoses: _____

   _____

3. Procedures: _____

   _____

4. Issues to clarify with physician: _____

   _____

Case 2

Discharge Summary

Patient is a 78-year-old female. She saw the doctor recently with abdominal pain and constipation. A barium enema showed diverticulosis and perhaps a stricture near the sigmoid and rectal junction. She was scoped by the doctor, who saw a stricture at that point and said he couldn't rule out a carcinoma. Upper GI showed a hiatal hernia and duodenal diverticulum. Ultrasound showed gallstones. The patient had some bladder incontinence. She has had atrial fibrillation, diabetes, and takes Lanoxin. Otherwise, she is doing quite well. She has had a previous right total hip.

At the time of admission, it was thought that she had a stricture, rule out carcinoma, diabetes mellitus, exogenous obesity, past history of atrial fibrillation, previous abdominal hysterectomy, previous right total hip. Her chest film showed some chronic blunting of the right costophrenic angle, but otherwise was negative. Her admission EKG showed what was thought to be a normal sinus rhythm. Her blood type was AB-positive. Urinalysis was negative. Hemoglobin was 13.3, white blood cell count 7,600. Prothrombin time 12, PTT was 23. The CEA, which came back several days later, was quite high at 856. Glucose is 127, albumin is 3.4. Other labs were normal.

After mechanical and chemical bowel prep, she was taken to surgery. First, we laparoscoped her to see if we could do this resection with the scope. When we found that it was adherent to loops of adjacent small bowel, she had an open resection. A large carcinoma of the rectosigmoid junction was found and resected with an end-to-end anastomosis. A segment of small bowel that was stuck to the tumor was also resected, and a functional end-to-end anastomosis was done. At least four separate liver metastases were noted. Needle biopsy of that was done as well. The pathology report showed moderate to poorly differentiated carcinoma, bases through the wall of the colon and into the perirectal fat. The small intestine was not involved. The liver metastases were also positive.

The patient had a rather smooth postoperative course. She was thought to be ready for discharge on the sixth post-operative day. She was seen in consultation prior to surgery by the doctor, who managed her medical problems and diabetes and will arrange for appropriate medication at the time of discharge. She was sent home on Darvocet for pain. Ferrous Gluconate 324 mg three times a day for a month to restore her blood count. She is to resume her other previous medications. She is to restrict her activities for 2 months and to see me in the office in 8 days.

Final Diagnosis:

1. Invasive adenocarcinoma of the rectosigmoid, metastatic to the liver
2. Type II diabetes mellitus
3. Exogenous obesity
4. Atrial fibrillation
5. Previous right total hip replacement
6. Previous abdominal hysterectomy

Surgical Procedure: Resection of rectosigmoid with low pelvic anastomosis with an EEA, small bowel resection, liver biopsy.

History

Patient is a 78-year-old female. She has been in to see the doctor recently with abdominal pain and complains that she was unable to move her bowels. She was admitted and subsequently had endoscopy following a number of x-rays.

The x-rays showed diverticulosis of the sigmoid and perhaps a stricture near the sigmoid rectal junction. This was difficult to delineate because of overlapping loops of bowel. The patient had an upper GI showing hiatal hernia and a duodenal diverticulum, and an ultrasound showing gallstones.

The patient was subsequently seen by the doctor. A week ago today, the doctor performed upper GI endoscopy, which showed a little antral gastritis. A sigmoidoscopic examination showed, at about 25 cm, a narrowed area of the bowel with edema and stricture, and some blood oozing from above. Doctor said that he could not be sure whether this was strictly a diverticular stricture or whether there was a tumor above this point. The patient has otherwise been pretty healthy.

She had a previous hysterectomy. She had a previous fracture in the right hip. She had pulmonary embolus secondary to thrombophlebitis in her legs on two different occasions. She is not a smoker and seldom drinks.

She has no known allergies.

She has three children. Both parents are deceased.

She has had type II diabetes for about 5 years and takes Tolinase 150 mg two times a day. She has had atrial fibrillation in the past and takes Lanoxin 0.125 mg a day for that condition. She has never had hypertension, heart disease (other than the atrial fibrillation), or stroke. She has no chest pain or shortness of breath.

She has had quite a bit of heartburn and indigestion, but this definitely has been improved by Zantac.

She has some bladder incontinence.

Physical Examination

She weighs 174. She is 5' 6½" tall. BP 152/84 on the right, 148/78 on the left. Pulse was 80.

Examination of the HEENT was negative. The patient seemed extremely alert. She has good carotid pulses without bruits. No goiter or nodes in the neck. Breasts were somewhat pendant, but there were no masses, no skin or nipple retraction, no axillary supraclavicular nodes.

The heart rate was regular. The heart was not enlarged. There was no murmur. The lungs were clear to auscultation and percussion.

There was a low midline scar. No hepatosplenomegaly. There was a little left lower quadrant tenderness.

Rectal and vaginal exams were not repeated.

She had good femoral, popliteal, and dorsalis pedis pulses. The ankles were quite thick. There was a scar on her right hip from previous surgery.

Neurologic function is normal.

Her skin tended to be sweaty and clammy, which she says is the normal case for her.

Impression:

1. Stricture of the sigmoid seen on barium enema and colonoscopy, probably secondary to diverticular disease, causing obstructive symptoms
2. Type II diabetes mellitus
3. Exogenous obesity
4. Past history of atrial fibrillation, past history of abdominal hysterectomy

Plan: Resection.

Consultation

It was a pleasure to see your patient, who is well known to me from my office. She is a pleasant 78-year-old white, obese female who, over the past 3 to 4 months, has had increasing amounts of difficulty with bowel movements. She has a complaint of small, pencil-thin bowel movements with some blood noted. The patient also had some difficulty with upper GI indigestion, as well as gastritis. She has been evaluated per gastroenterology at the hospital and diagnosed with antral gastritis as well as diverticulosis, diverticulitis with narrowing of the sigmoid colon, approximately 25 cm via colonoscopy. The patient has had a workup that included an upper GI series and endoscopies that have shown the above problem, etiology yet to be determined. The patient has a rather strong family history of having similar type of etiologies. Apparently, her three sisters have had similar surgeries, surgery-like etiology secondary to narrowing of sigmoid colon, and difficulties with irritable bowel–type symptoms. The patient has had difficulty with her bowel movements for many years. However, during the past 3 months they have become somewhat more bloody, as well as worsened in types. The patient came to my office approximately 3 months ago with the above etiology. Workup was done then and is on previous chart for review.

Her past medical history is consistent with type II diabetes mellitus. She is currently on Tolinase bid with fairly good control at home when the patient follows her diet. The patient does not have a history of smoking, nor does she drink. She currently lives alone. The patient had a hip replacement approximately a year or year and half ago with no sequelae. The patient has previous history of pulmonary embolus. However, she has had no difficulty with the previous surgery noted.

The medication protocol at home includes one-a-day aspirin and Tolinase bid basis. She is also taking Lanoxin 0.125 mg for previous history of atrial fibrillation, which has currently been controlled with normal sinus rhythm for the last 1-year period of time noted.

The patient has been evaluated for urinary incontinence secondary to a low-lying bladder. Surgical history includes a hysterectomy many years ago. The patient has been in fairly good health except for mild diabetes mellitus, which is controlled with diet as well as oral medications. Otherwise, she has done well and has been in fairly stable condition up to the recent history with her colon problems.

On physical examination, the patient's general HEENT, eyes, ears, nose, and throat are basically clear. Neck does not show any cervical nodes. Neck is clear for adenopathy. Lungs are clear to auscultation; no rales, rhonchi, or friction rubs. No wheezing. The heart rate is regular rate and rhythm. Abdomen is soft, not overtly tender at this time. Extremities do not show any edema. Cranial nerves are grossly intact as tested.

The patient's EKG shows that of normal sinus rhythm, as evaluated by the consultant. The lab work shows a glucose of 127. BUN and creatinine are within normal limits, as are the electrolytes. Albumin is slightly low at 3.4, with a total protein of 6.0. The liver function profile, SGOT, alk. phos., and bilirubin are within normal limits, as well as triglycerides.

Diagnostic Impressions:

1. Diverticulosis/diverticulitis with sigmoid constriction, etiology to be determined, rule out primary disease, that of diverticulosis or diverticulitis versus overt tumor
2. Diabetes mellitus
3. Atrial fibrillation by history, current normal sinus rhythm
4. Generalized obesity

Recommendation:

1. Will put the patient on medication protocol, Lanoxin for control of atrial fibrillation, normal sinus rhythm.
2. Will start a sliding scale Iinsulin, with regular Humulin Iinsulin while she is undergoing surgery. Back on Tolinase postsurgery if control is indicated at that time.

Surgical Record

Preoperative Diagnosis: Probable diverticular stricture of the sigmoid, rule out carcinoma

Postoperative Diagnosis: Carcinoma of the sigmoid invading into adjacent small bowel with metastases to the liver

Procedure: Attempted laparoscopic bowel removal, open exploration with resection of the sigmoid colon and end-to-end anastomosis with 28 mm EEA. Resection of segment of small bowel with direct extension of the tumor into that area with the functional end-to-end anastomosis, doing a side-to-side anastomosis, biopsy of liver metastases.

Patient is a 78-year-old female who presented with abdominal pain and constipation. Barium enema suggested diverticular stricture. Patient was seen in consultation by the doctor, who sigmoidoscoped the patient and found a stricture at about 25 cm. Doctor could not see above the stricture, so we could not rule out carcinoma. Patient understood the nature of the problem, the proposed surgical risk, and its possible complications, and consented to it. She was given a mechanical and chemical bowel prep.

Patient was brought to surgery and an NG tube was placed in the stomach and a Foley in the bladder. She was placed in the lithotomy position; routine prep and drape were done. We made a small incision in the right upper quadrant, directly into the peritoneal cavity and inserted the Hasson cannula, insufflated the peritoneal cavity with CO_2. Once we had a good tent, we examined the peritoneal cavity and could not really see the liver because we were so close to it. We then dissected out the sigmoid after we put in three other cannulas, a 12-mm in the right lower quadrant, a 10-mm in the left lower quadrant, and a 5-mm in the left upper quadrant. These were put in under direct vision. We then grasped the sigmoid and dissected it off the left pelvic gutter, and dissected down toward the bladder. She had undergone a previous hysterectomy, but there were no anterior adhesions. We could not get the small bowel to easily come up out of the pelvis. We then put the colonoscope through the rectum and came up to 25 cm, where we saw not a diverticular stricture, but a carcinoma. We marked this point.

When we were dissecting, we found the small bowel to be adherent at this time and we elected to open, so the trocars and instruments were all removed. We then made a midline incision and, on inspection, found a large mass in the pelvis. We had already freed up the left side of the sigmoid colon with laparoscope. We identified the ureter and pushed it away, opened the right pelvic peritoneum and identified the right ureter, and then transected the bowel above the junction of the sigmoid and descending colon with the GIA. We then divided the mesentery between Kelly clamps, including the inferior mesenteric terminal branch. These were all divided and ligated with heavy silks. We pulled the small bowel off the side, but it did look like there was some direct invasion there, and then further mobilized the tumor and the upper rectum. We divided all the mesentery between Kelly clamps and ligated with heavy silk. We then transected the rectum through its middle and upper one thirds, with TA55 on the distal side and Kocher on the proximal side, and then removed the specimen. We brought the proximal end of the bowel out, cleaned it off of fat and mesentery, put a pursestring instrument on it, excised the bowel distal to the pursestring instrument, opened the pursestring instrument, and then incised it. The size was 28 mm. We then put the anvil of EEA in the proximal bowel and tightened it down with pursestring. We put the EEA instrument up through the rectum, pushed the trocar up through the suture line, then connected the anvil to the EEA instrument and tightened it down under direct vision, cut the bowel making the anastomosis and removed the EEA. We then filled the pelvis with saline, clamped the bowel proximally, and put in the colonoscope to obtain a good anastomosis with no bleeding and no leak of air.

We then aspirated the fluid in the pelvis. We resected the segment of the small bowel with GIA and did a functional end-to-end anastomosis and transected the bowel loop outside the anastomosis with a TA55. We actually had done this before we completed the rectal anastomosis, and when we went back we found a hematoma in the mesentery. We dissected through the hematoma to get it controlled, ligated the bleeders with heavy silk, but then we had to resect another 10 cm of small bowel and then did another functional end-to-end anastomosis and closed the enterotomy with TA55 and the mesentery with fine silks. This gave us a nice anastomosis with good pink bowel, pretty close to the cecum.

We then noted there to be at least three, maybe four, metastases scattered over different areas of the right lobe of the liver. One was biopsied with a Tru-cut needle and the biopsy site cauterized. We then had a correct sponge, instrument, and needle count. We closed the fascia of the right upper quadrant puncture wound with some interrupted silk

Vicryls and closed the muscles with interrupted Vicryls. The other smaller ports were closed by skin clips. We then closed the fascia of the peritoneum of the midline wound with running suture of #l Vicryl and the fascia with interrupted figure 8 #l Vicryl, closed the skin with clips, and applied sterile dressings. Sponge, instruments, and sharp counts were again correct. The patient tolerated the procedure well and we trust she will do well.

Pathology Report

Specimen—Origin:

I.   Small bowel sigmoid colon

II. Liver biopsy

Pathologic Diagnosis:

I.   Segments of small bowel: Serosal adhesions

Colon: Invasive adenocarcinoma, moderate to poorly differentiated, extending into pericolic adipose

Lymph nodes, small bowel mesentery: Negative for metastasis (0/6 nodes)

Lymph nodes, pericolic: Negative for metastasis (0/6)

Pericolic adipose: Metastatic adenocarcinoma

II. Liver (needle biopsy): Metastatic adenocarcinoma

Case 2: Solution

1.   Principal diagnosis: _____
_____

2.   Other diagnoses: _____
_____

3.   Procedures: _____
_____

4.   Issues to clarify with physician: _____
_____

Case 3

Emergency Department Record

Chief Complaint: Shortness of breath

History of Present Illness: This is a 72-year-old male with a long history of bullous emphysema. He has home breathing treatments and is on Aminophylline and Lanoxin and pO_2 11/2 liters pm at home. Patient presents with a 2-day history of increasing dyspnea, and became increasingly restless and short of breath tonight. He was brought in here by family for evaluation. He does complain of feeling hot but denies any chills or increasing cough recently. Patient also has a history of CHF per his wife.

Physical Examination: Vital signs, temperature not recorded, pulse 135, respirations 32, blood pressure 124/82. Patient is cyanotic at the fingertips and somewhat dusky. He is breathing with pursed lips at a rapid rate and sitting up. Lung exam demonstrated very poor air movement bilaterally. Cardiac exam was irregular rhythm without murmurs, rubs, or gallops, and was tachycardiac. The patient has extremely dry leatherlike skin with brownish discoloration in the pretibial area, along with some scaling and chronic skin changes.

Initial ABG, which was obtained immediately on 2 L of oxygen, showed a pH of 7.15, pCO_2 of 69.5, pO_2 of 50, and bicarb of 25.5 with 72% oxygen saturation. Initially we gave him two breathing treatments over 45 minutes consisting of Albuterol med/neb along with Solu-Medrol 125 mg IV push and 2 L of oxygen support, hoping that he would improve and we could avoid intubation. However, during this 45-minute period the patient started developing multi-focal PVCs and also had runs of 3, 4, and 5 PVCs at a time, but had no chest pain. Therefore, we increased the patient's oxygen and placed him on lidocaine of 75 mg IV push bolus along with lidocaine at 2 mg per minute, resulting in good resolution of his arrhythmia except for a rare PVC. We did repeat his ABG while on 40% mask, which showed a pH of 7.17, pCO_2 of 75, pO_2 of 72, and bicarb of 2.8 at 89%.

Due to the extreme acidosis and the tachypnea, I discussed with the family (the patient and his wife, two sons, and also a son over the phone) that we should intubate the patient before he had impending respiratory failure.

The patient was therefore intubated per respiratory with number 8 ET tube. Ventilation was initially set on tidal volume of 500 cc with a rate of 16. Repeat gases on this after a half hour showed a pH of 7.15, pCO_2 of 68, pO_2 of 66, bicarb of 25, and O_2 sat of 85%. We therefore increased his tidal volume of 600 cc and kept him on the vent. A portable chest x-ray was done after tube placement, which showed the tube to be in excellent placement. Laboratory data included a hemoglobin of 18.6, hematocrit 58.1, white blood cell count 7,400 with 4 bands, 54 segs, CPK was high at 259, and MB was pending. EKG showed multifocal PVCs and atrial fibrillation with a rapid ventricular rate. Theophylline level was 11.6, Lanoxin level was 1.

History

Chief Complaint: Shortness of breath, restlessness, tingling in the hands, swelling of the feet

History of Present Illness: This 72-year-old white male has a history of rather advanced chronic obstructive pulmonary disease for many years. He presented to the emergency department with progressive dyspnea of 2 days' duration, restlessness, and feeling hot and burning up. According to his wife, the patient had episodes where he suddenly became dyspneic, was turning red all over, and had tingling all over his body. He did not have a cold or fever. He was evaluated in the emergency department. Patient had evidence of respiratory acidosis with respiratory failure with a pH of 7.15, pCO_2 of 68, pO_2 of 66, bicarb of 12, O_2 saturation of 85%. The patient was markedly dyspneic with labored respirations. Hemoglobin was 18.6 g. EKG showed premature ectopic beats. Theophylline level was 7.6, Dig level was 1.0.

The patient was intubated and transferred to ICU for further care. It was thought at that time that respiratory acidosis may have contributed to the patient's ectopy and the deterioration of his clinical condition. The patient was initially given respiratory therapy in the emergency department without any significant improvement.

The patient has a history of rather advanced chronic obstructive pulmonary disease with bullous emphysema. He also has a history of congestive cardiac failure with cor pulmonale. The patient has been on home IPPB treatment. He has also been on bronchodilators, intermittent antibiotic therapy, and O_2 therapy at home. He also has venous insufficiency in the lower extremities and stasis ulcer in the left leg, which has been healing slowly with local treatment and systemic antibiotic therapy.

Past Medical History: The patient was hospitalized for prostate surgery many years ago. He also has had a cataract removed with intraocular implant. A year ago, he had a skin lesion removed from the nose, which was basal cell carcinoma. He was treated with local radiation therapy.

Family History: Noncontributory

Personal History: He is married. He quit smoking cigarettes approximately 12 years ago. Drinks alcohol occasionally. Drinks four to five cups of coffee a day.

Review of Systems: Unremarkable, except for present illness

Physical Examination

The patient is a well-developed, well-nourished white male in acute respiratory distress, markedly cyanotic with labored respirations. He is slightly lethargic. BP is 130/86, Pulse 110; respirations were 38.

Head: Unremarkable.

Eyes: Evidence of surgery from previous cataract surgery with intraocular implant. No other abnormalities.

ENT: The patient is intubated with ET tube inserted. Copious secretions from the oral cavity. Surgical scar on nose from previous surgery.

Neck: Shows no masses, no venous engorgement, no bruit.

Chest: Air entry is equal on both sides. Scattered rhonchi in both lung fields with minimal diffuse basilar rales.

Heart: Irregular rhythm with ectopy. A Grade H x VI apical murmur present.

Abdomen: Soft, no tenderness. No palpable masses. Bowel sounds active. Hernia. Orifices normal.

Rectal Exam: Deferred.

Extremities: Edema in both lower extremities with marked excoriation and scaling of the skin distal to the knee with an ulcerative lesion in the left leg with hyperpigmentation for the skin of both lower extremities without any signs of acute infection.

Impression: Clinically, the patient has stasis dermatitis; stasis ulcer also in the left leg.

Neurologic exam is consistent with mild peripheral neuropathy.

Consultation

Patient has several-day history of increasing amounts of shortness of breath, increasing sputum production, and increased complaints of feeling hot, but denied chills. Patient was admitted for acute shortness of breath, respiratory failure needing intubation, and respiratory and ventilator care now.

Apparently, the patient came to the hospital with no chest pain, but having occasional and/or frequent PVCs requiring lidocaine initiation as well as increased amounts of oxygen. Secondary to respiratory acidosis, the patient was intubated. ABGs are to follow. Patient has a long history of emphysema with bullous changes in his lungs. He has a history of congestive heart failure as well as potential cardiac dysrhythmia. The patient currently is on ventilator care and was extubated yesterday. Postextubation, apparently 8 hours later patient had fatigue requiring reintubation noted. Other past medical history is significant of having extremity varicosities as well as ulceration and senile dementia. Patient has no known allergies.

Laboratory investigations of ABGs show acute respiratory acidosis, hypoxemia increased AA gradient noted. Subsequent arterial blood gases have been done with the patient on the ventilator. Patient's EKG showed that of sinus tachycardia with sinus arrhythmia. Some PVCs noted on the occasional EKG.

Patient has been in atrial fibrillation intermittently. His x-rays show bilateral hyperinflated airways. The patient does have a large left heart with some nonspecific interstitial markings. Patient appears to have fibrotic changes. No pleural effusion in the patient's left base. Review of chest x-ray changes shows some increase in the interstitial markings. Left heart remains enlarged.

Consulting Diagnoses:

1. Acute exacerbation of COPD emphysema in stages leading to respiratory failure that of acute respiratory acidosis and hypoxemia
2. Probable superimposed upon respiratory failure with COPD emphysema is that of cardiac dysrhythmia and probable mild to moderate congestive heart failure
3. Probable significant coronary artery disease and cor pulmonale, II
4. Theophylline toxic at this time

Laboratory Tests

Test	1/9	1/9	1/9	1/9	Reference
ART BLOOD GASES					
pH	7.154 L		7.167 L	7.152 L	7.340–7.450
pCO$_2$	69.5 H		74.9 H	67.9 H	32.0–5.0
pO$_2$	50.2 L		72.0 L	66.1 L	75.0–100.0
Bicarb	23.4		26.1 H	22.8	20.0–26.0
Total CO$_2$	25.5		28.4 H	24.9	21.0–27.0
O$_2$ sat	72.5 L		88.5 L	85.2 L	95.0–98.0
CHEMISTRY					
Glucose		157 H			77–115
BUN		23			8–24
Creatinine		1.4 H			0.5–1.2
Sodium		141			137–147
Potassium		4.6			3.6–5.2
Chloride		103			97–111
CO$_2$		31			21–32
CK Total		259 H			55–215
CKMB		3.3			0.4–4.7
LDH		173			91–179
SGOT-AST		45 H			11–33
Magnesium		1.8			1.6–2.4
THERAPEUTIC DRUGS					
Digoxin		1.0			0.8–1.6
Theophylline		11.6			10.0–20.0

Laboratory Tests

Test	1/12	1/12	1/13	1/13	Reference
ART BLOOD GASES					
pH	7.419	7.434		7.477 H	7.340–7.450
pCO$_2$	42.6	41.3		41.0	32.0–45.0
pO$_2$	52.7 L	51.3 L		57.0 L	75.0–100.0
Bicarb	27.4 H	27.5 H		30.2 H	20.0–26.0
Total CO$_2$	28.7 H	28.7 H		31.5	21.0–27.0
O$_2$ sat	87.5 L	87.2 L		91.3 L	95.0–98.0
CHEMISTRY					
Potassium			3.2 L		3.6–5.2
THERAPEUTIC DRUGS					
Theophylline			34.1 H		10.0–20.0

Clinical Resume

This 72-year-old white male has history of fairly advanced chronic obstructive pulmonary disease for many years. He presented to the emergency department with progressive shortness of breath of several days' duration, associated with restlessness, feeling hot, and burning up. He did not have any history of recent cold, fever, or flu. He had several episodes of acute shortness of breath prior to admission. He was evaluated in the emergency department and was in acute respiratory failure with pH of 7.15, pCO_2 of 68, and pO_2 of 66. Saturation was 85%. The patient was intubated in the emergency department and transferred to ICU for further care. His hemoglobin was 18.6 g. EKG showed premature ventricular ectopic beats. Theophylline level was 11.6. Digoxin level was 1.0. The patient has history of chronic obstructive pulmonary disease with bullous emphysema. He also has history of congestive heart failure. He has been on bronchodilators, IPPB, intermittent antibiotic therapy at home. In addition to the above, he has venous insufficiency in both lower extremities with stasis dermatitis and stasis ulcers in the lower extremity.

On physical examination, he was a well-developed, well-nourished white male in acute respiratory distress with labored respiration, slightly lethargic. BP 130/86, pulse 110, resp 38. Examination of the HEENT, neck was unremarkable. Chest showed bilateral rhonchi in both lung fields with minimal diffuse basilar rales. Heart rhythm was irregular with ectopy. Grade II by VI apical murmur was present. Abdominal examination was unremarkable. Extremities showed edema in both lower extremities and marked excoriation and scaling of the skin distal to the knee, ulcerative lesions in the left leg with hyperpigmentation consistent with stasis dermatitis.

Laboratory Data: Chest x-ray showed no acute infiltrate. There was a suggestion of mild congestive cardiac failure. EKG showed atrial fibrillation with ventricular ectopic beats and showed lateral ischemia. Arterial blood gases showed pH of 7.15, pCO_2 of 69.5, and pO_2 of 50. Blood glucose was 157, BUN 23, and creatinine 1.4. Electrolytes were normal. Digoxin level was 1.0. Theophylline was 11.6.

Course in Hospital: The patient was intubated and transferred to ICU, where he was started on ventilatory support. He was seen later on the same day with marked improvement in his clinical condition. He was more alert and responsive, and there was also improvement in the acidosis. He was continued on the same therapy. On 1-11, the patient was reevaluated. He had significant improvement. His acidosis had been corrected, and ABGs showed a pO_2 of 55 and pCO_2 of 59 with good negative inspiratory effort. It was thought that the patient could tolerate extubation. He was extubated on 1-11. He tolerated it well for 6 hours. post extubation. Subsequent to that, he developed gradual increasing pCO_2 and decreasing pO_2 with acidosis. His respirations became labored and the patient became cyanotic. He was reintubated on January 11 and started on ventilatory support.

The next day, the patient was clinically improved. His vital signs were also improved. A consultation was obtained from a pulmonologist. In his opinion, the patient had respiratory failure with acute exacerbation of chronic obstructive pulmonary disease. When he examined the patient, the patient's Theophylline was higher than therapeutic level, at 34.1. He recommended that the patient be continued on ventilatory support. Electrolyte imbalance should be corrected and also his dose of Theophylline needed adjustment. All these orders were carried out. The patient started showing signs of improvement. When the patient's condition was stable, he was started on intermittent ventilation. He had signs of congestive cardiac failure, which were treated with diuretics. He was continued on Digoxin. Patient was extubated on January 15. This time he tolerated it well. His condition remained stable and he was transferred to a regular unit. He was initially placed on corticosteroids. The dose was gradually decreased, and he was switched to oral antibiotics and corticosteroids. He continued to improve but still was dyspneic. However, he was markedly improved since admission.

After he recovered to a significant level and his oral intake had improved, pulmonary rehabilitation was discussed with the patient. It is thought that the patient could be discharged at this time and be followed up as an outpatient. After the patient was informed that he would be discharged that morning, he became anxious, agitated, and very apprehensive. Arterial blood gases were still satisfactory for a patient who has chronic obstructive pulmonary disease. His pCO_2 level was 71.2, pO_2 was 77.3, and pH was 7.3. It was discovered that there was an element of anxiety on the patient's part, and he may require further supportive care. However, continuation of hospitalization would not benefit the patient. He was discharged on 1/23. At the time of discharge, the patient had mild dyspnea. However, he had significantly improved. His vital signs were stable.

Medications at Discharge:

1.   No-added-salt diet with high-fat and low-carbohydrate content
2.   Procardia SR 500 mg tid
3.   Slobid 200 mg bid
4.   Lasix 40 mg daily
5.   Zantac 150 mg daily
6.   Lanoxin 0.25 mg daily except on Sunday
7.   K-Dur 20 mg daily
8.   Prednisone 20 mg twice a day for 4 days; once a day for 1 week; and 10 mg daily for 1 week and 10 mg every day subsequent to that

Case 3: Solution

1. Principal diagnosis: _____
   _____

2. Other diagnoses: _____
   _____

3. Procedures: _____
   _____

4. Issues to clarify with physician: _____
   _____

Appendix A

Ethics in Coding

Preamble to the American Health Information Management Association Code of Ethics

The ethical obligations of the health information management (HIM) professional include the protection of patient privacy and confidential information; disclosure of information; development, use, and maintenance of health information systems and health records; and the quality of information. Both handwritten and computerized medical records contain many sacred stories—stories that must be protected on behalf of the individual and the aggregate community of persons served in the healthcare system. Healthcare consumers are increasingly concerned about the loss of privacy and the inability to control the dissemination of their protected information. Core health information issues include what information should be collected, how the information should be handled, who should have access to the information, and under what conditions the information should be disclosed.

Ethical obligations are central to the professional's responsibility, regardless of the employment site or the method of collection, storage, and security of health information. Sensitive information (genetic, adoption, drug, alcohol, sexual, and behavioral information) requires special attention to prevent misuse. Entrepreneurial roles require expertise in the protection of the information in the world of business and interactions with consumers.

Professional Values

The mission of the HIM profession is based on core professional values developed since the inception of the Association in 1928. These values and the inherent ethical responsibilities for AHIMA members and credentialed HIM professionals include providing service; protecting medical, social, and financial information; promoting confidentiality; and preserving and securing health information. Values to the healthcare team include promoting the quality and advancement of healthcare, demonstrating HIM expertise and skills, and promoting interdisciplinary cooperation and collaboration. Professional values in relationship to the employer include protecting committee deliberations and complying with laws, regulations, and policies. Professional values related to the public include advocating change, refusing to participate in or

---

Revised and adopted by AHIMA House of Delegates—July 1, 2004

conceal unethical practices, and reporting violations of practice standards to the proper authorities. Professional values to individual and professional associations include obligations to be honest, bringing honor to self, peers, and profession, committing to continuing education and lifelong learning, performing Association duties honorably, strengthening professional membership, representing the profession to the public, and promoting and participating in research.

These professional values will require a complex process of balancing the many conflicts that can result from competing interests and obligations of those who seek access to health information and require an understanding of ethical decision-making.

Purpose of the American Health Information Management Association Code of Ethics

The HIM professional has an obligation to demonstrate actions that reflect values, ethical principles, and ethical guidelines. AHIMA's Code of Ethics sets forth these values and principles to guide conduct. The code is relevant to all AHIMA members and credentialed HIM professionals and students, regardless of their professional functions, the settings in which they work, or the populations they serve.

The AHIMA Code of Ethics serves six purposes:

- Identifies core values on which the HIM mission is based.

- Summarizes broad ethical principles that reflect the profession's core values and establishes a set of ethical principles to be used to guide decision-making and actions.

- Helps HIM professionals identify relevant considerations when professional obligations conflict or ethical uncertainties arise.

- Provides ethical principles by which the general public can hold the HIM professional accountable.

- Socializes practitioners new to the field to HIM's mission, values, and ethical principles.

- Articulates a set of guidelines that the HIM professional can use to assess whether they have engaged in unethical conduct.

The code includes principles and guidelines that are both enforceable and aspirational. The extent to which each principle is enforceable is a matter of professional judgment to be exercised by those responsible for reviewing alleged violations of ethical principles.

The Use of the Code

Violation of principles in this code does not automatically imply legal liability or violation of the law. Such determination can only be made in the context of legal and judicial proceedings. Alleged violations of the code would be subject to a peer review process. Such processes are generally separate from legal or administrative procedures and insulated from legal review or proceedings to allow the profession to counsel and discipline its own members; in some situations, violations of the code would constitute unlawful conduct subject to legal process.

Guidelines for ethical and unethical behavior are provided in this code. The terms "shall and shall not" are used as a basis for setting high standards for behavior. This does not imply that everyone "shall or shall not" do everything that is listed. For example, not everyone participates in the recruitment or mentoring of students. A HIM professional is not being unethical if this is not part of his or her professional activities; however, if students are part of one's professional responsibilities, there is an ethical obligation to follow the guidelines stated in the code. This concept is true for the entire code. If someone does the stated activities, ethical behavior is the standard. The guidelines are not a comprehensive list. For example, the statement "protect all confidential information to include personal, health, financial, genetic, and outcome information" can also be interpreted as "shall not fail to protect all confidential information to include personal, health, financial, genetic, and outcome information."

A code of ethics cannot guarantee ethical behavior. Moreover, a code of ethics cannot resolve all ethical issues or disputes or capture the richness and complexity involved in striving to make responsible choices within a moral community. Rather, a code of ethics sets forth values and ethical principles, and offers ethical guidelines to which professionals aspire and by which their actions can be judged. Ethical behaviors result from a personal commitment to engage in ethical practice.

Professional responsibilities often require an individual to move beyond personal values. For example, an individual might demonstrate behaviors that are based on the values of honesty, providing service to others, or demonstrating loyalty. In addition to these, professional values might require promoting confidentiality, facilitating interdisciplinary collaboration, and refusing to participate in or conceal unethical practices. Professional values could require a more comprehensive set of values than what an individual needs to be an ethical agent in their personal lives.

AHIMA's Code of Ethics is to be used by AHIMA and individuals, agencies, organizations, and bodies (such as licensing and regulatory boards, insurance providers, courts of law, agency boards of directors, government agencies, and other professional groups) that choose to adopt it or use it as a frame of reference. AHIMA's Code of Ethics reflects the commitment of all to uphold the profession's values and to act ethically. Individuals of good character who discern moral questions and, in good faith, seek to make reliable ethical judgments, must apply ethical principles.

The code does not provide a set of rules that prescribe how to act in all situations. Specific applications of the code must take into account the context in which it is being considered and the possibility of conflicts among the code's values, principles, and guidelines. Ethical responsibilities flow from all human relationships, from the personal and familial to the social and professional. Further, AHIMA's Code of Ethics does not specify which values, principles, and guidelines are the most important and ought to outweigh others in instances when they conflict.

Code of Ethics 2004

Ethical Principles: The following ethical principles are based on the core values of AHIMA and apply to all HIM professionals.

HIM professionals:

> I. *Advocate, uphold, and defend the individual's right to privacy and the doctrine of confidentiality in the use and disclosure of information.*

> II. *Put service and the health and welfare of persons before self-interest and conduct themselves in the practice of the profession so as to bring honor to themselves, their peers, and to the health information management profession.*

> III. *Preserve, protect, and secure personal health information in any form or medium and hold in the highest regard the contents of the records and other information of a confidential nature, taking into account the applicable statutes and regulations.*

IV. *Refuse to participate in or conceal unethical practices or procedures.*

V. *Advance health information management knowledge and practice through continuing education, research, publications, and presentations.*

VI. *Recruit and mentor students, peers and colleagues to develop and strengthen professional workforce.*

VII. *Represent the profession accurately to the public.*

VIII. *Perform honorably health information management association responsibilities, either appointed or elected, and preserve the confidentiality of any privileged information made known in any official capacity.*

IX. *State truthfully and accurately their credentials, professional education, and experiences.*

X. *Facilitate interdisciplinary collaboration in situations supporting health information practice.*

XI. *Respect the inherent dignity and worth of every person.*

How to Interpret the Code of Ethics

The following ethical principles are based on the core values of AHIMA and apply to all HIM professionals. Guidelines included for each ethical principle are a noninclusive list of behaviors and situations that can help to clarify the principle. They are not to be meant as a comprehensive list of all situations that can occur.

I. *Advocate, uphold, and defend the individual's right to privacy and the doctrine of confidentiality in the use and disclosure of information.*

Health information management professionals **shall:**

1.1. Protect all confidential information to include personal, health, financial, genetic, and outcome information.

1.2. Engage in social and political action that supports the protection of privacy and confidentiality, and be aware of the impact of the political arena on the health information system. Advocate for changes in policy and legislation to ensure protection of privacy and confidentiality, coding compliance, and other issues that surface as advocacy issues as well as facilitating informed participation by the public on these issues.

1.3. Protect the confidentiality of all information obtained in the course of professional service. Disclose only information that is directly relevant or necessary to achieve the purpose of disclosure. Release information only with valid consent from a patient or a person legally authorized to consent on behalf of a patient or as authorized by federal or state regulations. The need-to-know criterion is essential when releasing health information for initial disclosure and all redisclosure activities.

1.4. Promote the obligation to respect privacy by respecting confidential information shared among colleagues, while responding to requests from the legal profession, the media, or other nonhealthcare-related individuals, during presentations or teaching and in situations that could cause harm to persons.

II. **Put service and the health and welfare of persons before self-interest and conduct themselves in the practice of the profession so as to bring honor to themselves, their peers, and to the health information management profession.**

Health information management professionals **shall:**

2.1. Act with integrity, behave in a trustworthy manner, elevate service to others above self-interest, and promote high standards of practice in every setting.

2.2. Be aware of the profession's mission, values, and ethical principles, and practice in a manner consistent with them by acting honestly and responsibly.

2.3. Anticipate, clarify, and avoid any conflict of interest, to all parties concerned, when dealing with consumers, consulting with competitors, or in providing services requiring potentially conflicting roles (for example, finding out information about one facility that would help a competitor). The conflicting roles or responsibilities must be clarified and appropriate action must be taken to minimize any conflict of interest.

2.4. Ensure that the working environment is consistent and encourages compliance with AHIMA's Code of Ethics, taking reasonable steps to eliminate any conditions in their organizations that violate, interfere with, or discourage compliance with the code.

2.5. Take responsibility and credit, including authorship credit, only for work they actually perform or to which they contribute. Honestly acknowledge the work of and the contributions made by others verbally or written, such as in publication.

Health information management professionals **shall not:**

2.6. Permit their private conduct to interfere with their ability to fulfill their professional responsibilities.

2.7. Take unfair advantage of any professional relationship or exploit others to further their personal, religious, political, or business interests.

III. **Preserve, protect, and secure personal health information in any form or medium and hold in the highest regard the contents of the records and other information of a confidential nature obtained in the official capacity, taking into account the applicable statutes and regulations.**

Health information management professionals **shall:**

3.1. Protect the confidentiality of patients' written and electronic records and other sensitive information. Take reasonable steps to ensure that patients' records are stored in a secure location and that patients' records are not available to others who are not authorized to have access.

3.2. Take precautions to ensure and maintain the confidentiality of information transmitted, transferred, or disposed of in the event of a termination, incapacitation, or death of a healthcare provider to other parties through the use of any media. Disclosure of identifying information should be avoided whenever possible.

3.3. Inform recipients of the limitations and risks associated with providing services via electronic media (such as computer, telephone, fax, radio, and television).

IV. **Refuse to participate in or conceal unethical practices or procedures.**

Health information management professionals **shall:**

4.1. Act in a professional and ethical manner at all times.

4.2. Take adequate measures to discourage, prevent, expose, and correct the unethical conduct of colleagues.

4.3. Be knowledgeable about established policies and procedures for handling concerns about colleagues' unethical behavior. These include policies and procedures created by AHIMA, licensing and regulatory bodies, employers, supervisors, agencies, and other professional organizations.

4.4. Seek resolution if there is a belief that a colleague has acted unethically or if there is a belief of incompetence or impairment by discussing their concerns with the colleague when feasible and when such discussion is likely to be productive. Take action through appropriate formal channels, such as contacting an accreditation or regulatory body and/or AHIMA's Professional Ethics Committee.

4.5. Consult with a colleague when feasible and assist the colleague in taking remedial action when there is direct knowledge of a health information management colleague's incompetence or impairment.

Health information management professionals **shall not:**

4.6. Participate in, condone, or be associated with dishonesty, fraud and abuse, or deception. A non-inclusive list of examples includes:

- Allowing patterns of retrospective documentation to avoid suspension or increase reimbursement

- Assigning codes without physician documentation

- Coding when documentation does not justify the procedures that have been billed

- Coding an inappropriate level of service

- Miscoding to avoid conflict with others

- Engaging in negligent coding practices

- Hiding or ignoring review outcomes, such as performance data

- Failing to report licensure status for a physician through the appropriate channels

- Recording inaccurate data for accreditation purposes

- Hiding incomplete medical records

- Allowing inappropriate access to genetic, adoption, or behavioral health information

- Misusing sensitive information about a competitor

- Violating the privacy of individuals

V. *Advance health information management knowledge and practice through continuing education, research, publications, and presentations.*

Health information management professionals **shall:**

5.1. Develop and enhance continually their professional expertise, knowledge, and skills (including appropriate education, research, training, consultation, and supervision). Contribute to the knowledge base of health information management and share with colleagues their knowledge related to practice, research, and ethics.

5.2. Base practice decisions on recognized knowledge, including empirically based knowledge relevant to health information management and health information management ethics.

5.3. Contribute time and professional expertise to activities that promote respect for the value, integrity, and competence of the health information management profession. These activities may include teaching, research, consultation, service, legislative testimony, presentations in the community, and participation in their professional organizations.

5.4. Engage in evaluation or research that ensures the anonymity or confidentiality of participants and of the data obtained from them by following guidelines developed for the participants in consultation with appropriate institutional review boards. Report evaluation and research findings accurately and take steps to correct any errors later found in published data using standard publication methods.

5.5. Take reasonable steps to provide or arrange for continuing education and staff development, addressing current knowledge and emerging developments related to health information management practice and ethics.

Health information management professionals **shall not:**

5.6. Design or conduct evaluation or research that is in conflict with applicable federal or state laws.

5.7. Participate in, condone, or be associated with fraud or abuse.

VI. *Recruit and mentor students, peers and colleagues to develop and strengthen professional workforce.*

Health information management professionals **shall:**

6.1. Evaluate students' performance in a manner that is fair and respectful when functioning as educators or clinical internship supervisors.

6.2. Be responsible for setting clear, appropriate, and culturally sensitive boundaries for students.

6.3. Be a mentor for students, peers, and new health information management professionals to develop and strengthen skills.

6.4. Provide directed practice opportunities for students.

Health information management professionals **shall not:**

6.5. Engage in any relationship with students in which there is a risk of exploitation or potential harm to the student.

VII. *Accurately represent the profession to the public.*

Health information management professionals **shall:**

7.1. Be an advocate for the profession in all settings and participate in activities that promote and explain the mission, values, and principles of the profession to the public.

VIII. *Perform honorably health information management association responsibilities, either appointed or elected, and preserve the confidentiality of any privileged information made known in any official capacity.*

Health information management professionals **shall:**

8.1. Perform responsibly all duties as assigned by the professional association.

8.2. Resign from an Association position if unable to perform the assigned responsibilities with competence.

8.3. Speak on behalf of professional health information management organizations, accurately representing the official and authorized positions of the organizations.

IX. *State truthfully and accurately their credentials, professional education, and experiences.*

Health information management professionals **shall:**

9.1. Make clear distinctions between statements made and actions engaged in as a private individual and as a representative of the health information management profession, a professional health information organization, or the health information management professional's employer.

9.2. Claim and ensure that their representations to patients, agencies, and the public of professional qualifications, credentials, education, competence, affiliations, services provided, training, certification, consultation received, supervised experience, and other relevant professional experience are accurate.

9.3. Claim only those relevant professional credentials actually possessed and correct any inaccuracies occurring regarding credentials.

X. *Facilitate interdisciplinary collaboration in situations supporting health information practice.*

Health information management professionals **shall:**

10.1. Participate in and contribute to decisions that affect the well-being of patients by drawing on the perspectives, values, and experiences of those involved in decisions related to patients. Professional and ethical obligations of the interdisciplinary team as a whole and of its individual members should be clearly established.

XI. *Respect the inherent dignity and worth of every person.*

Health information management professionals **shall:**

11.1. Treat each person in a respectful fashion, being mindful of individual differences and cultural and ethnic diversity.

11.2. Promote the value of self-determination for each individual.

Acknowledgement

Adapted with permission from the Code of Ethics of the National Association of Social Workers.

Resources

National Association of Social Workers. "Code of Ethics." 1999. Available at http://www.naswdc.org.

Harman, L.B. (Ed.). Ethical Challenges in the Management of Health Information. Gaithersburg, MD: Aspen, 2001.

AHIMA Code of Ethics, 1957, 1977, 1988, and 1998.

AHIMA Standards of Ethical Coding

AHIMA House of Delegates, September 2008

Introduction

The Standards of Ethical Coding are based on the American Health Information Management Association's (AHIMA's) Code of Ethics. Both sets of principles reflect expectations of professional conduct for coding professionals involved in diagnostic and/or procedural coding or other health record data abstraction.

A Code of Ethics sets forth professional values and ethical principles and offers ethical guidelines to which professionals aspire and by which their actions can be judged. Health information management (HIM) professionals are expected to demonstrate professional values by their actions to patients, employers, members of the healthcare team, the public, and the many stakeholders they serve. A Code of Ethics is important in helping to guide the decision-making process and can be referenced by individuals, agencies, organizations, and bodies (such as licensing and regulatory boards, insurance providers, courts of law, government agencies, and other professional groups).

The AHIMA Code of Ethics (available on the AHIMA web site) is relevant to all AHIMA members and credentialed HIM professionals and students, regardless of their professional functions, the settings in which they work, or the populations they serve. Coding is one of the core HIM functions, and due to the complex regulatory requirements affecting the health information coding process, coding professionals are frequently faced with ethical challenges. The AHIMA Standards of Ethical Coding are intended to assist coding professionals and managers in decision-making processes and actions, outline expectations for making ethical decisions in the workplace, and demonstrate coding professionals' commitment to integrity during the coding process, regardless of the purpose for which the codes are being reported. They are relevant to all coding professionals and those who manage the coding function, regardless of the healthcare setting in which they work or whether they are AHIMA members or nonmembers.

These Standards of Ethical Coding have been revised in order to reflect the current healthcare environment and modern coding practices. The previous revision was published in 1999.

Revised and approved by the AHIMA House of Delegates 09/08.

Standards of Ethical Coding

Coding professionals should:

1. Apply accurate, complete, and consistent coding practices for the production of high-quality healthcare data.

2. Report all healthcare data elements (e.g. diagnosis and procedure codes, present on admission indicator, discharge status) required for external reporting purposes (e.g. reimbursement and other administrative uses, populat ion health, quality and patient safety measurement, and research) completely and accurately, in accordance with regulatory and documentation standards and requirements and applicable official coding conventions, rules, and guidelines.

3. Assign and report only the codes and data that are clearly and consistently supported by health record documentation in accordance with applicable code set and abstraction conventions, rules, and guidelines.

4. Query provider (physician or other qualified healthcare practitioner) for clarification and additional documentation prior to code assignment when there is conflicting, incomplete, or ambiguous information in the health record regarding a significant reportable condition or procedure or other reportable data element dependent on health record documentation (e.g. present on admission indicator).

5. Refuse to change reported codes or the narratives of codes so that meanings are misrepresented.

6. Refuse to participate in or support coding or documentation practices intended to inappropriately increase payment, qualify for insurance policy coverage, or skew data by means that do not comply with federal and state statutes, regulations and official rules and guidelines.

7. Facilitate interdisciplinary collaboration in situations supporting proper coding practices.

8. Advance coding knowledge and practice through continuing education.

9. Refuse to participate in or conceal unethical coding or abstraction practices or procedures.

10. Protect the confidentiality of the health record at all times and refuse to access protected health information not required for coding-related activities (examples of coding-related activities include completion of code assignment, other health record data abstraction, coding audits, and educational purposes).

11. Demonstrate behavior that reflects integrity, shows a commitment to ethical and legal coding practices, and fosters trust in professional activities.

Resources

AHIMA Code of Ethics: Available at http://www.ahima.org/about/ethics.asp

ICD-9-CM Official Guidelines for Coding and Reporting: http://www.cdc.gov/nchs/datawh/ftpserv/ftpicd9/icdguide07.pdf

AHIMA's position statement on Quality Health Data and Information: Available at http://www.ahima.org/dc/positions

AHIMA's position statement on Uniformity and Consistency of Healthcare Data (DRAFT)

AHIMA Practice Brief titled "Managing an Effective Query Process:" Available at http://www.ahima.org/infocenter/briefs.asp

How to Interpret the Standards of Ethical Coding

The following ethical principles are based on the core values of the American Health Information Management Association and the AHIMA Code of Ethics and apply to all coding professionals. Guidelines for each ethical principle include examples of behaviors and situations that can help to clarify the principle. They are not meant as a comprehensive list of all situations that can occur.

1. ***Apply accurate, complete, and consistent coding practices for the production of high-quality healthcare data.***

   Coding professionals and those who manage coded data shall:

   1.1. Support selection of appropriate diagnostic, procedure and other types of health service related codes (e.g. present on admission indicator, discharge status).

   Example: Policies and procedures are developed and used as a framework for the work process, and education and training is provided on their use.

   1.2. Develop and comply with comprehensive internal coding policies and procedures that are consistent with official coding rules and guidelines, reimbursement regulations and policies and prohibit coding practices that misrepresent the patient's medical conditions and treatment provided or are not supported by the health record documentation.

   Example: Code assignment resulting in misrepresentation of facts carries significant consequences.

   1.3. Participate in the development of institutional coding policies and ensure that coding policies complement, and do not conflict with, official coding rules and guidelines.

   1.4. Foster an environment that supports honest and ethical coding practices resulting in accurate and reliable data.

   Coding professionals **shall not:**

   1.5. Participate in improper preparation, alteration, or suppression of coded information.

2. ***Report all healthcare data elements (e.g. diagnosis and procedure codes, present on admission indicator, discharge status) required for external reporting purposes (e.g. reimbursement and other administrative uses, population health, public data reporting, quality and patient safety measurement, research) completely and accurately, in accordance with regulatory and documentation standards and requirements and applicable official coding conventions, rules, and guidelines.***

   Coding professionals **shall:**

   2.1. Adhere to the ICD coding conventions, official coding guidelines approved by the Cooperating Parties, the CPT rules established by the American Medical Association, and any other official coding rules and guidelines established for use with mandated standard code sets. (The Cooperating Parties are the American Health Information Management Association, American Hospital Association, Centers for Medicare & Medicaid Services, and National Center for Health Statistics.)

   Example: Appropriate resource tools that assist coding professionals with proper sequencing and reporting to stay in compliance with existing reporting requirements are available and used.

2.2. Select and sequence diagnosis and procedure codes in accordance with the definitions of required data sets for applicable healthcare settings.

2.3. Comply with AHIMA's standards governing data reporting practices, including health record documentation and clinician query standards.

3. ***Assign and report only the codes that are clearly and consistently supported by health record documentation in accordance with applicable code set conventions, rules, and guidelines.***

Coding professionals **shall:**

3.1. Apply skills, knowledge of currently mandated coding and classification systems, and official resources to select the appropriate diagnostic and procedural codes (including applicable modifiers), and other codes representing healthcare services (including substances, equipment, supplies, or other items used in the provision of healthcare services).

> **Example:** Failure to research or confirm the appropriate code for a clinical condition not indexed in the classification, or reporting a code for the sake of convenience or to affect reporting for a desired effect on the results, is considered unethical.

4. ***Query provider (physician or other qualified healthcare practitioner) for clarification and additional documentation prior to code assignment when there is conflicting, incomplete, or ambiguous information in the health record regarding a significant reportable condition or procedure or other reportable data element dependent on health record documentation (e.g. present on admission indicator).***

Coding professionals **shall:**

4.1. Participate in the development of query policies that support documentation improvement and meet regulatory, legal, and ethical standards for coding and reporting.

4.2. Query the provider for clarification when documentation in the health record that impacts an externally reportable data element is illegible, incomplete, unclear, inconsistent, or imprecise.

4.3. Use queries as a communication tool to improve the accuracy of code assignment and the quality of health record documentation, not to inappropriately increase reimbursement or misrepresent quality of care.

> **Example:** Policies regarding the circumstances when clinicians should be queried are designed to promote complete and accurate coding and complete documentation, regardless of whether reimbursement will be affected.

Coding professionals **shall not:**

4.4. Query the provider when there is no clinical information in the health record prompting the need for a query.

> **Example:** Query the provider regarding the presence of gram-negative pneumonia on every pneumonia case, regardless of whether there are any clinical indications of gram-negative pneumonia documented in the record.

5. *Refuse to change reported codes or the narratives of codes so that meanings are mis-represented.*

   Coding professionals **shall not:**

   5.1. Change the description for a diagnosis or procedure code or other reported data element so that it does not accurately reflect the official definition of that code.

   Example: The description of a code is altered in the encoding software, resulting in incorrect reporting of this code.

6. *Refuse to participate in or support coding or documentation practices intended to inappropriately increase payment, qualify for insurance policy coverage, or skew data by means that do not comply with federal and state statutes, regulations and official rules and guidelines.*

   Coding professionals **shall:**

   6.1. Select and sequence the codes such that the organization receives the optimal payment to which the facility is legally entitled, remembering that it is unethical and illegal to increase payment by means that contradict regulatory guidelines.

   Coding professionals **shall not:**

   6.2. Misrepresent the patient's clinical picture through intentional incorrect coding or omission of diagnosis or procedure codes, or the addition of diagnosis or procedure codes unsupported by health record documentation, to inappropriately increase reimbursement, justify medical necessity, improve publicly reported data, or qualify for insurance policy coverage benefits.

   Example: A patient has a health plan that excludes reimbursement for reproductive management or contraception; so rather than report the correct code for admission for tubal ligation, it is reported as a medically necessary condition with performance of a salpingectomy. The narrative descriptions of both the diagnosis and procedures reflect an admission for tubal ligation and the procedure (tubal ligation) is displayed on the record.

   A code is changed at the patient's request so that the service will be covered by the patient's insurance.

   Coding professionals **shall not:**

   6.3. Inappropriately exclude diagnosis or procedure codes in order to misrepresent the quality of care provided.

   Example: Following a surgical procedure, a patient acquired an infection due to a break in sterile procedure; the appropriate code for the surgical complication is omitted from the claims submission to avoid any adverse outcome to the institution.

   Quality outcomes are reported inaccurately in order to improve a healthcare organization's quality profile or pay-for-performance results.

7. *Facilitate interdisciplinary collaboration in situations supporting proper coding practices.*

   Coding professionals **shall:**

   7.1. Assist and educate physicians and other clinicians by advocating proper documentation practices, further specificity, and re-sequence or include diagnoses or procedures when needed to more accurately reflect the acuity, severity, and the occurrence of events.

Example: Failure to advocate for ethical practices that seek to represent the truth in events as expressed by the associated code sets when needed is considered an intentional disregard of these standards.

8. *Advance coding knowledge and practice through continuing education.*

Coding professionals **shall:**

8.1. Maintain and continually enhance coding competency (e.g., through participation in educational programs, reading official coding publications such as the Coding Clinic for ICD-9-CM, and maintaining professional certifications) in order to stay abreast of changes in codes, coding guidelines, and regulatory and other requirements.

9. *Refuse to participate in or conceal unethical coding practices or procedures.*

Coding professionals **shall:**

9.1. Act in a professional and ethical manner at all times.

9.2. Take adequate measures to discourage, prevent, expose, and correct the unethical conduct of colleagues.

9.3. Be knowledgeable about established policies and procedures for handling concerns about colleagues' unethical behavior. These include policies and procedures created by AHIMA, licensing and regulatory bodies, employers, supervisors, agencies, and other professional organizations.

9.4. Seek resolution if there is a belief that a colleague has acted unethically or if there is a belief of incompetence or impairment by discussing their concerns with the colleague when feasible and when such discussion is likely to be productive. Take action through appropriate formal channels, such as contacting an accreditation or regulatory body and/or the AHIMA Professional Ethics Committee.

9.5. Consult with a colleague when feasible and assist the colleague in taking remedial action when there is direct knowledge of a health information management colleague's incompetence or impairment.

Coding professionals **shall not:**

9.6. Participate in, condone, or be associated with dishonesty, fraud and abuse, or deception. A non-exhaustive list of examples includes:

- Allowing inappropriate patterns of retrospective documentation to avoid suspension or increase reimbursement

- Assigning codes without supporting provider (physician or other qualified healthcare practitioner) documentation

- Coding when documentation does not justify the diagnoses and/or procedures that have been billed

- Coding an inappropriate level of service

- Miscoding to avoid conflict with others

- Adding, deleting, and altering health record documentation

- Copying and pasting another clinician's documentation without identification of the original author and date
- Knowingly reporting incorrect present on admission indicator
- Knowingly reporting incorrect patient discharge status code
- Engaging in negligent coding practices

10. *Protect the confidentiality of the health record at all times and refuse to access protected health information not required for coding-related activities (examples of coding-related activities include completion of code assignment, other health record data abstraction, coding audits, and educational purposes).*

Coding professionals **shall:**

10.1. Protect all confidential information obtained in the course of professional service, including personal, health, financial, genetic, and outcome information.

10.2. Access only that information necessary to perform their duties.

11. *Demonstrate behavior that reflects integrity, shows a commitment to ethical and legal coding practices, and fosters trust in professional activities.*

Coding professionals **shall:**

11.1. Act in an honest manner and bring honor to self, peers, and the profession.

11.2. Truthfully and accurately represent their credentials, professional education, and experience.

11.3. Demonstrate ethical principles and professional values in their actions to patients, employers, other members of the healthcare team, consumers, and other stakeholders served by the healthcare data they collect and report.

Appendix B

AHIMA Practice Brief: Managing an Effective Query Process

In today's changing healthcare environment, health information management (HIM) professionals face increased demands to produce accurate coded data. Therefore, establishing and managing an effective query process is an integral component of ensuring data integrity. A query is defined as a question posed to a provider to obtain additional, clarifying documentation to improve the specificity and completeness of the data used to assign diagnosis and procedure codes in the patient's health record. Documentation can be greatly improved by a properly functioning query process.

This practice brief offers HIM professionals important components to consider in the management of an effective query process. It is intended to offer guiding principles to implement the query process while in no way prescribing what must be done.

Background

The "ICD-9-CM Official Guidelines for Coding and Reporting" are the official rules for coding and reporting ICD-9-CM. They are approved by the four organizations that make up the ICD-9-CM Cooperating Parties: the American Hospital Association, the American Health Information Management Association, the Centers for Medicare and Medicaid Services, and the National Center for Health Statistics. The guidelines may be used as a companion document to the official current version of the ICD-9-CM coding conventions and instructions.

The guidelines state:

A joint effort between the healthcare provider and the coding professional is essential to achieve complete and accurate documentation, code assignment, and reporting of diagnoses and procedures. These guidelines have been developed to assist both the healthcare provider and the coding professional in identifying those diagnoses and procedures that are to be reported. The importance of consistent, complete documentation in the medical record cannot be overemphasized. Without such documentation, accurate coding cannot be achieved. The entire record should be reviewed to determine the specific reason for the encounter and the conditions treated.[1]

Note: This practice brief updates the 2001 practice brief "Developing a Physician Query Process," with a continued focus on compliance.

A provider is defined as any physician or other qualified healthcare practitioner who is legally accountable for establishing the patient's diagnosis. The guidelines apply to all healthcare providers, organizations, facilities, and entities (referred to throughout this document collectively as "healthcare entities"), regardless of size and function. They are clear in their directive regarding the relationship between documentation and the accurate, consistent coding and reporting of healthcare services.

Individuals who perform the query function should be familiar with AHIMA's Standards of Ethical Coding, which direct coders to "assign and report only the codes and data that are clearly and consistently supported by health record documentation in accordance with applicable code set and abstraction conventions, rules, and guidelines."[2] The standards further state:

> Query provider (physician or other qualified healthcare practitioner) for clarification and additional documentation prior to code assignment when there is conflicting, incomplete, or ambiguous information in the health record regarding a significant reportable condition or procedure or other reportable data element dependent on health record documentation (for example, present on admission indicator).

Organizations should establish a process for "ensuring that the physician documents in the health record any clarification or additional information resulting from communication with coding staff," according to Sue Bowman, AHIMA's director of coding policy and compliance, in the book *Health Information Management Compliance: A Model Program for Healthcare Organizations*. "Communication tools between coding personnel and physicians, such as coding summary sheets, attestation forms, or coding clarification forms (e.g., physician query forms), should never be used as a substitute for appropriate physician documentation in the health record."[3]

The electronic health record creates new challenges for compliance in clinical documentation. The issues to address include the use of electronic templates, generating and responding to electronic queries, and input from the appropriate staff regarding the electronic record documentation process.

The Expectations for Documentation

The primary purpose of health record documentation is continuity of patient care, serving as a means of communication among all healthcare providers. Documentation is also used to evaluate the adequacy and appropriateness of quality care, provide clinical data for research and education, and support reimbursement, medical necessity, quality of care measures, and public reporting for services rendered by a healthcare entity.[4]

Documentation and Coding

As a result of the disparity in documentation practices by providers, querying has become a common communication and educational method to advocate proper documentation practices. Queries may be made in situations such as the following:

- Clinical indicators of a diagnosis but no documentation of the condition

- Clinical evidence for a higher degree of specificity or severity

- A cause-and-effect relationship between two conditions or organisms

- An underlying cause when admitted with symptoms

- Only the treatment is documented (without a diagnosis documented)

- Present on admission (POA) indicator status

Lack of accurate and complete documentation can result in the use of nonspecific and general codes, which can impact data integrity and reimbursement and present potential compliance risks.

Expectation of the Provider

According to the Centers for Medicare and Medicaid Services and the Joint Commission, providers are expected to provide legible, complete, clear, consistent, precise, and reliable documentation of the patient's health history, present illness, and course of treatment. This includes observations, evidence of medical decision-making in determining a diagnosis, and treatment plan, as well as the outcomes of all tests, procedures, and treatments. This documentation should be as complete and specific as possible, including information such as the level of severity, specificity of anatomical sites involved, and etiologies of symptoms.

Providers are expected to follow medical staff bylaws and assist in developing documentation and query policies and procedures. The query policy may include a statement regarding timely response and consequences for noncompliance or lack of response to queries.

Expectation of Individuals Performing the Query Function

Individuals performing the query function should follow their healthcare entity's internal policies related to documentation, querying, coding, and compliance, keeping in mind that data accuracy and integrity are fundamental HIM values. Only diagnosis codes that are clearly and consistently supported by provider documentation should be assigned and reported. A query should be initiated when there is conflicting, incomplete, or ambiguous documentation in the health record or additional information is needed for correct assignment of the POA indicator.

Expectation of the Healthcare Entity

The query process improves the quality of documentation and coding for complete clinical data capture. Queries may be initiated for all payer types regardless of the impact on reimbursement or quality reporting. The healthcare entity's documentation or compliance policies can address situations such as unnecessary queries, leading queries, repetitive overuse of queries without measureable improvement in documentation, and methods for provider education.

A provider's response to a query can be documented in the progress note, discharge summary, or on the query form as a part of the formal health record. Addendums to the discharge summary or the progress note should include appropriate date and authentication.

Permanence and retention of the completed query form should be addressed in the healthcare entity's policy, taking into account applicable state and quality improvement organization guidelines. The policy should specify whether the completed query will be a permanent part of the patient's health record. If it will not be considered a permanent part of the patient's health record (e.g., it might be considered a separate business record for the purpose of auditing, monitoring, and compliance), it is not subject to health record retention guidelines.

It is recommended that healthcare entities employ, educate, and train qualified individuals to perform the query process who have strong competencies in the following areas:

- Knowledge of healthcare regulations, including reimbursement and documentation requirements

- Clinical knowledge with training in pathophysiology

- Ability to read and analyze all information in a patient's health record

- Established channels of communication with providers and other clinicians

- Demonstrated skills in clinical terminology, coding, and classification systems

- Ability to apply coding conventions, official guidelines, and *Coding Clinic* advice to health record documentation

The Query Process

Who to Query

A healthcare entity's query policy should address the question of who to query. The query is directed to the provider who originated the progress note or other report in question. This could include the attending physician, consulting physician, or the surgeon. In most cases, a query for abnormal test results would be directed to the attending physician.

Documentation from providers involved in the care and treatment of the patient is appropriate for code assignment; however, a query may be necessary if the documentation conflicts with that of another provider. If such a conflict exists, the attending physician is queried for clarification, as that provider is ultimately responsible for the final diagnosis.

When to Query

Providers should be queried whenever there is conflicting, ambiguous, or incomplete information in the health record regarding any *significant* reportable condition or procedure.

Queries are not necessary for every discrepancy or unaddressed issue in physician documentation. Healthcare entities should develop policies and procedures that clarify which clinical conditions and documentation situations warrant a request for physician clarification. Insignificant or irrelevant findings may not warrant a query regarding the assignment of an additional diagnosis code, for example. Entities must balance the value of collecting marginal data against the administrative burden of obtaining the additional documentation.

Healthcare entities could consider a policy in which queries may be appropriate when documentation in the patient's record fails to meet one of the following five criteria:

- **Legibility.** This might include an illegible handwritten entry in the provider's progress notes, and the reader cannot determine the provider's assessment on the date of discharge.

- **Completeness.** This might include a report indicating abnormal test results without notation of the clinical significance of these results (e.g., an x-ray shows a compression fracture of lumbar vertebrae in a patient with osteoporosis and no evidence of injury).

- **Clarity.** This might include patient diagnosis noted without statement of a cause or suspected cause (e.g., the patient is admitted with abdominal pain, fever, and chest pain and no underlying cause or suspected cause is documented).

- **Consistency.** This might include a disagreement between two or more treating providers with respect to a diagnosis (e.g., the patient presents with shortness of breath. The pulmonologist documents pneumonia as the cause, and the attending documents congestive heart failure as the cause).

- **Precision.** This might include an instance where clinical reports and clinical condition suggest a more specific diagnosis than is documented (e.g., congestive heart failure is documented when an echocardiogram and the patient's documented clinical condition on admission suggest acute or chronic diastolic congestive heart failure).

Healthcare entities may design their query programs to be concurrent, retrospective, post-bill, or a combination of any of these. Concurrent queries are initiated while the patient is still present. Retrospective queries are initiated after discharge and before the bill is submitted; post-bill queries are initiated after the bill has been submitted.

Concurrent queries are initiated "real time," during the course of the patient encounter or hospitalization, at the time the documentation is naturally done. They thus encourage more timely, accurate, and reliable responses. Retrospective queries are effective in cases where additional information is available in the health record, in short stays where concurrent review was not completed, or whenever a concurrent query process is not feasible.

Post-bill queries are initiated after the claim is submitted or remittance advice is paid. Post-bill queries generally occur as a result of an audit or other internal monitor. Healthcare entities can develop a policy regarding whether they will generate post-bill queries and the timeframe following claims generation that queries may be initiated. They may consider the following three concepts in the development of a post-bill (including query) policy:

- Applying normal course of business guidelines[5]

- Using payer-specific rules on rebilling timeframes

- Determining reliability of query response over time

When Not to Query

Codes assigned to clinical data should be clearly and consistently supported by provider documentation. Providers often make clinical diagnoses that may not appear to be consistent with test results. For example, the provider may make a clinical determination that the patient has pneumonia when the results of the chest x-ray may be negative. Queries should not be used to question a provider's clinical judgment, but rather to clarify documentation when it fails to meet any of the five criteria listed above—legibility, completeness, clarity, consistency, or precision.

A query may not be appropriate simply because the clinical information or clinical picture does not appear to support the documentation of a condition or procedure (e.g., documentation of acute respiratory failure in a patient whose laboratory findings do not appear to support this diagnosis). In situations where the provider's documented diagnosis does not appear to be supported by clinical findings, a healthcare entity's policies can provide guidance on a process for addressing the issue without querying the attending physician.

The Query Format

It is recommended that the healthcare entity's policy address the query format. A query generally includes the following information:

- Patient name

- Admission date and/or date of service

- Health record number

- Account number

- Date query initiated

- Name and contact information of the individual initiating the query

- Statement of the issue in the form of a question along with clinical indicators specified from the chart (e.g., history and physical states urosepsis, lab reports WBC of 14,400. Emergency department report fever of 102)

It is not advisable to record queries on handwritten sticky notes, scratch paper, or other notes that can be removed and discarded. The preferred formats for capturing the query include facility-approved query form, facsimile transmission, electronic communication on secure e-mail, or secure IT messaging system.

Verbal queries have become more common as a component of the concurrent query process. The desired result of a verbal query is documentation by the provider that supports the coding of a condition, diagnosis, or procedure. Therefore entities should develop specific policies to clearly address this practice and avoid potential compliance risks.

It is recommended that queries be written with precise language, identifying clinical indications from the health record and asking the provider to make a clinical interpretation of these facts based on his or her professional judgment of the case. Queries that appear to lead the provider to document a particular response could result in allegations of inappropriate upcoding. The query format should not sound presumptive, directing, prodding, probing, or as though the provider is being led to make an assumption.

Examples of leading queries include:

Dr. Smith	Based on your documentation, this patient has anemia and was transfused 2 units of blood. Also, there was a 10 point drop in hematocrit following surgery. Please document "Acute Blood Loss Anemia," as this patient clearly meets the clinical criteria for this diagnosis.
Dr. Jones	This patient has COPD and is on oxygen every night at home and has been on continuous oxygen since admission. Please document "Chronic Respiratory Failure."

In these examples the provider is not given any documentation option other than the specific diagnosis requested. The statements are directive in nature, indicating what the provider should document, rather than querying the provider for his or her professional determination of the clinical facts. In the first example, the statement "the patient has anemia" may be presumptive, and the statement "please document 'acute blood loss anemia'" is directive and clearly leading the provider. In the second example, the provider is inappropriately asked to document chronic respiratory failure.

Examples of the above queries correctly written could include the following:

Dr. Smith   In your progress note on 6/20, you documented anemia and ordered transfusion of 2 units of blood. Also, according to the lab work done on xx/xx, the patient had a 10 point drop in hematocrit following surgery. Based on these indications, please document, in the discharge summary, the type of anemia you were treating.

Dr. Jones   This patient has COPD and is on oxygen every night at home and has been on continuous oxygen since admission. Based on these indications, please indicate if you were treating one of the following diagnoses:

- Chronic Respiratory Failure
- Acute Respiratory Failure
- Acute on Chronic Respiratory Failure
- Hypoxia
- Unable to determine
- Other:_____

The introduction of new information not previously documented in the medical record is inappropriate in a provider query. For example:

Dr. Harvey   According to the patient's emergency room record from last week, the patient was placed on antibiotics for cellulitis of her leg. If the patient is still taking antibiotics, please document the cellulitis.

In this case, if this diagnosis was not documented in the current admission and is not affecting the patient's care, it does not meet the definition of a secondary diagnosis. [6] Querying for this new information, which does not meet coding and reporting requirements, is inappropriate.

In general, query forms should not be designed to ask questions about a diagnosis or procedure that can be responded to in a yes/no fashion. The exception is present on admission (POA) queries when the diagnosis has already been documented.

It is recommended that healthcare entities should address the issue of yes/no queries in their policies. When setting this policy, the entity should consider the compliance risk. In general, it is a much safer practice to ask the provider to document the diagnosis he or she is agreeing to. Concerns about yes/no queries are less of an issue if the entity requires the provider to document the diagnosis in the health record rather than relying on the query form for the final documentation.

Multiple choice formats that employ checkboxes may be used as long as all clinically reasonable choices are listed, regardless of the impact on reimbursement or quality reporting. The choices should also include an "other" option, with a line that allows the provider to add free text. Providers should also be given the choice of "unable to determine." This format is designed to make multiple choice questions as open ended as possible.

A single query form can be used to address multiple questions. If it is, a distinct question should be asked for each issue (e.g., if three questions exist based on clinical indications in the health record, there should be three distinct questions clearly identified on the query form).

For example, insulin-dependent diabetes with high blood sugars on admission is documented in a patient with renal failure. The three questions identified on the query might be related to type of diabetes (type I or II, or secondary); relationship of diabetes to renal failure; and whether the diabetes is controlled or uncontrolled.

Finally, the query should never indicate that a particular response would favorably or unfavorably affect reimbursement or quality reporting.

Methods of Auditing and Monitoring

Healthcare entities should consider establishing an auditing and monitoring program as a means to improve their query processes. They can consider several methods for this ongoing process.

Queries can be reviewed retrospectively to ensure that they are completed according to documented policies. This might include reviewing:

- That the query was necessary

- That the language used in the query was not leading or otherwise inappropriate

- That the query did not introduce new information from the health record

Based on the results of this review, the healthcare entity may need to identify follow-up actions. For example, cases identified as inappropriate queries resulting in inaccurate code assignment will require that codes be corrected at the level supported by the documentation without the leading query. Inappropriate queries should be tracked and trended, followed by appropriate education and training.

In order for the query process to be effective, auditing and monitoring should be conducted on a regular basis. This process can include a representative sample of total queries as well as a sampling by individuals initiating the query. Effective elements of an auditing and monitoring program include:

- Auditing for percentage of negative and positive provider responses. A high negative response rate may indicate overuse of the query by the coding staff; a high positive response rate may indicate a pattern of incomplete documentation that needs further investigation.

- Auditing the format of query forms. Discovery of inappropriate query formats can be used as an educational tool for coding staff.

- Auditing of individual providers to indicate improvement in health record documentation. Improvement in documentation should result in a decreased number of queries for an individual provider.

- Auditing of high-risk or problem diagnoses. The results may determine whether additional education resulted in a decreased number of queries for a particular diagnosis.

Auditing and monitoring programs should establish the data fields to be collected and reported. When reviewing both performance measures and compliance monitors, the errors related to documentation will become apparent.

Healthcare entities should have a process in place to support and educate the staff involved in conducting provider queries. Ongoing education and training is a key component of the auditing and monitoring process.

Conclusion

HIM professionals are constantly challenged to improve the accuracy of coded data to meet regulatory, state, and federal requirements. In addition, electronic records pose new challenges in the collection and maintenance of quality data.

The quality of coding is driven directly by the documentation contained in the patient's health record. Establishing and managing a query process can be an effective tool to improve clinical documentation and thereby increase the accuracy of coded data. Typically, both concurrent and retrospective query processes are needed. An effective query process, using an appropriate format, will enable the facility to obtain needed documentation without compromising coding compliance standards.

Since the query process has become a tool to improve provider documentation, it is critical that the design of these processes be maintained with legal, regulatory, and ethical issues in mind. Healthcare entities can create and maintain a compliant query process by:

- Creating comprehensive policies and procedures for query processes

- Generating queries only when documentation is conflicting, incomplete, or ambiguous

- Conducting auditing and monitoring activities to determine the effectiveness of the query process

- Providing education and training for the staff involved in conducting provider queries

Notes

1. Centers for Medicare and Medicaid Services and the National Center for Health Statistics. "ICD-9-CM Official Guidelines for Coding and Reporting." Available online at www.cdc.gov/nchs/datawh/ftpserv/ftpicd9/ftpicd9.htm#guidelines.

2. American Health Information Management Association. "Standards of Ethical Coding." 2008. Available online at www.ahima.org/infocenter/guidelines.

3. Prophet, Sue. *Health Information Management Compliance: A Model Program for Healthcare Organizations.* 2d edition. Chicago, IL: AHIMA, 2002.

4. For the purposes of this practice brief, *healthcare entity* encompasses all providers: short-term acute care hospitals; long-term acute care hospitals; skilled nursing facility and hospice; inpatient and outpatient psychiatric and rehabilitation; home-health; hospital-based outpatient and clinic; and all professional providers such as physician practice as well as any other healthcare entity or professional provider that serves patient care solo or part of a corporation. The healthcare entity uses the same policies and procedures throughout the components of the organization.

5. Normal course of business guidelines include ensuring that the post-bill query process is conducted in the healthcare entity's normal timeframe for completing health records in accordance with medical staff bylaws and rules and regulations for health record completion.

6. For reporting purposes, the term *other diagnoses* is interpreted as additional conditions that affect patient care in terms of requiring clinical evaluation, therapeutic treatment, diagnostic procedures, extended length of hospital stay, or increased nursing care and/or monitoring. UHDDS item 11-b defines other diagnoses as "all conditions that coexist at the time of admission, that develop subsequently, or that affect the treatment received and/or the length of stay. Diagnoses that related to an earlier episode which have no bearing on the current hospital stay are to be excluded."

Reference

Prophet, Sue. "Developing a Physician Query Process." *Journal of AHIMA* 72, no. 9 (Oct. 2001): 88I–M.

Prepared by

Sue Bowman, RHIA, CCS

Patricia Collins Smith, RHIA

Kathy DeVault, RHIA, CCS

Linda Hyde, MA, RHIA

Teri Jorwic, MPH, RHIA, CCS

Christine Lewis, MHA, RHIA, CCS, CCS-P

Krystal Lloyd, RHIA, CCS

Anita Majerowicz, MS, RHIA

Janie Miller, RHIT, CCS

Ruthann Russo, PhD, JD, MPH, RHIT

Shelley Safian, CCS-P, NCICS, CHA

Carol Spencer, RHIA

Acknowledgment

Lisa M. Horning, Esq.

The information contained in this practice brief reflects the consensus opinion of the the professionals who developed it. It has not been validated through scientific research.

AHIMA. 2008. Managing an Effective Query Process. *Journal of AHIMA* 79(10):83–88.

Clinical Documentation Query for Physician Progress Note

Patient Name: _____ Physician Queried: _____

MR# _____ Query Date: _____

The Clinical Documentation Coordinator has reviewed the medical record in order to ensure that the principal diagnosis and all secondary diagnoses are accurately documented in the medical record. The record needs to reflect the severity of illness and expected risk of mortality for the patient.

It appears that additional clinical documentation may be necessary. Please review the query/queries below. **If you agree with the documentation query, please document the diagnosis/diagnoses in the Physician Progress Notes.**

_____
_____
_____
_____
_____
_____
_____
_____
_____
_____
_____
_____
_____
_____
_____
_____
_____

Thank you in advance for reviewing this record and documenting additional definitive diagnosis/diagnoses.

For questions, please contact: _____ *phone* _____

If you agree with the documentation query please initial here and check the appropriate physician box. _____ • **Attending Physician** • **Resident**	**If you disagree with the query please specify on this sheet why the query was not appropriate and initial here.** _____

• **ALL RESPONSES AND NO RESPONSES WILL BE REVIEWED BY THE DIVISION CHIEFS**

DO NOT DISCARD—SEND WITH THE MEDICAL RECORD AT DISCHARGE

Source: Vanderbilt University Medical Center.

Appendix C

Managing Coding Compliance
Leadership, Collaboration Keep Processes from Derailing

by Cathy Bodnar, MS, RN, CHC, and Dianne Willard, MBA, RHIA, CCS-P, CHC

The key to ensuring coding compliance in the ever-changing world of healthcare is to have a solid foundation. This includes ensuring effective processes throughout all departments in the organization.

Coding managers can visualize each process that contributes to correct coding as a track—a data input track, a documentation track, a query track, a coding track, a billing track. Each track enables records to be properly coded and moved from one department to the next. A network of well-run, efficient tracks can ensure that records are properly coded and processed.

For example, coding managers should look for all registration information, admitting source, diagnoses, and physician orders on the data input track. On the documentation track, they should look for information that clearly supports the diagnoses, procedures, and services performed. On the query track, managers should look for clear and concise questions and keep a record to identify patterns and trends. Trending can reveal opportunities for additional education.

Ensuring a Smooth Ride

Once the tracks are in place, coding managers must maintain each process to keep records moving between departments, making sure everyone does his or her job properly. There will be times when there are problems on the track, but when problems arise, managers with leadership skills and good processes in place can identify and work with necessary stakeholders throughout the organization to get records moving properly again.

Coding managers can keep the record moving by homing in on problems and working with departments to resolve them. For example, if registration is not providing accurate admission source codes, staff may not be referring to policy or guidelines. Coding managers can pinpoint the concerns and work with the admitting manager to correct any issues.

CPT infusion coding, which has been a challenge for coding departments over the last two years, is another example. Correctly coding CPT infusions requires significant change in documentation, thorough understanding of the coding guidelines, and clear communication of the changes.

Annual coding changes and the move from paper to electronic records may affect the codes organizations can report due to a change in documentation. When moving to an EHR, the data fields or data format can change significantly. It is crucial to make certain all data needed for coding is included in any process changes. For example, in time documentation, clinicians may document a.m. or p.m., yet the electronic system may use military time. This can affect the electronic time calculations.

Missed start or stop times, unclear route of administration, or unclear understanding of coding guidelines can make coding these services difficult, if not impossible. Coding departments may have encountered major concerns if infusion codes are hard-coded in the charge master.

Resolving these issues may require significant changes to the tracks. Coding managers may need to help implement documentation improvement changes in clinical areas to achieve the correct coding. They may need to share guidance from official sources. They should network with colleagues on best practices for implementing the coding changes in busy clinical areas.

For specific questions that are not clearly addressed in the official coding sources, coding managers can seek input from other coding professionals in forums such as AHIMA's Coding Community of Practice. They can seek further understanding of the documentation process from managers of the areas involved in the services. Coding managers should also provide input on the forms or other tools used by the clinical areas and become involved in educating clinical areas on coding guidelines.

Once these changes are implemented, coding managers should help assess and manage the changes, continuing to work with stakeholders to ensure everyone stays on track. Ongoing feedback and follow-up are key to ensuring that an issue has been resolved.

Proactive coding compliance helps organizations stay on track. Coding managers should identify new codes or coding changes and speak with operational areas that may use the codes, educating those areas on the key documentation needed to support the codes. They should also recommend that departments take into consideration all work steps and systems involved in the coding process. This may include modifying the charge master, notifying billing of coding changes, and ensuring that new coding and billing edits are updated. Coding managers should present the information broadly and remind the operational areas that correct coding affects quality reporting and reimbursement.

It takes more than the coding manager to keep records moving. Coding managers should partner with operational areas on practices that affect coding. They can help identify an area of focus for department review—for instance, a key documentation challenge—and then circle back to discuss the results.

Coding managers should also conduct proactive coding compliance reviews, starting with a probe sample and looking for trends and patterns. Another method is to perform a focused review, considering the codes that are more difficult to support in documentation or recall during the initial rollout of the codes.

The results of the review may identify potential coding issues that need further investigation and education. By staying vigilant through operational or coding reviews coding managers will identify loose wheels before they result in major derailments.

It is important that coding managers communicate the review process to all stakeholders within the organization. It is easy for managers to focus on the staff directly involved in the coding process, but many other healthcare professionals may have an important stake in coding issues.

Consider physician documentation and its impact on professional coding versus facility coding. A coding review may ask these questions: Does the facility-coded data correlate to the professional coded data? Does other clinical documentation impact coding decisions? Are there coding guidelines that affect coding decisions? Do Medicare or other third-party payers have reimbursement guidelines that may determine what services can be coded together or where services can be performed?

When meeting with stakeholders, coding managers should be prepared to define the coding compliance process and all aspects of the coding review. Identifying the specific focus of the review is key to investigating and following up on the issue.

Repairing Broken Rails

Once a potential coding compliance problem has been identified, coding managers will need to determine the 5 Ws:

- Who is involved in the issue?

- What occurred and how does it affect coding or billing?

- Where did the issue originate?

- When did the issue occur?

- Why did it occur?

Answers to these questions may involve several rapid-fire meetings to determine if your compliance or legal department should be involved. Coding managers should focus on resolutions. Meetings should stress the coding-documentation issue and include education on specific coding guidelines, if needed.

If systems or other processes are affected by the coding documentation change, coding managers should ensure that appropriate stakeholders are involved. Once a resolution is agreed upon, a management action plan should resolve the coding documentation issue. The action plan should include specific work steps with goals, dates, and responsible parties.

As corrective actions are jointly agreed upon and put into place, financial consideration should be explored. Were accounts incorrectly billed? Did the organization receive incorrect reimbursement? Account correction to reflect compliant coding is critical.

Cathy Bodnar (cbodnar@nmh.org) is director of the office of corprorate integrity and **Dianne Willard** (dwillard@nmh.org) is coding integrity program administrator at Northwestern Memorial Hospital in Chicago, IL.

Bodnar, C. and D. Willard. 2009. Managing Coding Compliance: Leadership, Collaboration Keep Processes from Derailing. *Journal of AHIMA* 80(4):74–75.

Appendix D

AHIMA Practice Brief: Collecting Root Cause to Improve Coding Quality Measurement

Each healthcare organization has its own coding quality review and reporting program. Most programs aim to improve the quality of coded data by improving the accuracy of codes assigned by the coding staff. However, without a reference standard for accuracy or standardized coding performance measurement, it is impossible for organizations to compare their coding measurements against industry benchmarks and determine if the quality of administrative coded data is indeed improving.

Organizations must begin measuring and collecting coding quality review data consistently throughout the profession. Measuring coding quality performance by tracking, trending, and reporting by the root cause of coding errors is an important first step in standardizing coding quality measurement.

This practice brief explores methods for reporting coding quality and shares highlights from a survey on coding quality measurement. It provides a model for reporting coding errors by root cause.

Methods for Reporting Coding Accuracy

It is important for organizations to report individual coder accuracy uniformly. However, it is also important that organizations understand and correct the root causes for coding errors, more appropriately characterized as coding variances.[1]

An important component of coding quality reviews is evaluating the quality of coding at the code level, reviewing for consistency among a team of coders. Coder variation, also known as inter-rater reliability, is the extent to which the same sets of codes are applied to the same source documentation by independent coders (i.e., "raters").

For example, if four coders assign codes to the same documentation, ideally all four coders would produce the same set of codes. This would reflect 100-percent inter-rater agreement; anything less than 100 percent reflects coder variation.[2] One obvious root cause for coder variation is the quality of documentation, including the degree of specificity, consistency, completeness, and timeliness of documentation.

Facility-specific policies and procedures such as medical record completion and query policies, though often necessary for consistency within the facility, ultimately contribute to coding variance nationally, as do payer-specific coding policies.

A common method for reporting coding accuracy is to report it as a percent accuracy; for example, MS-DRG accuracy, principal diagnosis accuracy, or overall coding accuracy. Many facilities set performance goals and report coding quality performance results based on accuracy targets (e.g., 95 percent or greater, 90–94 percent, 85–89 percent, etc.). If the results of the review miss the target, then action steps are developed, follow-up reviews are performed, and incremental improvements in percent accuracy are monitored.

Kim Streit, vice president of healthcare research and information for the Florida Hospital Association, states:

> Everyone needs to understand what is being reported, how the data are being used, and how to make sure the information is captured clearly in the medical record. It's not only the responsibility of the coders, it's the HIM professionals, and even the physician community.[3]

It is time to eliminate the vagueness about what is counted as coding accuracy. Reporting an accuracy rate of 97 percent is not meaningful if there is no clear understanding of what was wrong with the 3 percent of cases that failed to achieve the "accuracy" stamp of approval. The root causes contributing to coding variance must be collected in order to improve the quality of coded data. Without that information, there is no clear understanding of what comprises the error rate.

At face value, it may appear that a variance is due to mistakes made in applying coding convention and guidelines; however, the variance may instead be due to the fact that the coder did not have the discharge summary at the time of coding. This would not be a "coder error" but an unintended consequence of a process that some hospitals have instituted in an effort to meet unbilled targets.

Some organizations adjust the coder accuracy rate, removing these cases from the final accuracy rate reported, while others do not. This illustrates why accuracy rates cannot be compared across organizations. The coding accuracy rate, commonly reported today, is incomplete at best and often misleading.

Root Cause: A More Reliable Measure

Coder accuracy, although important for internal coder performance tracking, is not the ideal measure for reporting the overall quality of coded data. Tracking and trending the underlying root causes for code variation is a more reliable method for measuring the consistency of coded data that results from an entire healthcare system. Once the underlying causes for code variations are understood, then system-wide improvements can be made to the process, technology, education, or training.

This type of method for measuring is more consistent with the Hospital Payment Monitoring Program (HPMP), which was created by the Department of Health and Human Services and Office of Inspector General (OIG) to monitor the accuracy of payments made in the Medicare Fee for Service Program.

In a recent report that reflects Medicare discharges in the 12-month period ending December 31, 2006, the national error rate, reported as 3.9 percent, is broken down into five root causes for errors: no documentation, insufficient documentation, medically unnecessary, incorrect coding, and other.[4] The data for paid claims error rate are further refined and reported by incorrect coding; for example, 5 percent error rate due to DRG 551, Permanent cardiac pacemaker implant with major cardiovascular diagnosis or AICD lead or generator; 2.6 percent due to DRG 416, Septicemia (FY 2006). The data for paid claims error rate for no documentation are 9.9 percent on DRG 217, Wound debridement and skin graft except hand for musculoskeletal and connective tissue disease (FY2006). This is an effective reporting method for HPMP's focus on reducing paid claims errors.

The performance target, national improper payment error rate, is adjusted from year to year. In 2007, it was 4.3 percent, and next year's performance target is 3.8 percent. The national paid claims error rate has significantly dropped from 14.2 percent reported in 1996 to 3.9 percent in 2007.[5]

OIG has been tracking and trending underlying root causes for error rates for many years. A 1988 report breaks down the 20.8 percent DRG total error rate by root cause.[6] It found that 39 percent of the total error rate was related to principal diagnosis assignment not supported by the physician documentation in the medical record; 27 percent was related to incorrect sequencing of principal diagnosis; 12 percent was related to incorrect code selection based on coding convention and rules; and 13 percent was based on physician documentation of vague or nonspecific diagnostic language, patient status, data entry errors, and coding from an incomplete record.

As these examples illustrate, understanding the cause for coding errors provides insight that can lead to improvements in the processes that support code assignment. Research conducted by Pavani Rangachari on coding accuracy supports this as well:

> Studies investigating factors contributing to coding accuracy have found that a majority of the coding errors occur due to inadequate physician documentation . . . [F]ederal and state investigations into issues of physician documentation have suggested that there is an overall lack of knowledge exchange and communication between hospital administrators, physicians, and coders, which may be playing an important role in adversely impacting documentation, and correspondingly, coding accuracy . . . This suggests that neither professional subgroup, physicians or coders, may have a proper understanding of the role of documentation and coding with respect to organizational outcomes such as hospital reimbursement and comparative quality results.[7]

The report shows that more detailed analysis of this gap between coding and documentation is required at the individual hospital level to reduce the inconsistency and variation in coding and the impact to quality reporting.

Rangachari cites studies that have demonstrated that nearly 20 percent of payments based on codes on hospital bills are incorrect and that there is considerable variation in coding accuracy by geographic location and bed size. Without having detailed information about the root causes for coding errors, it is difficult to respond to such statistics and make improvements.

Survey Results on Underlying Causes

Healthcare organizations must disseminate and adopt a standardized terminology for measuring coding quality performance, standardized definitions for how to count coding variance, and a standardized method for classifying and reporting coding variance. HIM and coding professionals must be educators and advocates concerning the use of standards.

In an effort to begin evaluating the current state of coding performance measurement, the AHIMA Work Group on Benchmark Standards for Clinical Coding Performance Measurement convened in 2007. A subgroup was charged with addressing coding quality measurement.

One aspect of the subgroup's work was to search for a standardized metric for measuring the quality of coded data or a regulatory requirement for consistency in reporting data quality, which it did not identify. The subgroup also conducted a survey on coding quality measurement to collect the contributing causes to coding error and variation. "Survey on Coding Quality Measurement: Hospital Inpatient Acute Care" further aimed to collect data on coding quality review outcomes to understand how coding review data are used to improve the coding quality, reduce coder variation, and develop best practices for national coding consistency.[8] A total of 668 surveys were e-mailed to AHIMA members, with 68 responses returned.

Survey responses indicated coding errors are reported by the following error type (listed in order from the most common to the least common):

- Accuracy by coder

- Accuracy by MS-DRG, DRG, APC (reimbursement)

- Total coding accuracy

- Reported as overcoding or undercoding (reimbursement)

- Reported by coding guideline, coding convention, or coding clinic

- Reported by documentation issue

- Accuracy by query

- Reported by root cause of the coding error

A Framework for Reporting Root Causes of Coding Variation

This framework may be universally applied across all organizations in collecting and reporting quality measurement data. The root causes of coding variation are grouped under six general error types.

Coder

- Insufficient clinical knowledge of disease processes, pathophysiology, and treatment
- Insufficient knowledge of coding conventions and application of official coding guidelines and coding advice
- Incorrect application of hospital-specific policies and procedures, including query policies
- Ineffective work habits, continuing education, use of resources, and communication

Provider (Physician Documentation)

- Ambiguous or nonspecific documentation
- Conflicting documentation
- Incomplete or late documentation
- Illegible documentation
- Lack of or inadequate response to queries

Administrative (Policy and Procedures)

- Insufficient medical record completion requirements
- Retrospective query and concurrent clinical documentation improvement query policies
- Coding without key documents such as discharge summary
- Facility-specific coding guidelines
- Payer-specific coding guidelines

Computer Systems

- Degree of electronic health record implementation
- Degree of embedded clinical terminologies and computer-assisted coding applications
- Accuracy of chargemaster code assignment
- Interface between clinical, coding, and billing systems

Leadership (Education and Training)

- Insufficient involvement in the development of electronic health record systems and their impact on coded data
- Insufficient accountability by the medical staff
- Lack of standardized HIM workflow model
- Inadequate tracking, trending, reporting, and follow up on coding quality review results
- Lack of regular coder education and training
- Insufficient external review of the facility's coding quality review program

Other

- Other (cannot be categorized above)
- No reason identified

Coder and provider (physician documentation) comprise the two main reasons for coding error. The survey results report the leading reason for coder error is due to complication/comorbidity code assignment, followed by principal diagnosis code assignment and secondary diagnosis code assignment.

The top three reasons for coder error related to query policies are lack of a clear understanding of clinical indicators for the condition being queried, writing unnecessary queries, and lack of follow-up for inappropriate queries initiated by clinical documentation specialist.

The number-one reason for missing coding quality performance targets (accuracy) is the challenge of meeting productivity standards while balancing quality expectations.

Survey results related to coding errors due to provider (physician documentation) find the leading reason for coding errors is vague documentation that leads to nonspecific code assignment or the need to query. This is followed by a lack of documentation to support a cause-and-effect relationship between two conditions, attending physician not concluding with a definitive diagnosis (after study) as the reason for admission, and conflicting or inconsistent documentation.

The top two reasons for coding errors related to physician response to queries are a delayed response followed by no response to queries.

Systems, policies, and procedures are another cause for coding errors. The survey asked members to list reasons for insurance denials due to coding and noncoding reasons; for example, codes not crossing to the UB-04, codes assigned by chargemaster incorrectly, payers who do not follow official coding guidelines or payer contract, or insurance companies that do not have updated codes or use old groupers. These types of coding errors should not be attributed to the coder or physician.

The survey also collected data on contributing root causes for coding errors. These are factors that indirectly impact the quality of coded data. Contributing root causes as reported in the responses include coding leadership, HIM leadership, and administrative support.

The primary reason for coding leadership contributing to coding error is that the coding lead is consumed with the day-to-day operations, followed by the priority for productivity over quality. HIM leadership contributions to coding errors relate to an ineffective workflow process to support quality coding and lack of electronic or computerized tools to support coders.

Other respondents reported that administrative support is not holding the medical staff accountable to medical record completion requirements including query requirements. Administrative staff is also focused on the financial aspects of coded data, which can contribute to root causes.

Based on the survey results, the work group created a framework for reporting root causes for coding variation that may be universally applied across all organizations in collecting and reporting quality measurement data. The root causes for each error type are outlined in the table above.

Coding variance may be classified and reported in one of six categories in an effort to eliminate or reduce coding variation. The total coding variance may be reported as one number; for example, 10 percent. However, the real value is in the reporting by root cause to explain what comprises the 10 percent coding variance—3 percent due to coder (misapplication of a coding guideline), 4 percent due to physician documentation (conflicting documentation led to inaccurate code assignment), 2 percent due to administrative (coding without a discharge summary), and 1 percent due to a system issue (code did not transfer from abstracting to billing), for example. For reporting purposes, a pie chart may be an excellent illustration of the data.

The top three departments in support of coding quality efforts, according to the survey, are medical staff, HIM leadership, and the quality department. "Survey on Coding Quality Measurement: Hospital Inpatient Acute Care" is available in the FORE Library: HIM Body of Knowledge at www.ahima.org.

Formulas for Reporting Coder Accuracy

The quality subgroup also developed formulas for reporting coder accuracy at the code level, including overall coding accuracy, principal diagnosis or first listed diagnosis accuracy, secondary diagnosis accuracy, principal procedure accuracy, secondary procedure accuracy, and DRG/APC accuracy. The subgroup also created formulas for reporting present on admission and patient status accuracy. Definitions for coding variance were established and formulas were developed for consistent reporting of coder accuracy.

A tool reflecting these formulas and definitions is available on CD-ROM as part of the AHIMA book Benchmarks for Performance Improvement in Coding Quality and Productivity.

The Goal: Consistent, Reliable Coded Data

There are many independent variables that affect the selection of administrative code sets linked to a health service encounter. Coding professionals rarely work with perfect documentation correctly aligned with the language used in the classification systems. The use of code set conventions and official coding guidelines must be applied to achieve the highest level of reliability and consistency for clinical coded data.

The translation of a case into a correctly coded data set is a matter of professional and ethical pride to those who perform this service. As healthcare moves into an era of increased scrutiny of coded data, accompanied by an expectation that administrative coded data reflect quality of care, it is in the profession's best interest to adopt standardized coding processes and use best practices for quality measurement.

It is important to classify coding variance by root cause and measure the improvement over time. Furthermore, HIM professionals may need to stretch beyond reporting individual coder accuracy rates to reporting coding variance reflective of the entire system. Furthermore, HIM professionals may begin to focus on reducing coder variation (inter-rater reliability) among a team of coders by understanding the reasons for code variation.

Reporting root cause consistently is a first step in moving to performance metrics that reflect the quality and consistency of administrative coded data. Moving from measuring individual coder accuracy to measuring organizational coding consistency of diagnostic and procedural coded data using standardized performance measures is a critical next step for HIM professionals.

Notes

1. Wilson, Donna, et al. "A New Focus on Process and Measure." *Journal of AHIMA* 79, no. 3 (Mar. 2008): 54–58.
2. Osborn, Carol. *Statistical Applications for Health Information Management.* Boston, MA: Jones and Bartlett Publishers, 2006.
3. Healthcare Financial Management Association. "A Hospital's Tale: Understanding Challenges and Strategies Associated with Data Reporting Is Key to Effectively Communicate Performance." February 2007. Available online at www.hfma.org/NR/rdonlyres/C865A076-F35E-4E2F-91C6-16125A4DC685/0/400545AHospitals Tale.pdf.
4. Centers for Medicare and Medicaid Services. "Improper Medicare Fee-For-Service Payments Report: November 2007 Long Report." Available online at www.cms.hhs.gov/apps/er_report/preview_er_report_print.asp?from=public&which=long&reportID=7#330.
5. Ibid.
6. Office of Inspector General, Office of Analysis and Inspections. "National DRG Validation Study Special Report on Coding Accuracy." February 1988. Available online at http://oig.hhs.gov/oei/reports/oai-05-88-00740.pdf.
7. Rangachari, Pavani. "Coding for Quality Measurement: The Relationship between Hospital Structural Characteristics and Coding Accuracy from the Perspective of Quality Measurement." *Perspectives in Health Information Management* 4, no. 3 (2007). Available online at www.ahima.org/perspectives.
8. D'Amato, Cheryl, et al. "Survey on Coding Quality Measurement: Hospital Inpatient Acute Care." Final report. AHIMA Foundation of Research and Education. February 2008. Available online in the FORE Library: HIM Body of Knowledge at www.ahima.org.

References

Hanna, Joette. "Constructing a Coding Compliance Plan." *Journal of AHIMA* 73, no. 7 (July–Aug. 2002): 48–56.

Olsen, Jack. *Data Quality: The Accuracy Dimension.* San Francisco, CA: Morgan Kaufman Publishers, 2003.

O'Malley, Kimberly J., et al. "Measuring Diagnoses: ICD Code Accuracy." *Health Services Research* 40, no. 5, part 2 (Oct. 2005): 1620–39.

Schedel, Ellen, and Beth Parker. "Coding Compliance and Operations: Can the Marriage Survive?" AHIMA's 78th National Convention and Exhibit Proceedings, October 2006.

Prepared by

e-HIM Work Group on Benchmark Standards for Clinical Coding Performance Measurement quality subgroup:

Cheryl D'Amato, RHIT, CCS
Kim Bagshaw, BSBM, CCS
Gwen Blackford, BS, RHIA
Susan Fenton, PhD, RHIA
Terri Hall, MHA, RHIT, CPC, CAC
Kathy Johnson, RHIA
Mary Johnson, RHIT, CCS-P
Genia Isaacs Kelley, RHIA, CCS, CCS-P
Carol Spencer, RHIA
Donna Wilson, RHIA, CCS

Acknowledgments

Sue Malone, MA, MBA, RHIA, FAHIMA

This work is sponsored in part by a grant to FORE from 3M Health Information Systems.

---

e-HIM Work Group on Benchmark Standards for Clinical Coding Performance Measurement quality subgroup. "Collecting Root Cause to Improve Coding Quality Measurement." *Journal of AHIMA* 79, no.3 (March 2008): 71–75.

Appendix E

A New Focus on Process and Measure

Raising Data Quality with a Standard Coding Workflow and Benchmarks

by Donna Wilson, RHIA, CCS; Kim Hampton-Bagshaw, BSBM, CCS; Therese M. Jorwic, MPH, RHIA, CCS, CCS-P; Jean Bishop, CCA; and Elizabeth Giustina, CCS-P

> Establishing a standard coding workflow that incorporates continuous improvement and creating performance benchmarks is key to improving the quality of coded data.

HIM professionals who assign codes or manage coded data take responsibility for translating clinical documentation and health services information into bytes consumable by today's information systems. Each seeks to be a champion of data integrity, doing his or her best to stay above the fray of competing interests for data use.

The data they code can have far-reaching effects beyond provision of care. Administrative code sets are used for a variety of reporting requirements, including registries, indexing of disease and operations, prospective payment systems, fee schedule building, health plan insurance coverage, medical necessity justification, quality measurement, vital statistics, public health, and much more.

Providing quality healthcare requires that this encoded data meet established quality standards.[1] The performance measures and work process flow behind these data, however, have yet to be standardized, making both automation difficult and unreliable and making current industry comparisons imprecise and variable.

The lack of standardization hinders communication related to clinical coding performance and work processes, and it impedes future development. The use of a common language or vocabulary is a fundamental component of performance measure and workflow. Re-engineering the work process and evaluation measures seeks to facilitate use of informatics tools to make the coding process more reliable and efficient.

Workflow process varies by purpose, practice setting, and organizational factors, among other variables. Formidable challenges remain for defining measurement benchmarks, standardization, and continuous quality improvement models that will improve data integrity and code assignment.

To address these challenges, HIM professionals came together through AHIMA in 2007 to re-engineer the coding workflow and performance benchmarks and establish useful tools for a better way to accomplish coding's ultimate goal—data everyone can count on. The group created a model for the coding workflow process and developed standard tools and best practices for measurement of code assignment reliability and productivity. They laid a foundation for change designed to make the coding process better.

A Universal Coding Workflow

The need for change has been building over several years, accelerated by the increased use of technology for data mining, a quest for automation, use of the code systems for quality of care measures tied to payment incentive, and scrutiny of reimbursement accuracy.

The volunteers were charged with developing processes and measurement systems that can assist in both the identification and subsequent revision or elimination of problem codes, data models, and guidelines or other elements that add cost, complexity, and confusion to coded data results.

The work began with evaluating the traditional coding work process to create an incremental model simple enough to be universally understood and wide-ranging enough to create a continuous quality improvement cycle. The seven-step model can be used in any healthcare setting where codes are assigned for data processing. Coding managers should compare this model to their current workflow and determine if their coding process includes all seven steps, completing the circle with quality assurance.

Two work groups developed standard methods of reliability and productivity measurement. The methods are designed to help both individuals and organizations monitor data integrity. Read about standard methods that take the guesswork out of the coding quality assessment process in the practice brief "Collecting Root Cause to Improve Coding Quality Measurement" on page 71 [*Journal of AHIMA* 79, no. 3 (Mar. 2008)].

Building measures for evaluation, benchmarking, and documentation improvement at the point of service is a critical factor. Data quality is impossible if the source document is inadequate, ambiguous, inaccurate, or incomplete at the time of coding. Improving source documentation involves clinical documentation improvement programs focused on the results important to patient care and data management.

Scanning the Coding Landscape

All process change requires an understanding of the current environment. To assess the challenges ahead, the teams scanned the field to identify what's "out there" now:

- Code assignments are prone to error due to a variety of factors.

- Inter-rater reliability between even expert coders is lower than we would like it to be.

- Coding is most often performed the "old fashioned way," where text documents are read by coding professionals from paper charts or computer screens and the codes are entered in data fields by coding professionals.

- There is no recognized or official "right" way to measure cost, productivity, and accuracy of code assignment and associated data abstraction. A reference standard (sometimes referred to as a "gold standard") does not exist.

A Model for the Coding Workflow Process

This model can be used in any healthcare setting where codes are assigned for data processing. It is intended to be simple enough to be universally understood yet comprehensive enough to help create a continuous quality improvement cycle.

Detail on each step in the process may be found in the conference proceedings for the AHIMA 2007 Computer Assisted Coding Standards Workshop and in the resources section of the CAC Standards Community of Practice at www.ahima.org.

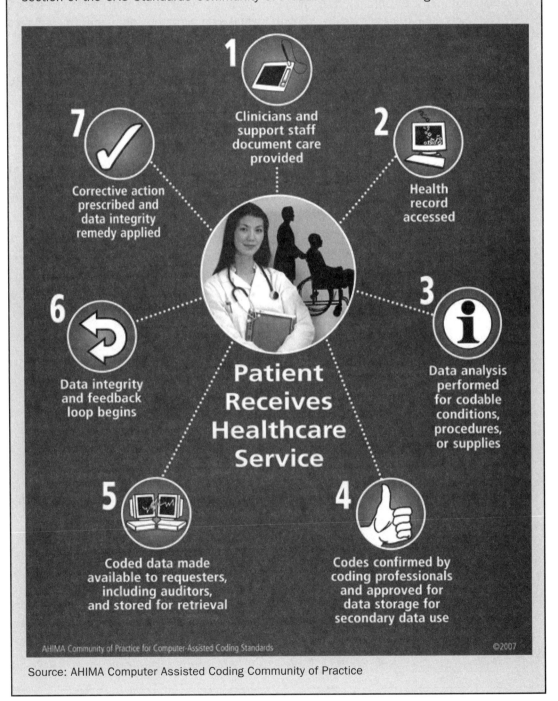

Source: AHIMA Computer Assisted Coding Community of Practice

- Existing coding workflows do not always include a quality review and improvement component (steps 6 and 7 in the coding workflow process figure). These steps include comparing code assignment variances between individuals from the same source data, tracking deficiencies in the codes or code sets to influence change to reduce variability, and correcting the root causes of variance that affect data quality and integrity.

- Automation is possible for some tasks, but there are existing barriers in the current process that make it difficult to accomplish (most often due to external regulatory factors).

- National metrics would uncover "points of pain and weakness" in the existing HIPAA code sets and transactions by allowing valid comparability and uniform variance tracking.

- Rather than require multiple layers of evaluation and review for accuracy checking, healthcare organizations should use tools similar to those used by payers to identify coder performance, specific code, or code set performance.

- Review processes must include the application of appropriate data integrity remedies so variances do not continue to replicate.

- Standardized metrics used for individual performance assessment create fairness and transparency for coding professionals and foster career growth and reduce compliance risk.

Choosing Words with Care

Coding quality initiatives often cross into financial and regulatory compliance territories, where words may carry different and exact definitions. In the table below, the words to the left may in some situations invoke special meaning or an unintended standard to others. They should be used with care or avoided in favor of more neutral terms. The terms on the right are frequently used in review processes involving clinical code assignment to help decrease the potential for misunderstanding.

Words to Use with Care or to Avoid Completely	Alternate, Neutral Terms
Audit	Trace, monitor, evaluate, assess, inspect, check, analyze, measure performance
Errors, error rates	Variance, inconsistent with reference standard, consistency rate
Undercoding	Codes omitted, level of care lower than documentation guidelines allow
Overcoding	Unnecessary or otherwise inappropriate codes assigned, level of care higher than documentation guidelines allow
Incentive targets	Production benchmark, performance measure, performance standard
Gold standard	Reference standard, benchmark
Accuracy	Variance, comparison to standard
Precision	Specificity

A "Controlled Vocabulary" for Process Improvement

There are many ways HIM professionals can express their organization's intent to follow recognized best practices and compliance standards in process improvement. However, they should be conscious of the words they choose, because some words have sensitive and highly specific meanings depending on the audience.

Coding measurement often cross into an organization's financial and regulatory compliance territories. It is helpful to remember that some words may imply different things in different departments. When discussing, documenting, or planning coding process re-engineering or performance assessment, HIM professionals should use certain words with care or even avoid them completely. The coding profession should consider creating its own controlled vocabulary to communicate clearly to others about measurements, their purpose, and their effectiveness.

The terms shown on the right in the table above are typically neutral terms in a process involving clinical code assignment. The terms on the left, however, should be used with care. It may be preferable that they be avoided altogether.

In some situations, for example, the assertion that a coding manager conducted an "audit" may invoke an unintended standard that the legal entity or professional providing the service (e.g., the coding manager or consultant reviewer) is neither qualified nor authorized to perform. That is especially true if the associated financial transactions are affected, such as in claims submission or resubmission for reimbursement.

Auditing and monitoring as a joint concept were introduced by the Federal Sentencing Guidelines and related Office of the Inspector General compliance program guidance.[2] Use of this phrase has special meaning since the enactment of the Sarbanes-Oxley legislation.[3]

There are two formal types of auditing that are generally understood—financial statement auditing and internal auditing for controls and risk assessment. Each type is governed by professional standards that predate corporate compliance plans for healthcare organizations. In both cases, the concept of auditing is specific and includes the concepts of independence and objectivity.

Standards such as the Generally Accepted Auditing Standards for financial statement audits and Standards for the Professional Practice of Internal Auditing for internal audits also refer to objectivity-related concepts such as professional care and professional skepticism.[4,5] It is generally understood that to be referred to as an "audit" the activity should have been conducted by the internal audit department, a division of a healthcare enterprise, or another independent party with reporting responsibility to the CEO or the organization's board of directors. It is possible that a coding compliance review conducted under the authority and at the direction of the chief compliance officer, who reports to the CEO or board of directors, may be properly named as an audit.

All other actions that support management activities designed to ensure compliance with regulatory requirements for code assignment, including selected activities completed as part of a work plan, should be generally labeled as monitoring. This is a conservative approach that focuses on the data quality, education, or training aspect without introducing the overlaying financial implications.

Using alternative terms builds a more meaningful and positive rapport between reviewer and coder toward consistency and compliance with both internal and external rules. Another benefit leads to reduction of risks associated with the project findings by placing focus on the continuous quality improvement process rather than the punitive aspects of not "getting it right," when the definition of "right" involves multiple factors, some beyond the control of the individual selecting codes.

Information Guardians

HIM professionals have been referred to as "information guardians" in the healthcare delivery system. Standard methods of measurement serve that higher purpose and protect the integrity of translations from clinical data into codes for other important, secondary uses.

Reliable information for medical research, biosurveillance, decision support, consumer use, health policy development, and patient safety assurance depends on those responsible for code assignment or management of the process. They must take this role seriously and constantly watch for ways to make the process better.

This standards work began with workflow design and performance measures. Now it needs the scrutiny of HIM professionals and other industry stakeholders who use coded data for refinement and confirmation of "goodness of fit."

This work is a vital step in making the coding process better by embracing a standard workflow, using standard performance measures for coding accuracy, consistency reviews, and production. Together healthcare can create reliable coding results and valid measures for performance assessment.

Notes

1. AHIMA. "Quality Healthcare Data and Information." Position statement. December 2007. Available online at www.ahima.org/dc/positions.
2. U.S. Federal Sentencing Guidelines. Available online at www.ussc.gov/guidelin.htm.
3. Sarbanes-Oxley Act of 2002. Public law. Available online at http://thomas.loc.gov/cgi-bin/query/z?c107:H.R. 3763.ENR:.
4. Generally Accepted Accounting Standards. Available online at www.gao.gov/govaud/ybk01.htm.
5. Institute of Internal Auditors. International Standards for the Professional Practice of Internal Auditing. Available online at www.theiia.org/guidance/standards-and-practices.

Donna Wilson (donna.wilson@rsfh.com) is revenue integrity manager for Roper St. Francis Healthcare in Charleston, SC. **Kim Hampton-Bagshaw** is director of coding services for Pyramid Healthcare Solutions. **Therese M. Jorwic** is an assistant professor at the University of Illinois at Chicago and a consultant for MC Strategies in Atlanta. **Jean Bishop** is senior manager with Deloitte Financial Advisory Services LLP (the views expressed in this article are those of the authors, and do not necessarily reflect the views of Deloitte Financial Advisory Services LLP). **Elizabeth Giustina** is with MedPartners in Jacksonville, FL. The authors would like to acknowledge the assistance of **Rita Scichilone,** MHSA, RHIA, CCS, CCS-P, and **Carol Spencer,** RHIA.

Wilson, Donna, et al. "New Focus on Process and Measure: Raising Data Quality with a Standard Coding Workflow and Benchmarks." *Journal of AHIMA* 79, no.3 (March 2008): 54–58.

Appendix F

Developing an Effective Compliance Audit Process

Introduction

The dictionary definition of an audit is "a methodical examination and review." To monitor is to "watch, observe, or check, especially for a special purpose." Because of a variety of reasons in the current healthcare delivery market, assessment and monitoring of information gathering and reporting processes to ensure compliance with organizational and customer needs is a critical function. This paper will discuss the structure and process of conducting audits for compliance related to coding, reimbursement, and related documentation issues.

Background

The Payment Error Protection Program (PEPP) has resulted in a number of excellent manuals and structures for coding and reimbursement evaluation. HIM professionals can look to this resource prepared by the Peer Review Organizations (PROs) under contract with government agencies for reliable means to improve processes and minimize risk of noncompliance. The first time an audit or review process is undertaken it can be more resource intensive than subsequent review activities. A first-time look at any process is generally referred to as a "baseline assessment." It is impossible to initiate performance improvement until it is known where most problems occur. Areas for investigation must be determined, processes must be developed and documented, personnel must be identified to conduct the audit, and the audit must be performed. Baseline audits demand that a wider net be cast to ensure important deficiencies are recognized. Unidentified coding problems translate into reimbursement not received or potential liability for compliance problems. To be sure there are no surprises, the first audit must be comprehensive. Subsequent audits will be much less time-consuming because processes will have already been established, and it will be clear which areas do not require focused attention or additional review resources and time.

Source: Scichilone, Rita. 2001 (October). *AHIMA National Convention Proceedings*. Chicago: AHIMA.

Note: The appendixes mentioned in this document refer to the appendixes of the original work. When possible, URLs for these resources are included for ease of use.

Audit Strategy

Subsequent audits will start the monitoring and evaluation process. Frequency of review is facility specific, and may depend on who is reviewing the information and what action will be taken from the results. Assessments should be conducted at regular intervals (monthly, quarterly, semiannually, annually), with the results used to monitor the effectiveness of the compliance program.

Reviews performed subsequent to the baseline measurement seek answers to the following questions:

1. For problem areas, did improvement occur since the last review?

2. For nonproblem areas, was the initial baseline level maintained, or did significant deviations occur?

3. Does any result of review require immediate referral to the compliance office for investigation of noncompliance that involves overpayments or fraudulent activity?

4. Are there any findings that require immediate referral to the business services unit or clinical department management for underreporting or missed charges?

Some organizations choose to review coding accuracy and conduct claims review separately. Coding accuracy requires individual record assessment, while some aspects of claims review are based on aggregate data analysis. Any coding assessment should include verification that the codes selected for the case are the same codes reported for any external purpose, such as reimbursement from a third party.

Section I: Coding Assessment

Code assignment review should be performed to ensure that coding is being done in compliance with coding rules and official guidelines. The baseline audit should be extensive enough to establish baseline performance (coding accuracy) in distinct areas considered to be important (e.g., settings, departments, and types of coding). As stated previously, subsequent audits, which may be smaller in scope, should be performed at regular intervals to compare the current accuracy level with the baseline accuracy level. More frequent audits may be performed in areas identified as requiring improvement. Coding audits will generally involve reviewing a sample of the population as opposed to auditing all claims. A coding audit compares the clinical documentation to the codes assigned and evaluates whether all possible codes were reported, whether they were correct, whether the documentation is inadequate for complete coding, or whether coding principles were not followed. In addition, it includes a tracking of the codes assigned on the resulting claim form to make sure the information is accurate and complete.

Selecting an Approach to a Coding Audit

A variety of means are useful to structure and approach the assessment of coding accuracy. The first step is to establish when during the coding or billing process you wish to conduct the review. Reviews may be conducted prior to billing, or after billing has occurred and payment has been received. There are advantages and disadvantages to each approach. The next step is to establish the approach you will use for selecting cases for review. Every coding staff member should have records included in the sample, and if physician documentation is under scrutiny, each physician should also have records in the sample for at least the baseline review. Once documentation adequacy has been established, this can be suspended. Most facilities review this in a cyclic fashion and make the results available at the time of medical staff reappointment or performance evaluation for employed physicians. Reviewing adequacy of documentation at the same time a coding assessment is performed is one way of keeping the process efficient and avoiding duplication of effort in pulling records and conducting review.

It is also recommended that particular areas identified as problematic are reviewed. This will be based on past audit results or on the current OIG Workplan[1] that identifies high-risk areas. By doing both, you should not miss persistent coding errors in low-risk areas or errors in areas that are known to be problematic in other facilities and that represent significant risk of external review and subsequent compliance problems.

Typical Facility Coding Audit Approaches

- A facility performs quarterly retrospective coding reviews as part of its quality improvement plan. Records from each coding staff member are selected randomly for all payers. The Data Quality Coordinator performs the review by selecting 10 records for each person. Coding errors are discussed with the persons responsible and are trended to track future improvement and suggest training needs. Cases with errors that affect reimbursement are referred to the business office for rebilling when appropriate.

- A facility monitors claims containing selected DRGs and APCs that have been identified as problematic prior to billing. Any revisions are made prior to billing, thus allowing the hospital to be paid correctly the first time. This reduces the amount of rebilling and minimizes the risk of external agency focused review. The population for sample selection is limited to payers that use the reimbursement system under review.

- A facility conducts studies of remittance advices received by the billing office for trends and patterns that involve coding issues. The facility looked for inconsistencies between the DRGs assigned by the hospital coders and what was paid by the Fiscal Intermediary or insurance plan. Rebills are submitted as appropriate within the required time frame. The facility quantifies underpayments and overpayments, as well as denials. These results are logged over time to identify problem areas. Summary information is provided to the compliance committee.

- A facility conducts monthly coding accuracy reviews by using the manager of clinical data as the auditor. Samples of each coding staff member's work are pulled from all patient types-inpatient acute care, outpatient surgery, outpatient ancillary, endoscopy, emergency room, observation, and skilled care. UB-92s are pulled to make sure codes are transferring correctly. Errors are reviewed at a coding staff meeting where at least one educational topic is presented to improve skills in coding and record analysis. Each quarter, an external consulting firm conducts an independent coding review by using the same population. The consulting group also provides an in-service in conjunction with their report on areas of concern or new topics requiring special knowledge or application of unfamiliar coding guidelines.

- In addition to auditing coding accuracy, you should also review adequacy and completeness of physician medical record documentation to support optimal coding. Some facilities make this part of the medical record review function and review not only for adequacy to support code selection and justify billing but also for application of clinical pertinence criteria defined by medical staff. Records that fail the screens are referred to committee for peer review and medical staff follow-up. Documentation inadequacies for coding purposes are trended, and educational programs are provided to improve processes. For example, a hospital may choose to monitor the presence or absence of final diagnoses on the record at the time of discharge, according to medical staff rules and regulations. Another indicator may be to measure the inclusion of complications and comorbidities in the diagnostic statements or the persistent need for clarification from the coding staff because of ambiguous documentation.

Establishing Who Will Conduct the Reviews

Each facility must establish the person(s) responsible for performing the coding audits. This should begin with deciding whether to use internal or external resources. Objectivity demands that someone independent of the actual coding function conduct the reviews. Coder-to-coder peer review is effective only when the identity of the coder is concealed. It can also hide inappropriate coding practices that are universally applied even though they are incorrect. Perhaps a workshop presenter gave questionable advice or a previous supervisor instructed the coders to apply a certain interpretation of coding rules. This would not be picked up until an objective review was undertaken by a disinterested party.

The designated reviewers must all have coding expertise and credible training background. Some facilities choose to use a panel of auditors, with each providing expertise in a particular area or healthcare setting. For example, one auditor specializes in CPT coding and another specializes in ICD-9-CM coding; others may fully understand physician professional fee reporting or home health data sets or skilled nursing requirements.

A physician advisor should be available to field clinical questions or questions about the application of clinical pertinence criteria or documentation adequacy.

Documenting the Process

As with all compliance activities, it is important to develop detailed written policy and procedures for conducting audits and maintaining the results. As appropriate, the policy should identify when and how audits should be performed, what forms and criteria are used in the review process, and what is done with the results. Some compliance plans require all coding audits to be performed under the direction of legal counsel to qualify for the attorney-client privilege, work-product immunity, or other protections. Appendix B (http://library.ahima.org/xpedio/groups/secure/documents/graphic/bok2_001447.pdf) includes some sample audit forms and tools. [*These forms are also included in Appendix G of this book.*]

Establishing a Review Plan

The written audit plan should be in force for a specified period and reviewed at the end of its life. A written audit plan should contain at least the following elements:

1. A discussion of the established frequency for performing the audit.

2. A discussion of the established period covered by each audit.

3. A description of the population eligible for review should be specified in the audit plan, if the audit processing is ongoing and selected departments or patient types are reviewed in rotation.

4. An explanation of how the sample size will be determined, which will depend on the type of audit being conducted. Various resources provide recommendations for various types of samples; for example, a routine review is suggested to sample five percent or 30 records, whichever number is greater. A discussion of the established sample design, in most cases a simple random sample, is sufficient, though the source of the random numbers must be documented if used for self-disclosure. For self-disclosure, the OIG recommends the use of its Office of Audit Services Statistical Sampling Software, also known as RAT-STATS (currently available free of charge through the Internet at www.hhs.gov/progorg/oas/ratstat.html). *A Guide to Auditing Health Care Billing Practices,* published by Atlantic Information Services, Inc.,[2] also contains a good example form for the documentation of a sample selection plan, among other tools.

5. A description of the indicators (see the next section of this paper for more details).

6. A description of the planned analysis techniques.

Defining Indicators

Appropriate indicators must be defined to measure accuracy of code reporting in a consistent and fair process. One type of indicator will be the coding error rate. This must be defined by the number of records with coding errors, as compared with the number of records without coding errors. Some facilities also collect data in greater detail by comparing the number and accuracy of the codes assigned to the omissions or incorrect code assignment. This is more complicated to administer but may be more meaningful depending on what analysis is needed.

Two types of error rate categories are recommended: errors that affect reimbursement by causing a grouping error or fee-schedule payment error and errors that do not affect reimbursement. Both are important, since they affect the reliability of data in many systems, not just the payment process. Reimbursement errors are critical because they increase risk of fraud or abuse allegations and can trigger overpayments that must be returned and impact the financial health of the organization. In developing the coding compliance program, standards for coding accuracy are clearly stated. In a perfect world, standards will be 100 percent accuracy for all coders, but each organization must consider the degree of risk associated with errors and decide for itself the level of accuracy that must be maintained. If you expect 100 percent accuracy in code assignment, you must find a way to produce 100 percent adequacy and completeness in physician documentation. Asking a coding professional to identify all reportable procedures from an incomplete record and then attributing errors to that person after review of a completed record is not fair. A defined indicator will allow you to evaluate compliance with coding accuracy standards and benchmarks. Other common indicators include areas such as accuracy of grouping assignment, selection of the principal diagnosis for inpatients, and correct selection of the discharge status.

After completion of the baseline audit, the facility should have identified problems or opportunities for improvement in the coding process. The next step is to define indicators that will show how the coding process and outcome is expected to improve by the next audit. For example, after a comprehensive training program concerning correct coding of spinal fusion procedures, you may expect the percentage of certain DRGs to decrease. Another result might be an expectation that the number of FI rejections for a particular reason will decrease or maybe the expectation is to show an increase in the case mix index (CMI). A selected indicator could be a quantitative measure of these processes that can be measured over time, such as a percentage of discharges with FI rejections or the ratio of one DRG to another in Medicare or other defined financial classes that show DRG payment impact. Sampling protocols may be used to determine when additional record review may be needed in vulnerable areas. Often, serious problems can be prevented if an effective monitoring process is in place to catch coding aberrations early and allow immediate intervention.

Designing Reports, Compiling Results, and Effecting Change

Report formats for tracking and analyzing coding audit results must be customized to the audience. Reports should allow tracking overall coding accuracy and the accuracy of individual employees. They should also allow monitoring of those areas you have determined to be problematic so improvement or backsliding is evident and can be addressed. In general, charts and graphs are worth 10 text descriptions, especially with management-level users or physicians. Any employee or physician results should be encrypted for public display, with details available for authorized and appropriate personnel.

An example format is included as Appendix C (http://library.ahima.org/xpedio/groups/secure/documents/graphic/bok2_001448.html).

Using Audit Results

The results of coding assessments and any corrective action implemented as a result should be summarized and submitted to the compliance officer for consideration and maintenance. Legal counsel should be consulted in deciding how results will be documented and who is authorized access to the reports.

Section II: Claims Auditing

Because the coding process and the billing process for third-party reimbursement are so integrated and dependent on each other, claims audits should be performed to ensure that claims are processed in accordance with required healthcare program and billing regulations.

Electronic databases of paid claims enable an organization to access the entire universe of their claims in aggregate. Compare this to coding audits for which it is practical to review only samples of the population. Any facility without an electronic database should consider reviewing each claim process along with the coding review and perhaps selecting additional cases purely for claims processing review.

Selecting an Approach to a Claims Audit

Auditing of claims can be approached from three different perspectives. Use of reimbursement methods such as the DRG and APC can provide frequency reports, so a "big picture" view can be created about the nature of the services being reported. Some claims reviews include an audit to determine completeness of medical record documentation in supporting the services billed. Finally, any claims review process must consider the codes selected by the coding staff or physician and include those dropped in the charge description master, as compared with the codes submitted to the FI or carrier to ensure that they are exactly the same.

The second and third perspectives are actually extensions of the coding audit, and the same guidelines provided in the previous section apply to the claims review process. Some facilities choose to separate the reviews, since they focus on different objectives, while others choose to combine the reviews to minimize pulling of records and overlapping tasks. To meet market demand, vendors have created software programs that profile facilities' claims data and/or search for upcoding or trends requiring further study. Some of these programs may be very valuable in helping you audit because of the amount of analysis they can provide, but exercise caution in their selection. The OIG recently tested software designed to detect upcoding and achieved only modest success.[3] The analyses proposed in this section are simple to conduct if a facility can perform basic queries of their database systems and do not require purchase of additional software.

Establishing Who Will Conduct Claims Audits

As with the coding reviews, it is important to establish who will perform the audits and how the review process interacts with the coding assessment process. Each facility needs to evaluate whether the organization has the internal resources to perform the work or if an auditing firm with the required expertise should be hired. Both options have advantages, and a blend of the two strategies is preferred. The use of internal staff should represent cost-savings over hiring an outside contractor. For billing reviews, additional expertise is required to identify missed charges or billing process errors, and some coding experts may not have this knowledge without specific training or experience. An experienced auditing firm can bring knowledge of other clients' situations to identify risk areas. Ideally, a facility would acquaint itself with its data and data systems before bringing in an outside contractor. Some health systems employ internal auditors that fill this role. They must work closely with the HIM or coding personnel in a facility to ensure optimal review results.

Documenting the Process of Claims Audits

As with the coding assessment, a detailed policy and procedure for conducting the audits is prepared. The policy should identify when and how audits should be conducted and the circumstances of working under the direction of legal counsel to maintain legal protection under the attorney-client or work-product privileges. Report formats are developed that will be used to compile results to meet the objectives of a claims-processing review.

Establishing the Audit Plan

The audit plan should include:

- Audit frequency
- Time period
- Review population
- Sample size and sample design (if using sampling)
- Indicators
- Indicator specifications
- Time frames
- Comparative data or benchmarks
- Analysis techniques

Identifying the Necessary Personnel for Claims Audits

A team of individuals from various departments may be assembled to assist with developing claims-auditing procedures. Generally, a project of this scope requires individuals from various disciplines throughout the organization because of the widespread use of chargemasters and/or charge tickets for many items. HIM staff will be called on to identify important coding issues and develop coding accuracy and/or grouping assignment indicators, while billing department staff will be called on to guide the selection of appropriate claims and their data sources. When working with aggregate data, information services staff will be helpful in creating automated tools and programs for retrieving all the necessary data.

The compliance officer and the compliance committee should oversee the process and provide input into how it is conducted and who should be in charge of the analysis of the process.

Defining Indicators

Indicators to be examined in claims audits are different from those used in coding reviews. The detailed work of defining the appropriate indicators is a crucial step that must be completed before any data is retrieved. Analysis of multiple indicators allows a facility to prioritize areas for further examination. To begin with, each organization should establish simple descriptive indicators such as the most frequently billed (top 10, top 50, and so on) APCs and DRGs, average length of stay for each DRG, or number of short-stay admissions. These indicators may be further stratified, or broken out into smaller groups by payer or unit, depending on the needs of the individual facility.

CMI as assigned by HCFA can be used as a crude indicator. CMI for APC is possible but requires attention to appropriate grouping because of wide disparity in APC relative weights and associated resource use and costs.

CMI for inpatient analysis is an indicator of a facility's overall resource use and is driven by ICD-9-CM coding. If complications and comorbidities are either not being coded as they should, or are being coded without supporting documentation, this will result in either an artificially low or high CMI. Comparison of a facility's CMI with those of other similar facilities, or comparison of the CMI in the previous year with the CMI in the current year, may indicate a need to examine the facility's coding accuracy in more depth. There are other factors that affect case mix, but all significant increases or decreases should be closely examined and the reason confirmed. APC case mix is driven by HCPCS/CPT coding and is not affected currently by the selection of the diagnosis code.

Denial or rejection rates also serve as an indicator of how the claims processing system and front-end edits in a facility are working.

Using Comparative Data and Designing Claims Audit Reports

Comparative data is used to assist in the evaluation of indicator results and serve as a guide in determining whether an area should be examined in greater depth.

For example, if 42 percent of an organization's total pneumonia cases are reported as complex pneumonia (DRG 079), and 75 percent of the hospitals in the state, or the nation, bill no more than 30 percent of their pneumonia cases as complex pneumonia, then the organization would be wise to examine the coding of their pneumonia records. In some cases, this may be traced to misinterpretation of coding guidelines or misguided advice provided by a reimbursement optimization consultant about what constitutes bacterial pneumonia.

Comparative data from a state or group of similar facilities will help determine whether an indicator merits further examination. Additional sources of comparative data may include the local PRO, the state hospital association or data commission, state medical societies, or consulting firms.

Many hospitals produce comparative data through the use of HCFA's Medicare Provider Analysis and Review (MEDPAR) file. The MEDPAR file contains data for 100 percent of Medicare beneficiaries using hospital inpatient services. A file of services in one year for a state is available from HCFA for a little more than $1,000.

Ordering information for this file is available from HCFA's Web site at www.hcfa.gov/ stats/pufiles.htm in the Public Use Files catalog. Also available from HCFA's Web site are two files that may be downloaded at no cost. Summary statistics of several years of MEDPAR data are available at www.hcfa.gov/stats/medpar/medpar.htm. The most recent year's CMI values for all hospitals in the nation are available at www.hcfa.gov/stats/pufiles.htm under Payment Rates-Institutional Providers.

Meaningful reports should be developed for displaying and analyzing results of the claims review. After design is completed, specifications for indicators are submitted to the individual or department to be responsible for the extraction of the data from the database used for the claims review. These individuals are often in the information services department or the billing or accounting department.

Compiling the Results

Information systems programs can be written for extraction of the data from appropriate databases. You should consider a time period of at least six months (preferably a year) for an initial claims audit. Extraction of claims information from archived claims may be difficult. To obtain information from claims processed in the preceding 12 to 15 months, you may need to restore data from backup tapes or other media. This requires advance planning and collaboration with the information systems department well in advance of the review.

Most hospitals use indicators that measure performance in areas of investigation by federal agencies. This type of indicator is usually a proportion in which the numerator represents a potentially problematic area, such as a commonly miscoded DRG or a short-stay admission. The denominator represents an appropriate larger group of admissions from which the numerator is drawn. The proportion is then multiplied by 100 to obtain the percentage.

An example of an indicator used to examine an area frequently under federal investigation is the DRG pair. The first DRG in the pair is a higher-weighted DRG susceptible to upcoding. The second DRG in the pair is the DRG that more commonly should have been coded instead of the first DRG. This may occur if coding staff inappropriately designates complications and comorbidities not fully supported by clinical documentation or without concurrence with the physician's diagnostic statement. It can also occur if the physician is "coached" or led by an inappropriate query process to add information to the record that indicates these conditions, although the resource use by the hospital did not increase.

This type of indicator would be calculated to produce the proportion of the first DRG to the sum of the first and second DRG. Examples of these calculations are provided in Appendix D (http://library.ahima.org/xpedio/groups/secure/documents/graphic/bok2_001449. html) and illustrated in practice in the *Journal of AHIMA* article, "DRG Analysis Reveals Potential Problems, Trends."[4] The table in Appendix E (http://library.ahima.org/xpedio/groups/ secure/documents/graphic/bok2_001450.html) provides a listing of some suggested DRG pairs for examination.

A one-day stay for a medical DRG may be suspect for medical necessity and admission appropriateness, but a consistent problem may exist if the proportion of one-day stays is very high in a particular DRG or group of related DRGs. Other ideas for indicators can be found in the Medicare Fiscal Intermediary newsletters, the OIG's Workplans, OIG fraud alerts, and materials from your local PRO.

Once the preliminary list of indicators is agreed upon by the organization stakeholders, the specifications for each indicator are delineated. Specifications are instructions regarding what data elements are required to define the numerator and denominator and where to locate each data element in the information system or database.

Specifications should be thoroughly documented and understood for several reasons. This allows an outside auditing firm to understand how a facility obtained results so they can be compared to the external reviewer's results. This also allows the audit team to consistently replicate the indicators when the time comes for the next auditing period, and it also allows new staff to consistently replicate the indicators.

Appendix F (http://library.ahima.org/xpedio/groups/secure/documents/graphic/bok2_001455.pdf) shows a model for producing a compliance audit report.

Interpreting the Results of a Claims Audit

After data collection, analysis must take place to interpret the findings and produce meaningful results. One important fact to remember is that indicators with smaller denominators (less than 30) will yield results that are less stable, meaning they are more subject to random fluctuation. A high percentage in one year could be followed by a very low percentage in the following year. Indicators with denominators greater than or equal to 30 are more stable from year to year, and they represent a facility's more commonly rendered services.

By using the data from the model report (Appendix F, http://library.ahima.org/xpedio/groups/secure/documents/graphic/bok2_001455.pdf), it is possible to make some interpretations of the indicator results for this facility. The comparison data provided represents the median, 10th percentile, and 90th percentile values of the indicator percentages from one large state's group of hospitals for 1999. The median value is the value in the middle of the range of values. The l0th and 90th percentile values define the range in which 80 percent of the group's values fall. Values higher or lower than these percentiles should automatically identify an indicator for further examination.

All four indicators from the example facility are worthwhile for further examination because the denominators are larger than 30. All three DRG-related indicators for the example facility exceed the comparison group's median value, but they are still within the range of values representing 80 percent of facilities in the comparison group. Of the three DRG-related indicators, this facility's proportion of DRG 087 (15 percent) is highest relative to the median of the comparison group (6.3 percent). Further investigation is recommended, which may take the form of a coding audit of a sample or all of the 44 claims billed to DRG 087. The one-day stay indicator result is below the median of the comparison group; however, a problem may exist within a single DRG or group of DRGs, and the data should be stratified according to DRG. There may be a high proportion of one-day stays for DRG 127 (congestive heart failure), for example.

Trend Analysis

Initial audits, whether they are focused on coding practices or claims, will provide a baseline or starting point value that can be used to compare to all subsequent measurements. To compare subsequent measurements to the baseline, you should develop a process to allow collection and analysis of measurements made over time. Collecting the measurements made over time in a spreadsheet and plotting them on a line graph is one technique that may be used. Statistical process control charts represent another tool for this task. Control charts to be monitored on a regular basis can be constructed for each indicator, and the calculation of upper and lower control limits will signal when a process is "out of control."

Using Audit Tools for Coding or Claims Review

Use of an audit tool provides consistency in data collection and facilitates collection of required data. Samples are provided in Appendix B (http://library.ahima.org/xpedio/groups/secure/documents/graphic/bok2_001447.pdf). [*These forms are also included in Appendix G of this book.*]

Audit tools for coding review can be used to evaluate simple coding errors and complex errors that affect the DRG assignment. They can be used to identify problems in coding, DRG, or APC assignments or to monitor improvement in such assignments identified previously. Although the instructions are written as if you are performing a postpayment review, you could also adapt the form to a prepayment review.

Preparation for Use of Audit Tools

When review of a group of similar cases (like diagnoses and procedures) is planned, auditors are recommended to review related coding conventions and guidelines specific to that clinical area. It is helpful to be aware of any coding problems that can occur by reviewing the OIG fraud alerts or looking at past areas of concern.

Recording Record, Claim Review, and Findings Using the Audit Tools

Auditors compare the medical record to the claim to ensure that the documentation matches what was reported on the claim form.

If the medical record does not match the claim in terms of the patient name, admission date, physician orders, or provider number, further action is necessary. Consultation with the physician may be needed, and a request to provide an addendum to the medical record, correct the claim, and rebill the services, or take other action, may also be required. Documentation after discharge for the express purpose of seeking reimbursement and not contributing to patient care may be a questionable practice.

The auditor should review the medical record to ensure that the diagnosis reported as the principal diagnosis meets UHDDS definitions. It must have been present at admission, been a principal reason for admission, and received treatment or evaluation during the stay. If several diagnoses meet all of these requirements, and sequencing guidelines do not require you to code one over the others, you may select any one of the diagnoses as the principal diagnosis. If the principal diagnosis was chosen incorrectly, the correct diagnosis should be determined. If this can be determined by using official coding conventions and guidelines, you do not necessarily have to obtain physician consultation, as long the record clearly supports this action. If the documentation in the medical record is unclear, consultation with the attending physician is mandatory to obtain answers to questions about the appropriateness of the codes reported. Best practices suggest that physicians be notified any time the code reporting is at variance with the final diagnostic statement at discharge. If any changes affect the DRG, resubmission of the claim is required. The hospital must ensure that physician clarification is documented in the medical record in an addendum. If a pattern of rebilling is noted for specific physicians or for specific types of cases, an indicator should be established and a corrective action plan implemented.

In addition to diagnosis and procedure verification with the medical record to determine if the patient's age and discharge status were billed correctly, incorrect designation of discharge status or age can result in incorrect DRG assignment. Problems in this area should also be trended and corrective action taken. Discharge status errors sometimes occur owing to a mapping error between the abstracting system and the claims generation process.

For outpatient records, the reason for the visit should be reported and corresponding diagnoses indicated to support justification of the medical necessity for each service rendered. Modifiers should be applied appropriately when indicated, and all CPT and Level II HCPCS codes assigned should be verified, whether they are selected by coding staff or posted by the chargemaster.

When coding affects the DRG or APC payments, auditors should classify the cause of changes by using the problem areas provided on the audit form. Also, note the original and revised DRG or APCs and the difference in reimbursement. This will allow you to track whether your coding errors involving claims are resulting in over- or underpayments.

Follow-up of Audit Tool Completion

Individual audit results are maintained to identify any undesirable patterns and trends. Once a problem or opportunity for improvement has been identified, an organization is expected to implement corrective action to protect its corporate integrity. After improvement has been noted, it is important to focus on new areas, being sure to periodically check old problems to ensure that improvement is sustained.

Credibility demands that the person completing the audit form sign and date it. This demonstrates that qualified staff is performing audits to ensure an effective compliance program committed to following regulatory requirements and payment rules. It also allows accountability tracking and facilitates quality review of the audit process. Also, should a government investigation occur in the future, this documentation would demonstrate that auditing predated the investigation, and there was a process in place to identify problems and take corrective action. Consultation with legal counsel is recommended regarding how to structure and document this type of information.

Results and Recommendations

Audits must result in corrective action specific to the problems identified in the reviews. Any problem involving significant overpayment, confirmed upcoding, questionable medical necessity trends, or any issues with potential for inaccurate payment must be referred to the compliance office or compliance committee for follow-up. On the basis of audit outcomes, corrective action may include designing a form to be used by physicians for documenting final diagnoses, providing physician education on medical record documentation and coding, updating coding books, providing feedback to the coding staff involved, implementing prebilling coding validation, or other steps specific to the problem.

Conclusion

Following the suggestions and guidelines set forth in this paper will produce an effective compliance audit process for coding and reimbursement and the related documentation supporting those activities.

Notes

1. The OIG Workplan is available at http://www.dhhs.gov/progorg/wrkpln/2001/hcfa.pdf.
2. Russo, R. and F. Fernald, ed. *A Guide to Auditing Health Care Billing Practices*. Washington, DC: Atlantic Information Services, Inc.
3. www.dhhs.gov/progorg
4. Osborne, C.E. 2001. DRG Analysis Reveals Potential Problems, Trends. *Journal of AHIMA* 72(7):78–83.

References

"2001 OIG Workplan" is available at www.dhhs.gov/progorg/wrkpln/2001/hcfa.pdf.

"Improper Fiscal Year 2000 Medicare Fee-for-Service Payments" is available at www.dhhs.gov/progorg/oas/reports/afma/a0002000.pdf.

Osborne, C.E. 2001. DRG analysis reveals potential problems, trends. *Journal of AHIMA* 72(7):78–83.

Payment Error Prevention Program. Arkansas Foundation for Medical Care, 2001. (Many states have similar reference materials available from the PRO under contract by the Medicare Intermediary.)

Practice Brief. 2001. *Journal of AHIMA* 72(7):64A–64C.

Prophet, S. 2000. *Health Information Management Compliance: A Model Program for Healthcare Organizations.* Chicago: AHIMA.

Russo, R. and F. Fernald, ed. 2001. *A Guide to Auditing Health Care Billing Practices.* Washington, DC: Atlantic Information Services, Inc.

Appendix G

Sample Audit Worksheets, Forms, and Tools

Inpatient Review
Variations by Coding Professional

Date of Review: _____

Variation Type

Inaccurate sequencing or specificity prin Dx, affect DRG   _____

Inaccurate sequencing or specificity prin Dx, no affect DRG   _____

Omission CC, affect DRG   _____

Omission CC, no affect DRG   _____

Inaccurate prin procedure, affect DRG   _____

Omission procedure, affect DRG   _____

More specific coding of Dx or proc, no affect DRG   _____

Inaccurate coding   _____

Source: Bowman, Sue. 2008. *Health Information Management Compliance: Guidelines for Preventing Fraud and Abuse,* 4th ed. Chicago: AHIMA.

Assessment Reference Date (ARD) Scoring Review

Resident Name

Activities of Daily Living (ADLs)	ARD:		ARD:		ARD:		ARD:		Comments
	MDS	REC	MDS	REC	MDS	REC	MDS	REC	
Bed Mobility Self Performance									
Bed Mobility Staff Support									
Bed Mobility—Other									
Transfer Self Performance									
Transfer Staff Support									
Transfer—Other									
Toileting Self Performance									
Toileting Staff Support									
Toileting—Other									
Eating Self Performance									
Eating Staff Support									
Eating—Other									

Completed By: _____   **Date:** _____

Audit of Therapy Services

Resident Name: _____

Admission Date: _____

5-Day Assessment			Assessment Reference Date (ARD)		
	MDS Days	**MDS Minutes**	**Chart Days**	**Minutes**	**UB-92**
PT					
OT					
SP					

14-Day Assessment			ARD:		
	MDS Days	**MDS Minutes**	**Chart Days**	**Minutes**	**UB-92**
PT					
OT					
SP					

30-Day Assessment			ARD:		
	MDS Days	**MDS Minutes**	**Chart Days**	**Minutes**	**UB-92**
PT					
OT					
SP					

_____-Day Assessment			ARD:		
	MDS Days	**MDS Minutes**	**Chart Days**	**Minutes**	**UB-92**
PT					
OT					
SP					

_____-Day Assessment			ARD:		
	MDS Days	**MDS Minutes**	**Chart Days**	**Minutes**	**UB-92**
PT					
OT					
SP					

Findings:

□ MDS/Medical Record and UB-92 are all in agreement
□ Problems noted as follows: _____

_____
_____
_____

Completed By: _____   Date:_____

Audit Summary Sheet

Audit topic: _____

Dates of service covered by the audit _____ to _____

Number of medical records or claims audited _____

Methodology used for sample selection _____

Physician(s) audited in this sample _____

☐ All physicians included in the sample

Accuracy percentage: _____

Findings:

1. _____

2. _____

3. _____

4. _____

5. _____

(Attach a copy of all audit tools used in this audit)

Recommendations:

1. _____

2. _____

3. _____

4. _____

5. _____

Follow-up audit date: _____

Reviewer: _____ Date completed: _____

Audit Date: _____
Reviewer: _____

Behavioral Compliance Audit Worksheet

Record # _____ Staff _____

Manager _____ **Mandatory Return Date** _____

The above record was reviewed for billing and documentation compliance and the following problems were found.

_____ Activity code error _____

Recommended Resolution _____

_____ Activity not on report of services _____
_____ Specify activity and date _____

Recommended Resolution (submit log) _____

_____ Documentation of activity billed missing or incorrect (including correct date and signature of individual providing services). Specify:
_____
_____
_____

Recommended Resolution (addendum note) _____

_____ Documentation in progress notes do not match interventions

Recommended Resolution _____

_____ Misdate ☐ Progress Note ☐ Activity Log ☐ Other

Recommended Resolution _____

_____ Comments

Recommended Resolution _____

_____ Tx Plan Issue

☐ Expired ☐ Not in chart ☐ Missing Signatures ☐ Content ☐ Other

Recommended Resolution _____

Source: The Kent Center, 2006.

Other QI Comments _____
_____

Signature _____

To be completed by supervisor and staff

_____ Corrective Action Plan (check one)

☐ Level One (Verbal Warning, plan of correction)

☐ Level Two (Written warning, plan of correction)

☐ Level Three (Written warning, plan of correction, probation)

Document action taken or any additional comments _____
_____
_____

_____ Date corrective action completed

_____
Staff signature

_____
Supervisor signature

To be completed by QI department

Further follow-up required   ☐ Y   ☐ N

If yes, specify_____
_____

Fiscal Office Response (if necessary) _____
_____

_____
Fiscal staff signature/date

_____   _____
Date filed   QI staff signature

Coding Audit Review Sheet

Coder: _____ _____
Type of Review (IP,OP,ER): _____
Date of Review: _____
Health Record #: _____
Discharge Date: _____

Initial Coding	Reviewer's Recommendations

Principal Diagnosis
   A. Chosen and coded correctly   _____
   B. Chosen correctly, coded incorrectly _____
   C. Chosen incorrectly, coded correctly _____
   D. Chosen and coded incorrectly   _____

Secondary Diagnoses
   A. Chosen and coded correctly   _____
   B. Chosen correctly, coded incorrectly _____
   C. Chosen incorrectly, coded correctly _____
   D. Chosen and coded incorrectly   _____

Principal Procedure
   A. Chosen and coded correctly   _____
   B. Chosen correctly, coded incorrectly _____
   C. Chosen incorrectly, coded correctly _____
   D. Chosen and coded incorrectly   _____

Secondary Procedures
   A. Chosen and coded correctly   _____
   B. Chosen correctly, coded incorrectly _____
   C. Chosen incorrectly, coded correctly _____
   D. Chosen and coded incorrectly   _____

DRG
   A. Chosen and coded correctly   _____
   B. Chosen correctly, coded incorrectly _____
   C. Chosen incorrectly, coded correctly _____
   D. Chosen and coded incorrectly   _____

Note: A form can also be constructed to monitor CPT coding information instead of DRG.

Coding Audit Summary

Date: _____ Reviewed by: _____

Review Type: _____   MR #: _____
Name: _____   Account #: _____
FC: _____   Admit/DC Date: _____
LOS: _____   Disposition: _____
Attending Physician: _____   Surgeon/Consult: _____

Original Dx Codes	**Revised Dx Codes**	**Type of Change**		
1. _____	1. _____	Pr Dx	/_____/	
2. _____	2. _____	CC Dx	/_____/	
3. _____	3. _____	2nd Dx	/_____/	
4. _____	4. _____	Add Dx	/_____/	
5. _____	5. _____	Del Dx	/_____/	
6. _____	6. _____	Other	/_____/	
7. _____	7. _____			
8. _____	8. _____			
9. _____	9. _____			

Original Procedure Codes	**Revised Procedure Codes**	**Type of Change**		
1. _____	1. _____	Pr Proc	/_____/	
2. _____	2. _____	Sig Proc	/_____/	
3. _____	3. _____	2nd Proc	/_____/	
4. _____	4. _____	Add Proc	/_____/	
5. _____	5. _____	Del Proc	/_____/	
6. _____	6. _____	Other	/_____/	
7. _____	7. _____			
8. _____	8. _____			
9. _____	9. _____			

Date Coded: _____   Date of D/S: _____   Coder: _____

Documentation Issues: _____   Physician(s): _____
                 _____   _____
                 _____   _____

Findings/Recommendations: _____
_____
_____
_____
_____
_____

DRG Change: ☐ Yes   ☐ No

Original DRG: _____   Weight: _____   Reimbursement: _____
Revised DRG: _____   Weight: _____   Reimbursement: _____
Rebilling Date: _____   Wt. Diff: _____   Adjustment: _____

Coding Compliance Review Daily Worksheet
Inpatient Cases

Date of Review: _____

Name	Health Record #	D/C Date	Coder	Date Coded	Original DRG	Revised DRG	Positive Impact	Negative Impact	Comment	Variation Type

Coding Compliance Review
Inpatient Summary

Name: _____ Age: _____ ADM: _____

MR #: _____ Sex: _____ DISCH: _____

ACCT #: _____ MD: _____ Facility: _____

HIC #: _____ LOS: _____ Payer: _____

Original Description and Codes **Revised Description and Codes**

Diagnosis   DRG _____   Diagnosis   DRG _____

1. _____	1. _____	*Variance Type*
2. _____	2. _____	PrDx Chg /___/
3. _____	3. _____	ReSeq PrDx /___/
4. _____	4. _____	Add 2nd Dx /___/
5. _____	5. _____	Chg 2nd Dx /___/
6. _____	6. _____	PrProc Chg /___/
7. _____	7. _____	Chg 2nd Proc /___/
8. _____	8. _____	Add Proc /___/
9. _____	9. _____	Other /___/
10. _____	10. _____	

Operative Description and Codes **Operative Description and Codes**

1. _____   1. _____

2. _____   2. _____

3. _____   3. _____

4. _____   4. _____

5. _____   5. _____

6. _____   6. _____

Disposition Code: _____   Disposition Code: _____

Summary Findings: _____

_____

_____

Recommendations: _____

_____

_____

_____

Date Reviewed: _____   Date Sent to Rebill HIM: _____

Reviewer: _____

Orig. DRG Wt.: _____   Revised DRG Wt.: _____

Pmt: _____   Pmt.: _____

                                               Diff.: _____

Dictation

DxSum (dict): _____   H+P (dict): _____   Oper. (dict): _____

Typed: _____   Typed: _____   Typed: _____

Coding and DRG Variation Form

Payer: _____

As part of the DRG management program, selected records of Medicare patients are being reviewed for the documentation, coding, and DRG assignment to ensure that we are receiving the most equitable reimbursement. Please review the following change:

If you concur with the following, please make the changes. We will rebill this through Medicare. If you do not feel the changes are justified and appropriate, please comment at the bottom of this form.

Patient Name: _____   Account #: _____

Health Record #: _____   Discharge Date: _____

Original Diagnoses/Procedures	**Recommended Change**

Principal Dx: _____   _____

Additional Dx: _____   _____

_____   _____

Procedure: _____   _____

_____   _____

Additional documentation to support these recommended changes are found as listed below:

_____ Discharge Summary   Circle one or more
_____ History & Physical   A = 1st Dx, affect DRG
_____ Progress Notes   B = 1st Dx, not affect DRG
_____ Consults   C = Proc/CC, affect DRG
_____ Operative Reports   D = Other Dx, Proc code
_____ Lab   E = Attest
_____ X ray   F = Other: _____
_____ Other: _____

Action Needed for Change: _____

_____

_____

Original DRG: _____   New DRG: _____   Coder: _____

Reimbursement: _____   Reimbursement: _____   Difference: _____

Reviewer's Comments: _____

_____

_____

_____

Coding Services Review Tool

Physician Name: _____

Health Record #: _____

Place of Service: _____

Hospital ID#: _____

Date of Service: _____

Type		HPI	ROS	PFSH
Pf	=	1–3	–	–
Exp	=	1–3	1	–
Det	=	4+	2–9	1
Comp	=	4+	10+	2–3

■ HISTORY

CC: _____

DPI: Brief = 1–3
  Extended = 4+ or status of 3
    chronic or inactive conditions

___ Location
___ Quality
___ Severity
___ Duration
___ Timing
___ Context
___ Mod Factors
___ Signs/Sxs

___ Office visit – prev. exam
___ Consult – postop
___ 2nd opinion – proc-only

ROS (14):   (1 = PP; 2 to 9 = ext; 10+ = comp)

___ Constitutional
___ Eyes
___ ENT
___ CV
___ Respiratory
___ GI
___ GU

___ M/S
___ Integument
___ Neuro
___ Psych
___ Endocrine
___ Heme/lymph
___ Allergic/immuno

PFSH:
___ Past
___ Family
___ Social

(1 = pp) (2–3 = comp)

Selected: _____
Reviewed: _____

HISTORY ERROR TYPES

(1) ___ History of present illness does not support level selected

(2) ___ Review of systems: documentation does not support level selected

(3) ___ Past, family, and social history: documentation does not support level selected

■ EXAM   (1 = pp) (2 to 7 = exp/det) (8+ = comp)

Body Areas:
___ Head
___ Neck
___ Chest
___ Abdomen
___ Genitalia
___ Back
Each extremity:
___ L. arm   ___ L. leg
___ R. arm   ___ R. leg

Organ Systems:
___ Constitutional
___ Eyes
___ ENT
___ CV
___ Respiratory
___ GI (rectal)
___ GU
___ M/S
___ Integument

___ Neuro
___ Psych
___ Heme/lymph/immuno

Selected: _____
Reviewed: _____

DEFINITIONS

Problem-focused exam: Examination of single system or body area

Expanded problem-focused exam: Limited exam of 2–7 body areas or organ systems

Detailed exam: Minimum of 2 areas/systems with 4 or more items identified for each of 2 area/systems

Comprehensive exam: Examination of 8 or more areas/systems

EXAM ERROR TYPE

(4) ___ Exam: documentation does not support level selected

ECS Initials: _____

■ MEDICAL DECISION MAKING

A. Dx/Management Options	B. Data	C. Risk
1 pt = Minor problem (max of 2)	1 pt = Labs	1 = 1 minor problem, basic lab and/or X ray, no meds
1 pt ea. = Established (stable)	1 pt = X rays	
2 pt ea. = Established (worsening)	1 pt = Other (EEG, TMT, etc)	2 = 2 minor problems, 1 chronic, 1 acute, Pfts, BE, Bx, OTC drugs
3 pt = New w/o additional workup (max. 1)	2 pt = Interp. image, etc.	3 = 1 chronic (worsening), 2 stable chronic, 1 potential serious, stress TMT/MRI, Rx, ref. to surg
4 pt ea. = New w/additional workup	2 pt = Review old records	4 = Chronic illness w/severe exacerbation, life threatening injury/illness, emergency surgery or referral
	1 pt = Contact other provider	
	1 pt = Send for old records	
Total points:	Total points:	Level:

Selected: _____
Reviewed: _____

Medical decision making
(2 of 3 required)

MDM Type	A. Dx	B. Data	C. Risk
☐ SF	1	1	1
☐ L	2	2	2
☐ M	3	3	3
☐ H	4+	4+	4

MDM ERROR TYPE

(5) _____ Documentation does not support level of medical decision making selected

OTHER ERROR TYPES

(6) _____ Level selected requires documentation

(7) _____ Level selected requires documentation of all 3 components (Hx, Ex, MDM)

(8) _____ Documentation supports higher level

(9) _____ Physical presence requirement not met

(10) _____ Time not documented

(11) _____ Documentation does not support consult

(12) _____ Documentation does not support consult follow-up

(13) _____ Documentation does not support initial hospital care

(14) _____ Documentation does not support discharge day management

(15) _____ Documentation does not support subsequent hospital care

(16) _____ Documentation does not support observation

(17) _____ Documentation does not support critical care

(18) _____ Documentation does not support preventive exam

(19) _____ Correct procedure code not selected

(20) _____ Correct diagnosis code not selected

(21) _____ Multiple errors

Documented Error Type:

Correct procedure code selected?	☐ Yes	☐ No
Correct diagnosis selected?	☐ Yes	☐ No
Correct modifiers selected?	☐ Yes	☐ No

CPT Code Selected: _____
Documentation Supports CPT Code: _____
RVU Selected: _____
RVU Reviewed: _____

☐ N/A

Coding Validation Worksheet
Medicare Coding Compliance—DRG/ICD-9-CM

Patient: _____
Health Record No.: _____
Account No.: _____
Disposition: _____ LOS: _____

Age/Sex: _____
Adm. Date: _____
Disch. Date: _____
Physician: _____

Financial Class: _____

Facility: _____

Date Reviewed: _____

FACILITY NARRATIVE	FACILITY CODE		REVIEWER NARRATIVE	REVIEWER CODE	TYPE OF CHANGE
1			1		Chg Pdx
2			2		Chg 2d dx
3			3		Add 2d dx
4			4		Chg Pr Proc
5			5		Chg 2d Proc
6			6		Add Proc
7			7		
8			8		
9			9		

1			1	
2			2	
3			3	
4			4	
5			5	
6			6	
7			7	
8			8	
9			9	
10			10	

DRG VARIANCES

Hospital DRG: _____
Relative Weight: _____
Reimbursement: _____

Reviewer DRG: _____
Relative Weight: _____
Reimbursement: _____

[ ] Difference

Rationale for Change: _____
_____
_____
_____
_____

Dictation: H&P: _____ D/C Summary: _____ Op: _____

Compliance Audit

Health Record #: _____ _____   Date of Surgery: _____

Procedure: _____   Diagnosis: _____

Reviewer agrees with codes assigned to record?   ☐ Yes   ☐ No

Revised ICD-9-CM Diagnosis Codes: _____

_____

Revised CPT Procedure Codes/ICD-9-CM Procedure Codes: _____

_____

Record Completeness (Medical necessity for procedure/treatment was documented?):

    ☐ All complete
    ☐ Areas not completed or deficient (documented below)

_____

_____

_____

BILLING REVIEW

Registration information complete and form signed by patient/other?   ☐ Yes   ☐ No

    Deficiencies: _____

If Medicare, CCI edits applied to case where applicable?   ☐ Yes   ☐ No

    Deficiencies: _____

If resubmitted to carrier based on code/CCI edit changes,
was payment appropriately refunded or additional billed? _____

Submit case to Compliance Committee for further review and discussion?   ☐ Yes   ☐ No

_____   _____
Reviewer   Date

Inpatient Rebilling Log

Date: _____   Hospital: _____

Patient		DRG/ASC Chg		$ Amount	Date of		Received		Comments
Account #	Name	From	To		RA	Rebill	Amount	Date	

LTCH Coding Audit

Case Number: _____

Date: Reviewed by:

Review Type:

Name: _____
MR #: _____   Age: _____   Admit Date: _____
Account #: _____   Sex: _____   DC Date: _____
                                        MD: _____   LOS: _____

Original Dx Codes:	**Revised Dx Codes:**	**Type of Change:**
1. _____	1. _____	
2. _____	2. _____	Pr Dx /_____/
3. _____	3. _____	CC Dx /_____/
4. _____	4. _____	2nd Dx /_____/
5. _____	5. _____	Add Dx /_____/
6. _____	6. _____	Del Dx /_____/
7. _____	7. _____	Other /_____/
8. _____	8. _____	
9. _____	9. _____	

Original Procedure Codes:	**Revised Procedure Codes:**	**Type of Change:**
1. _____	1. _____	
2. _____	2. _____	Pr Proc /_____/
3. _____	3. _____	Sig Proc /_____/
4. _____	4. _____	2nd Proc /_____/
5. _____	5. _____	Add Proc /_____/
6. _____	6. _____	Del Proc /_____/
7. _____	7. _____	Other /_____/
8. _____	8. _____	
9. _____	9. _____	

Date Coded: _____   Date of D/S: _____   Coder: _____

Documentation Issues: _____
_____
_____
_____
_____
_____

Findings/Recommendations: _____
_____
_____
_____
_____

DRG Change: Yes _____   No _____

Original DRG: _____   Weight: _____   Reimbursement: _____
Revised DRG: _____   Weight: _____   Reimbursement: _____
Rebilling Date: _____   Wt. Diff: _____   Adjustment: _____

LTCH audit spreadsheet
Date: _____

Case #	Coder	PT Last Name	PT First Name	MR #	Acc #	Principal Diagnosis	DRG	Age	Sex	MD Last Name	MD First Name	Admit Date	D/C Date	LOS	Facility	Comments
1	EJ	Smith	Jimmie	10101	1111111	Aftercare Dig. Surgery	466	75	M	Frank	Ed	7/11/05	7/15/05	4	HSC	Add secondary procedure
2	EJ	Wesson	Sam	10102	1111112	Resp. failure	475	82	M	Camp	Earl	9/1/05	9/26/05	26	HSC	Documented as acute and chronic respiratory failure 518.84
3																
4																
5																
6																
7																
8																
9																
10																
11																
12																
13																
14																
15																
16																
17																
18																
19																
20																

MINIMUM DATA SET (MDS) ASSESSMENT SCHEDULE

NAME	ROOM	ADM. DATE	ARD[1]	A8a[2]	A8b[3]	R2b[4]

MDS must be completed after ARD and before RN date in R2b.

[1]ARD: Assessment Reference Date. This date establishes common reference point (end date) for all data on the MDS.

[2]A8a: Primary reason for assessment or assessments required by CFR 483.20.

[3]A8b: Assessments required by Medicare PPS for payment.

[4]R2b: Date RN Assessment Coordinator signed as complete.

Coding Compliance Prebill Review Form

Date: _____

Patient #: _____   Last Name: _____   DOD: _____

Original DRG: _____   Reimbursement: _____

Principal Diagnosis: _____

Change: _____

Justification: _____

*   *   *   *   *   *   *   *   *   *   *

Additional Diagnoses/Procedures	**Justification**
Add: _____	_____
_____	_____
_____	_____
Change: _____	_____
_____	_____
_____	_____
Delete: _____	_____
_____	_____
_____	_____
	_____

New DRG: _____   Reimbursement: _____   Differences: _____

Attest: _____

*   *   *   *   *   *   *   *   *   *   *

Comments: _____   Coder #: _____

_____

*   *   *   *   *

_____   Circle one or more: A = 1st Dx, affect DRG

_____   B = 1st Dx, not affect DRG

_____   C = Proc/CC, affect DRG

_____   D = Other dx, proc, code

_____   E = Attest

                                                   F = Repeat

Rebilling Coding Change Summary

Name: _____   Age: _____   Adm: _____

MR #: _____   Sex: _____   Disch: _____

Acct #: _____   MD: _____   Facility: _____

HIC #: _____   LOS: _____

Disposition: _____

Original Codes: Diagnosis	Revised Codes: Diagnosis
1. _____	1. _____
2. _____	2. _____
3. _____	3. _____
4. _____	4. _____
5. _____	5. _____
6. _____	6. _____
7. _____	7. _____
8. _____	8. _____
9. _____	9. _____
10. _____	10. _____

Operative Codes	Operative Codes
1. _____	1. _____
2. _____	2. _____
3. _____	3. _____
4. _____	4. _____
5. _____	5. _____
6. _____	6. _____

CPT Codes	CPT Codes
1. _____	1. _____
2. _____	2. _____
3. _____	3. _____
4. _____	4. _____
5. _____	5. _____
6. _____	6. _____

The above account/record has been identified to have a coding change. Please rebill with the revised codes as soon as possible. If you have any questions, please contact: [enter contact name] @ [enter telephone number and extension].

Date rebilled: _____

Return this form to the HIM Department once rebill has been processed. Thank you.

Appendix G

Functional Independence Measure (FIM)
Audit Worksheet

Function Modifiers

Complete the following specific functional items prior to scoring the FIM instrument. Some items require the use of the following FIM levels:

    7 = No accidents
    6 = No accidents; uses devices such as a catheter
    5 = One accident in past 7 days
    4 = Two accidents in past 7 days
    3 = Three accidents in past 7 days
    2 = Four accidents in past 7 days
    1 = Five or more accidents in past 7 days

When assigning a level to an item, enter the lower (or more dependent) score from these FIM levels.

	Facility		Auditor	
	Admit	D/C	Admit	D/C

Score items 1–4 using FIM levels.

1. Bladder: Level of assistance

2. Bladder: Frequency of accidents

3. Bowel: Level of assistance

4. Bowel: Frequency of accidents

Score items 5 and 6 using FIM levels. Use 0 if activity does not occur.

5. Tub transfer

6. Shower transfer

Code items 7 and 8 using the following: 3 = 150 ft.; 2 = 50–149 ft.; 1 = less than 50 ft.; 0 = activity does not occur.

7. Distance walked

8. Distance traveled in wheelchair

Score items 10 and 11 using FIM levels. Use 0 if activity does not occur.

10. Walk

11. Wheelchair

FIM Instruments

Score the FIM instruments using the following FIM levels:

    7 = Complete independence (timely, safely)
    6 = Modified independence (device)
    5 = Supervision (subject = 100%)
    4 = Minimal assistance (subject = 75% or more)
    3 = Moderate assistance (subject = 50% or more)
    2 = Maximal assistance (subject = 25% or more)
    1 = Total assistance (subject less than 25%)
    0 = Activity does not occur

	Facility		Auditor	
	Admit	D/C	Admit	D/C

Self-Care
A. Eating
B. Grooming
C. Bathing
D. Dressing: Upper
E. Dressing: Lower
F. Toileting

Sphincter Control
G. Bladder
H. Bowel

Transfers
I. Bed, chair, wheelchair
J. Toilet
K. Tub, shower

Locomotion
L. Walk/wheelchair (W=walk; C=wheelchair; B=both)
M. Stairs

Total Motor Score

Communication
N. Comprehension (A=audio; V=visual; B=both)
O. Expression (V=vocal; N=nonvocal; B=both)

Social Cognition
P. Social interaction
Q. Problem solving
R. Memory

Total Cognition Score

©2002 Patricia Trela and Anna Tran. All rights reserved.

254

Patient Assessment Instrument (PAI)
Audit Worksheet

Identification Information

Patient Name: _____   Facility Name: _____

Patient Medicare (HICN) #: _____   Facility Medicare Provider #: _____

Patient Health Record #: _____   Discharge Date: _____

Patient's DOB: _____ Age: _____

Payer Information

Primary Payment Source: _____   Secondary Payment Source _____

Admission Information	Discharge Information
Admission Date: _____	Discharge Date: _____
Admit From: _____	Discharged To: _____
Admission Class: _____	Length of Stay if Transferred: _____

Program Interruptions Dates

1st Interruption Date: _____   1st Return Date: _____

2nd Interruption Date: _____   2nd Return Date: _____

3rd Interruption Date: _____   3rd Return Date: _____

Medical Information

		Facility		Auditor	
		Admit	D/C	Admit	D/C
1.	Impairment Group	_____	_____	_____	_____
2.	Etiologic Diagnosis	_____		_____	
3.	Date of Onset of Impairment	_____		_____	
4.	Comordid Conditions (Use ICD-9-CM codes to enter up to 10 conditions.)	A _____	B _____	A _____	B _____
		C _____	D _____	C _____	D _____
		E _____	F _____	E _____	F _____
		G _____	H _____	G _____	H _____
		I _____	J _____	I _____	J _____
5.	Diagnosis for Interruption or Death	_____		_____	
6.	Complications during Rehab Stay	A _____	B _____	A _____	B _____
		C _____	D _____	C _____	D _____
		E _____	F _____	E _____	F _____
7.	**Admission FIM**	**Motor** _____	**Cognitive** ___	**Motor** _____	**Cognitive** ___
8.	**CMG and Tier**	_____		_____	

255

SNF PPS Compliance Audit
Medicare Part A

Patient Name/Health Record #: _____   **UB-92 Claim Period Dates:** _____

MEDICARE ELIGIBILITY REQUIREMENTS

☐ Eligible for Medicare benefits   ☐ 3-day hospital stay/30-day transfer

☐ In Medicare-certified bed   ☐ Condition treated in hospital or developed after admission

MEDICARE CERTIFICATION/RECERTIFICATION

Are certification and applicable recertifications completed, signed, and dated?   ☐ Yes   ☐ No

Describe problem(s): _____

ICD-9-CM DIAGNOSIS CODES

	Principle Diagnosis on UB-92	Consistent with MDS	Coded Accurately	Relates to Coverage or Services Billed
1		☐ Yes ☐ No	☐ Yes ☐ No	☐ Yes ☐ No
	Secondary Diagnosis on UB-92	**Consistent with MDS**	**Coded Accurately**	**Relates to Coverage or Services Billed**
2		☐ Yes ☐ No	☐ Yes ☐ No	☐ Yes ☐ No
3		☐ Yes ☐ No	☐ Yes ☐ No	☐ Yes ☐ No
4		☐ Yes ☐ No	☐ Yes ☐ No	☐ Yes ☐ No
5		☐ Yes ☐ No	☐ Yes ☐ No	☐ Yes ☐ No
6		☐ Yes ☐ No	☐ Yes ☐ No	☐ Yes ☐ No
7		☐ Yes ☐ No	☐ Yes ☐ No	☐ Yes ☐ No

Should other diagnoses be on the UB-92?   ☐ *Yes*   ☐ *No*

Notes: _____

BILLING VERIFICATION

RUG Verification	
HIPSS code on UB-92	
HIPSS code after audit	
A-3 date on UB-92	
A-3 matches MDS	☐ Yes ☐ No

Rehab RUG Verification	
Total therapy days on MDS	
Days after audit	
Total therapy minutes on MDS	
Minutes after audit	

THERAPY VERIFICATION

Observation Period	Speech Therapy			Occupational Therapy			Physical Therapy		
	MDS	Therapy Documentation	Billing Logs	MDS	Therapy Documentation	Billing Logs	MDS	Therapy Documentation	Billing Logs
Day 1									
Day 2									
Day 3									
Day 4									
Day 5									
Day 6									
Day 7									
Total Days									
Total Minutes									

Was therapy plan of care completed, signed, and dated by the physician before billing?   ☐ Yes   ☐ No

Comments: _____

ADL VERIFICATION

	Bed Mobility	Transferring	Toileting	Eating
MDS column A				
Score based on charting				
MDS column B				
Score based on charting				

Is MDS scoring supported by health record documentation?   ☐ Yes   ☐ No

NONREHAB RUG VERIFICATION

Description of Nonrehab Service	Health Record Documentation Supports the Service
	☐ Yes ☐ No
	☐ Yes ☐ No
	☐ Yes ☐ No

SNF PPS Compliance Audit
Medicare Part A

BILLING VERIFICATION for ANCILLARY SERVICES and SUPPLIES

Service Billed on UB-92	Specific Service and Date Based on Vendor Invoice	Physician Order Present		Documentation of Medical Necessity Present		Documentation That Service Was Delivered	
Therapy		☐ Yes	☐ No	☐ Yes	☐ No	☐ Yes	☐ No
Pharmacy/IV		☐ Yes	☐ No	☐ Yes	☐ No	☐ Yes	☐ No
Laboratory and Radiology		☐ Yes	☐ No	☐ Yes	☐ No	☐ Yes	☐ No
Therapy services		☐ Yes	☐ No	☐ Yes	☐ No	☐ Yes	☐ No
Medical Supplies		☐ Yes	☐ No	☐ Yes	☐ No	☐ Yes	☐ No
Ambulance		☐ Yes	☐ No	☐ Yes	☐ No	☐ Yes	☐ No
Special Tests		☐ Yes	☐ No	☐ Yes	☐ No	☐ Yes	☐ No
Hospital Outpatient Services		☐ Yes	☐ No	☐ Yes	☐ No	☐ Yes	☐ No
"Incident to" Services		☐ Yes	☐ No	☐ Yes	☐ No	☐ Yes	☐ No
Other		☐ Yes	☐ No	☐ Yes	☐ No	☐ Yes	☐ No

Based on health record documentation, identify other services that should have been billed by the SNF but were not.

_____

_____

_____

_____

2 of 2

Statistics for Coding Quality Monitoring

Coder: _____   Type: _____

Total number of records in sample   _____

	#	%
Principal diagnosis (total)		
A. Chosen and coded correctly	_____	_____
B. Chosen correctly, coded incorrectly	_____	_____
C. Chosen incorrectly, coded correctly	_____	_____
D. Chosen and coded incorrectly	_____	_____
Secondary diagnoses found/total possible secondary diagnosis (total)		
A. All found	_____	_____
B. All not found: # missed	_____	_____
Secondary diagnoses coded/total possible secondary diagnosis (total)		
A. All coded correctly	_____	_____
B. All codes not correct: # missed	_____	_____
Principal procedure (total)		
A. Chosen and coded correctly	_____	_____
B. Chosen correctly, coded incorrectly	_____	_____
C. Chosen incorrectly, coded correctly	_____	_____
D. Chosen and coded incorrectly	_____	_____
Secondary procedures found/total possible secondary procedures (total)		
A. All found	_____	_____
B. All not found: # missed	_____	_____
Secondary procedures coded/total possible secondary procedures (total)		
A. All coded correctly		
B. All codes not correct: # missed		
DRG (total)		
A. DRG all correct	_____	
B. DRG not correct	_____	
1. Due to principal diagnosis	_____	
2. Due to secondary diagnosis	_____	
3. Due to principal procedure	_____	
4. Due to secondary procedure	_____	
CPT (total)		
A. All CPT codes correct	_____	
B. All CPT codes not correct: # wrong	_____	
Total records coded completely correctly	_____	_____
Total possible choices	_____	_____
Total actual correct	_____	_____

Appendix H

Developing a Coding Compliance Policy Document (Updated)

Organizations using diagnosis and procedure codes to report healthcare services must have formal policies and corresponding procedures in place that provide instruction on the entire process—from the point of service to the billing statement or claim form. Coding compliance policies serve as a guide to performing coding and billing functions and provide documentation of the organization's intent to correctly report services. The policies should include facility-specific documentation requirements, payer regulations and policies, and contractual arrangements for coding consultants and outsourcing services. This information may be covered in payer-provider contracts or found in Medicare and Medicaid manuals and bulletins.

Following are selected tenets that address the process of code selection and reporting. These tenets may be referred to as "coding protocols," a "coding compliance program," "organizational coding guidelines," or a similar name. These tenets are an important part of any organization's compliance plan and the key to preventing coding errors and resulting reimbursement problems. Examples are taken from both outpatient and inpatient coding processes for illustrative purposes only. This document cannot serve as a complete coding compliance plan but will be useful as a guide for creating a more comprehensive resource to meet individual organizational needs.

A coding compliance plan should include the following components:

- A general policy statement about the commitment of the organization to correctly assign and report codes

    Example: Memorial Medical Center is committed to establishing and maintaining clinical coding and insurance claims processing procedures to ensure, through accurate information system entries, that reported codes reflect actual services provided.

Source: Bielby, Judy A., et al. Developing a Coding Compliance Policy Document. *Journal of AHIMA* (Updated March 2010).

Editor's note: This update replaces the July 2001 practice brief "Developing a Coding Compliance Policy Document."

- The source of the official coding guidelines used to direct code selection

    Example: ICD-9-CM code selection follows the coding rules and conventions included with the ICD-9-CM code set; the *ICD-9-CM Official Guidelines for Coding and Reporting* developed by the cooperating parties; the American Hospital Association's (AHA) *Coding Clinic for ICD-9-CM,* the official publication for ICD-9-CM coding guidelines; and advice approved by the cooperating parties.

    Example: CPT or HCPCS code selection follows the guidelines set forth in the CPT manual and in *CPT Assistant,* published by the American Medical Association, and AHA *Coding Clinic for HCPCS,* the official coding clearinghouse for facility-based HCPCS coding questions.

- The parties delegated with responsibility for code assignment

    Example: For inpatient records, medical record analyst I staff are responsible for analysis of records and assignment of the correct ICD-9-CM codes on the basis of documentation by the attending physician or provider.

    Example: Emergency department evaluation and management levels for physician services will be selected by the physician and validated by outpatient record analysts using the Centers for Medicare and Medicaid Services and American Medical Association documentation guidelines. When a variance occurs, the following steps are taken for resolution (the actual document should follow with procedure details).

- The procedure to follow when the clinical information is not clear enough to assign the correct code

    Example: When the documentation used to assign codes is ambiguous or incomplete, the physician must be contacted to clarify the information and complete or amend the record, if necessary. Standard protocols for adding documentation to a record must be followed in accordance with the applicable laws and regulations.

- Specification of the policies and procedures that apply to specific locations and care settings. Official coding guidelines for inpatient reporting and outpatient or physician reporting are different. This means an organization that is developing a facility-specific coding guideline for emergency department services should designate that the coding rules or guidelines that apply only in this setting.

    Example: When a facility reports an injection of a drug provided in the emergency department to a Medicare beneficiary, the appropriate CPT or HCPCS code for the administration of the injection is reported in addition to the evaluation and management service code and drug code. CPT codes are reported whether a physician provides the injection personally or a nurse is carrying out a physician's order. This instruction does not always apply for reporting professional services in the clinics because administration of medication is considered bundled with the corresponding evaluation and management service for Medicare patients.

Example: When reporting diagnoses for outpatient claims, diagnoses that are documented as "probable," "suspected," "questionable," "rule-out," or "working diagnosis" are not to have a code assigned as a confirmed diagnosis. With such uncertain conditions, the code for the condition established to the highest degree of certainty at the close of the encounter should be assigned, such as a symptom, sign, abnormal test result, or clinical finding.

- Applicable reporting requirements required by specific agencies. The document should include where instructions on payer-specific requirements may be accessed.

  Example: For Medicare patients receiving immunization for both influenza virus and pneumococcus during the same visit, report ICD-9-CM diagnosis code V06.6 along with CPT or HCPCS codes G0008 and G0009 and the applicable vaccine codes for the specific type of influenza virus and pneumococcal vaccines administered.

  Many of these procedures will be put into software databases and would not be written as a specific policy. This is true with most billing software, whether for physician services or through the charge description master used by many hospitals.

- Procedures for correction of inaccurate code assignments in the clinical database and to the agencies where the codes have been reported

  Example: When an error in code assignment is discovered after bill release and the claim has already been submitted, this is the process required to update and correct the information system and facilitate claim amendment or correction (the actual document should follow with appropriate details).

- Areas of risk that have been identified through audits or monitoring. Each organization should have a defined audit plan for code accuracy and consistency review, and corrective actions should be outlined for problems that are identified.

  Example: A hospital might identify that urosepsis is being incorrectly reported as sepsis when there is no documentation in the medical record of sepsis. The specific reference to the *ICD-9-CM Official Guidelines for Coding and Reporting* and *Coding Clinic for ICD-9-CM* could be listed with instructions about correct coding of these conditions and the process to be used to correct the deficiency.

- Identification of essential coding resources available to and used by coding professionals

  Example: Updated ICD-9-CM, CPT, and HCPCS level II code books are used by all coding professionals. Even if the hospital uses automated encoding software, at least one printed copy of the coding manuals should be available for reference.

  Example: Updated encoder software, including the appropriate version of the National Correct Coding Initiative edits and DRG and APC grouper software, is available to the appropriate personnel.

  Example: *Coding Clinic for ICD-9-CM, Coding Clinic for HCPCS,* and *CPT Assistant* are available to all coding professionals.

- A process for coding new procedures or unusual diagnoses

  Example: When the coding professional encounters an unusual diagnosis, the coding supervisor or the attending physician is consulted. Follow the alphabetic index guidance when coding syndromes. In the absence of index guidance, assign codes for the documented manifestations of the syndrome. If, after research, a code cannot be identified, the documentation is submitted to the AHA for clarification.

- A procedure to identify any optional codes gathered for statistical purposes by the facility and clarification of the appropriate use of E codes

  Example: All ICD-9-CM procedure codes in the surgical range (ICD-9-CM Volume III codes 01.01–86.99) shall be reported for inpatients. In addition, codes reported from the nonsurgical section include the following (completed document should list the actual codes to be reported).

  Example: All appropriate E codes for adverse effects of drugs must be reported. In addition, this facility reports all E codes following the instructions outlined in the *ICD-9-CM Official Guidelines for Coding and Reporting.*

- Appropriate methods for resolving coding or documentation disputes with physicians

  Example: When the physician disagrees with the facility's interpretation and application of the official coding guidelines, the case is referred to the medical records committee after review by the designated physician liaison from that group.

- A procedure for processing claim rejections

  Example: All rejected claims pertaining to diagnosis and procedure codes should be returned to coding staff for review or correction. Any chargemaster issues should be forwarded to the chargemaster committee liaison. All clinical codes, including modifiers, must never be changed or added without review by coding staff with access to the appropriate documentation.

  Example: If a claim is rejected because of the codes provided in the medical record abstract, the billing department notifies the coding supervisor for a review rather than changing the code to a payable code and resubmitting the claim.

- A statement clarifying that codes will not be assigned, modified, or excluded solely for the purpose of maximizing reimbursement or avoiding reduced payment. Clinical codes will not be changed or amended merely because of either physicians' or patients' request to have the service in question covered by insurance. If the initial code assignment did not reflect the actual services, codes may be revised on the basis of supporting documentation

  Example: A patient calls the business office saying that her insurance carrier did not pay for her mammogram. After investigating, the HIM coding staff discover that the coding was appropriate for a screening mammogram and that this is a noncovered service with the insurance provider. The code is not changed, and the matter is referred back to the business office for explanation to the patient that she should contact her insurance provider with any dispute over coverage of service.

Example: Part of a payment is denied, and after review, the supervisor discovers that a modifier should have been appended to the CPT code to denote a separately identifiable service. Modifier -25 is added to the code set and the corrected claim is resubmitted.

Example: A physician approaches the coding supervisor with a request to change the diagnosis codes for a patient because the patient currently has a preexisting condition that is not covered by the current health plan. The coding supervisor must explain to the physician that falsifying insurance claims is illegal. If the physician insists, the physician liaison for the medical record committee is contacted, and the matter is turned over to that committee for resolution, if necessary.

Example: When a hospital-acquired condition is clearly documented and meets official coding guidelines as a reportable diagnosis, the coder must report the diagnosis code with the correct present on admission indicator even when it results in reduced payment for the facility.

- The use of and reliance on encoders within the organization. Coding staff cannot rely solely on computerized encoders. Current coding manuals must be readily accessible, and the staff must be educated appropriately to detect inappropriate logic or errors in encoding software. When errors in logic or code crosswalks are discovered, they are reported to the vendor immediately by the coding supervisor.

Example: During the coding process, an error is identified in the crosswalk between the ICD-9-CM Volume III code and the CPT code. This error is reported to the software vendor, with proper documentation and notification of all staff using the encoder to not rely on the encoder for code selection.

- Medical records are analyzed and codes selected only with complete and appropriate physician documentation available. According to coding guidelines, codes are not assigned without supporting documentation from the provider. The guidelines also state that the entire record should be reviewed to determine the specific reason for the encounter and the conditions treated.

Example: If records are coded without a discharge summary, they are flagged in the computer system. When the summaries are added to the record, the record is returned to the coding professional for review of codes. If there are any inconsistencies, appropriate steps are taken for review of the changes.

Additional Elements

A coding compliance document should include a reference to the AHIMA Standards of Ethical Coding. Reference to the data quality assessment procedures must be included in a coding compliance plan to establish the mechanism for determining areas of risk. Reviews will identify the need for further education and increased monitoring for those areas in which either coding variances or documentation deficiencies are identified.

Specific and detailed coding guidelines that cover the reporting of typical services provided by a facility or organization create tools for data consistency and reliability by ensuring that all coders interpret clinical documentation and apply coding principles in the same manner.

The format for facility-specific guidelines is most useful when organized by patient or service type and easily referenced by using a table of contents. If the facility-specific guidelines are maintained electronically, they should be searchable by key terms. Placing the coding guidelines on a facility intranet is a very efficient way to ensure their use and it also enables timely and efficient updating and distribution. References or live links should be provided to supporting documents such as Uniform Hospital Discharge Data Sets or other regulatory requirements outlining reporting procedures or code assignments. Facility-specific guidelines must be consistent with ethical coding practices, consistent with official coding guidelines, easily accessible, and updated on a regular basis.

References

AHIMA. "Managing an Effective Query Process." *Journal of AHIMA* 79, no. 10 (Oct. 2008): 83–88.

AHIMA Coding Practice Team. "Developing a Coding Compliance Policy Document." *Journal of AHIMA* 72, no. 7 (Jul. 2001): 88A–C.

AHIMA House of Delegates, "AHIMA Standards of Ethical Coding" September 2008. Available online at http://library.ahima.org/xpedio/groups/public/documents/ahima/bok2_001166.hcsp.

AHIMA Practice Councils (Clinical Terminology/Classification, Quality Initiatives/Secondary Data). "Understanding HACs and SREs for Quality Reporting and Reimbursement." *Journal of AHIMA* 80, no. 9 (Sept. 2009): 60–65.

Comfort, Angela D., and Linda Schwab. "Facility Specific ICD-9-CM Coding Guidelines." AHIMA audio seminar. October 30, 2008. Available online at https://www.ahimastore.org/ProductDetailAudioSeminars.aspx?ProductID=14012.

Prepared by

Judy A. Bielby, MBA, RHIA, CPHQ, CCS

Prepared by (original)

AHIMA's Coding Practice Team and reviewed by the Coding Policy and Strategy Committee and the Society for Clinical Coding Data Quality Committee

Appendix I

AHIMA Practice Brief: Internet Resources for Accurate Coding and Reimbursement Practices (Updated)

The availability of valuable information on the Internet has a positive effect on how the health information coding profession meets today's coding and reimbursement challenges. Coding professionals have access to Internet resources that assist with legislation, coding questions, coding education, payer policy, and clinical research. The Internet has also made it possible to network with coding professionals on a national level in virtual communities of practice.

This Internet resource guide was developed as a convenient resource for coding professionals in all settings. The list is not exhaustive, nor does inclusion on this list represent AHIMA's endorsement. All URLs were accurate at press time, but keep in mind the dynamic nature of Web content.

Editor's note: This update replaces the July 2004 practice brief "Internet Resources for Accurate Coding and Reimbursement Practices." The links provided were current at publication of this practice brief.

Recommended Resources	Description	Sponsoring Organization	Web Site
Health Insurance Portability and Accountability Act (HIPAA) Administrative Simplification			
Standards for Code Sets	Under HIPAA, this is any set of codes used to encode data elements, such as tables of terms, medical concepts, medical diagnostic codes, or medical procedure codes.	Centers for Medicare and Medicaid Services	http://www.cms.hhs.gov/ TransactionCodeSetsStands/ 02_TransactionsandCodeSets Regulations.asp#TopOfPage
Current Dental Terminology (CDT)	The official code set used to report medical services and procedures performed by dental professionals.	American Dental Association	www.ada.org/prof/resources/ topics/dentalcontent.asp
Healthcare Common Procedure Coding System (HCPCS) Level I —Current Procedural Terminology (CPT)	The official code set used to report procedures and services provided by healthcare professionals and outpatient institutions.	American Medical Association	www.ama-assn.org/ama/pub/ physician-resources/solutions- managing-your-practice/ coding-billing-insurance/ cpt.shtml
Healthcare Common Procedure Coding System (HCPCS) Level II—HCPCS National Codes	The official code set used by healthcare professionals and outpatient institutions to report products, supplies, and services not included in the CPT code set.	Centers for Medicare and Medicaid Services	www.cms.hhs.gov/ MedHCPCSGenInfo/
International Classification of Diseases, Ninth Revision, Clinical Modification (ICD-9-CM) Volumes I and II	Until October 1, 2013, the official coding classification system used by healthcare professionals and institutions to report diagnosis information.	National Center for Health Statistics	www.cdc.gov/nchs/icd/ icd9cm.htm
International Classification of Diseases Ninth Revision Clinical Modification (ICD-9-CM Volume III)	Until October 1, 2013, the official code set used by inpatient hospital institutions to report procedural information.	Centers for Medicare and Medicaid Services	www.cms.hhs.gov/ ICD9ProviderDiagnosticCodes/
International Classification of Diseases, Tenth Revision, Clinical Modification (ICD-10-CM)	Effective October 1, 2013, the official coding classification system to be used by healthcare professionals and institutions to report diagnosis information.	National Center for Health Statistics	www.cdc.gov/nchs/icd/ icd10cm.htm
International Classification of Diseases, Tenth Revision, Procedure Coding System (ICD-10-PCS)	Effective October 1, 2013, the official code set to be used by inpatient hospital institutions to report procedural information.	Centers for Medicare and Medicaid Services	www.cms.hhs.gov/ICD10/
National Drug Code (NDC)	A coding system for pharmacies to report services, supplies, drugs, and biologic information.	US Food and Drug Administration	www.fda.gov/Drugs/ InformationOnDrugs/ ucm142438.htm
Standards for Electronic Transactions	Under HIPAA, this is a transaction that complies with the applicable HIPAA standard.		
Designated Standard Maintenance Organization (DSMO)	The DSMO was established in the final HIPAA rule and is charged with maintaining the standards for electronic transactions and developing or modifying an adopted standard.	Secretary of the Department of Health and Human Services	www.hipaa-dsmo.org
Accredited Standards Committee X12 (ASC X12)	ASC X12 is a designated committee under the DSMO that develops uniform standards for cross-industry exchange of business transactions through electronic data interchange standards.	American National Standards Institute	www.x12.org

Recommended Resources	Description	Sponsoring Organization	Web Site
Health Insurance Portability and Accountability Act (HIPAA) Administrative Simplification (*continued*)			
Dental Content Committee (DeCC) of the American Dental Association	DeCC is the designated committee under the DSMO responsible for addressing standard transaction content on behalf of the dental sector of the healthcare community.	American Dental Association	www.ada.org/prof/resources/topics/dentalcontent.asp
Health Level Seven International (HL7)	HL7 is a designated organization under the DSMO that addresses issues at the seventh, or application, level of healthcare systems interconnections.	Health Level Seven International	www.hl7.org
National Council for Prescription Drug Programs (NCPDP)	A designated committee under the DSMO that specializes in developing standards for exchanging prescription and payment information.	NCPDP	www.ncpdp.org
National Uniform Billing Committee (NUBC)	A designated committee under the DSMO that is responsible for identifying data elements and designing the CMS-1450.	American Hospital Association	www.nubc.org
National Uniform Claim Committee (NUCC)	The national group that replaced the Uniform Claim Form Task Force in 1995 and developed a standard data set to be used in the transmission of noninstitutional provider claims to and from third-party payers.	American Medical Association	www.nucc.org
Other Electronic Transaction Resources			
Electronic Data Interchange (EDI)	A standard transmission format using strings of data for business information communicated among the computer systems of independent organizations.	Centers for Medicare and Medicaid Services	www.cms.hhs.gov/ElectronicBillingEDITrans/
National Provider Identifier (NPI)	An alphanumeric identifier used to identify individual healthcare providers for Medicare billing purposes and intended for use with all insurance plans.	Centers for Medicare and Medicaid Services	www.cms.hhs.gov/NationalProvIdentStand/
Washington Publishing Company (WPC)	WPC manages and distributes EDI from organizations that develop, maintain, and implement EDI standards. The WPC home page provides implementation guides such as the X12N HIPAA Implementation Guide, educational resources, and additional HIPAA tools.	Washington Publishing Company	www.wpc-edi.com/
Workgroup for Electronic Data Interchange (WEDI)	A consortium of leaders within the healthcare industry that has been involved in developing electronic data interchange standards for billing transactions.	Workgroup for Electronic Data Interchange	www.wedi.org
Versions 5010, D.0, and 3.0	Versions 5010, D.0, and 3.0 are required by the modifications made to HIPAA in January 2009 and to be implemented over the next few years.	Centers for Medicare and Medicaid Services	www.cms.hhs.gov/Versions5010andD0/

(Continued on next page)

Recommended Resources	Description	Sponsoring Organization	Web Site
Health Insurance Portability and Accountability Act (HIPAA) Administrative Simplification (*continued*)			
Official ICD-9-CM Resources			
American Hospital Association (AHA) Coding Clinic for ICD-9-CM	Official publication for ICD-9-CM coding guidelines and coding advice as approved by the four cooperating parties (AHA, AHIMA, CMS, NCHS).	American Hospital Association	www.ahacentraloffice.org/ahacentraloffice/html/icd9cm.html and www.ahacentraloffice.org/ahacentraloffice/html/products.html
ICD-9-CM Official Guidelines for Coding and Reporting	Official coding guidelines developed to assist coding professionals in situations in which ICD-9-CM does not provide instruction.	National Center for Health Statistics	www.cdc.gov/nchs/icd/icd9cm_addenda_guidelines.htm
ICD-9-CM Code Updates (Coordination and Maintenance Committee and addenda)	Addendum to the annual (biannual effective April 2005) diagnosis code updates and Coordination and Maintenance Committee reports.	National Center for Health Statistics	www.cdc.gov/nchs/icd/icd9cm_maintenance.htm and www.cdc.gov/nchs/icd/icd9cm_addenda_guidelines.htm
ICD-9-CM Volume III Code Updates (Coordination and Maintenance Committee and addenda)	Addendum to the annual (biannual effective April 2005) procedure code updates.	Centers for Medicare and Medicaid Services	www.cms.hhs.gov/ICD9ProviderDiagnosticCodes/
ICD-10-CM/PCS Resources			
ICD-10-CM	Official coding guidelines developed to assist coding professionals in situations in which ICD-10-CM does not provide instruction.	National Center for Health Statistics	www.cdc.gov/nchs/icd/icd10cm.htm
2009 ICD-10-PCS	This manual is written as a general introduction for data managers, payers, administrators, and medical record coders.	Centers for Medicare and Medicaid Services	www.cms.hhs.gov/ICD10/01m_2009_ICD10PCS.asp#TopOfPage
Diagnosis Code Set General Equivalence Mapping (GEM) Files ICD-10-CM to ICD-9-CM and ICD-9-CM to ICD-10-CM	Mappings between ICD-9-CM and ICD-10-CM attempt to find corresponding diagnosis codes between the two code sets, insofar as this is possible.	National Center for Health Statistics	www.cdc.gov/nchs/icd/icd10cm.htm
2009 Procedure Code Set General Equivalence Mapping (GEM) Files ICD-10-PCS to ICD-9-CM and ICD-9-CM to ICD-10-PCS	Mappings between ICD-9-CM and ICD-10-PCS attempt to find corresponding procedure codes between the two code sets, insofar as this is possible.	Centers for Medicare and Medicaid Services	www.cms.hhs.gov/ICD10/01m_2009_ICD10PCS.asp#TopOfPage
HCPCS Level I CPT Resources			
CPT Category I, II, III Updates	Category I codes are updated annually with vaccine codes updated twice a year. The process and frequency of updating category I, II, and III codes is described on the AMA Web site.	American Medical Association	www.ama-assn.org/ama/no-index/physician-resources/3882.shtml
CPT Assistant	A monthly newsletter that provides official CPT coding advice.	American Medical Association	https://catalog.ama-assn.org/Catalog/product/product_detail.jsp?productId=prod170136

Recommended Resources	Description	Sponsoring Organization	Web Site
Health Insurance Portability and Accountability Act (HIPAA) Administrative Simplification (*continued*)			
CPT Network	Resource for CPT coding answers.	American Medical Association	www.ama-assn.org/ama/no-index/physician-resources/16625.shtml
CPT Change Request Forms	CPT code modification process and request for changes.	American Medical Association	www.ama-assn.org/ama/pub/physician-resources/solutions-managing-your-practice/coding-billing-insurance/cpt/applying-cpt-codes/request-form-categories-i-iii.shtml
HCPCS Level II Resources			
Healthcare Common Procedure Coding System (HCPCS) Level II Coding Procedures	National codes are published annually and go into effect at the beginning of each year. Temporary codes can be revised quarterly, and the changes are made available electronically and published on an annual basis.	Centers for Medicare and Medicaid Services	www.cms.hhs.gov/MedHCPCSGenInfo/Downloads/LevelIICoding Procedures.pdf
AHA Coding Clinic for HCPCS	Official clearinghouse for advice on the proper use of level I HCPCS codes for hospital providers and certain level II HCPCS codes for hospitals, physicians, and other health professionals who bill Medicare.	American Hospital Association	www.ahacentraloffice.org/ahacentraloffice/html/products.html
CDT Resources			
CDT Updates	Code revisions are published and effective biannually at the beginning of odd-numbered years.	American Dental Association	www.ada.org/prof/resources/topics/cdt/index.asp
Additional Coding Classification Systems, Nomenclatures, and Vocabularies			
Diagnostic and Statistical Manual of Mental Disorders, Fourth Edition (DSM-IV)	A nomenclature to standardize the diagnostic process for patients with psychiatric disorders; includes codes that correspond to ICD-9-CM codes.	American Psychiatric Association	www.appi.org/dsm.cfx
Alternative Billing Concept (ABC) Codes	Contains more than 4,500 codes that describe what is said, done, ordered, prescribed, or distributed by providers of alternative medicine. Disciplines covered by this system include acupuncture, holistic medicine, massage therapy, homeopathy, naturopathy, ayurvedic medicine, chiropractors, and midwifery.	ABC Coding Solutions (formerly Alternative Link)	www.abccodes.com/ali/home/
Clinical Care Classification (CCC) System	A taxonomy of nursing diagnoses and nursing interventions.	The CCC System emerged from the federally funded Home Care Project conducted at Georgetown University School of Nursing.	www.sabacare.com
World Health Organization (WHO) International Classification of Diseases (ICD)	The ICD-10 version of the disease class-ification system developed by the World Health Organization is used to report morbidity and mortality information worldwide. Effective with deaths occur-ring in 1999, the United States replaced ICD-9 with ICD-10 for mortality reporting.	World Health Organization	www.who.int/classifications/icd/en/

(*Continued on next page*)

Recommended Resources	Description	Sponsoring Organization	Web Site
Health Insurance Portability and Accountability Act (HIPAA) Administrative Simplification (*continued*)			
World Health Organization (WHO) International Classification for Primary Care, Second Edition (ICPC-2)	A reliable classification system for primary care physicians that enables the labeling of the most prevalent conditions that exist in the community, as well as symptoms and complaints.	Published by the World Organization of Family Doctors (Wonca)	http://www.who.int/ classifications/icd/adaptations/ icpc2/en/index.html
International Classification of Diseases for Oncology, Third Edition (ICD-O-3)	The standard tool for coding diagnoses of neoplasms in tumor and cancer registrars and in pathology laboratories. ICD-O-3 is a dual classification with coding systems for both topography and morphology. The topography code describes the site of origin of the neoplasm and uses the same three- and four-character categories as in the neoplasm section of chapter II, ICD-10.	World Health Organization	www.who.int/classifications/ icd/adaptations/oncology/en/ index.html
International Classification of Functioning, Disability and Health (ICF)	The ICF is a health and health-related classification system that reports body functions and structures, activities, and participation.	World Health Organization	www.who.int/classifications/ icf/en/
Logical Observation Identifiers Names and Codes (LOINC)	The LOINC coding system electronically exchanges laboratory and clinical information.	The Regenstrief Institute maintains the LOINC database and its supporting documentation.	http://loinc.org/
MEDCIN	MEDCIN is a terminology and presentation engine. It includes more than 250,000 clinical data elements encompassing symptoms, history, physical examination, tests, diagnoses, and therapy.	Medicomp Systems, Inc.	www.medicomp.com
Medical Dictionary for Regulatory Activities (MedDRA)	MedDRA is a global standard medical terminology used to classify adverse event information associated with the use of biopharmaceuticals and other medical products (e.g., medical devices and vaccines).	Maintenance and Support Services Organization	www.meddramsso.com/index. asp
RxNorm	RxNorm is a clinical drug nomenclature that provides standard names for clinical drugs (active ingredient, strength, and dose forms).	National Library of Medicine	www.nlm.nih.gov/research/ umls/rxnorm/index.html
NANDA International (formerly North American Nursing Diagnosis Association)	NANDA International nursing diagnoses have evolved from an alphabetical listing in the mid-1980s to a conceptual system that guides the classification of nursing diagnoses in a taxonomy.	NANDA International	www.nanda.org/Home.aspx
Nursing Interventions Classification (NIC)	NIC is a comprehensive, research-based, standardized classification of interventions that nurses perform.	University of Iowa College of Nursing	www.nursing.uiowa. edu/excellence/nursing_ knowledge/clinical_ effectiveness/nic.htm
Nursing Outcomes Classification (NOC)	NOC is a comprehensive, standardized classification of patient/client outcomes developed to evaluate the effects of nursing interventions.	University of Iowa College of Nursing	www.nursing.uiowa. edu/excellence/nursing_ knowledge/clinical_ effectiveness/noc.htm

Recommended Resources	Description	Sponsoring Organization	Web Site
Health Insurance Portability and Accountability Act (HIPAA) Administrative Simplification (*continued*)			
Omaha System	The Omaha System is a research-based, comprehensive taxonomy designed to generate meaningful data after usual or routine documentation of client care.	Omaha System Advisory Committee	www.omahasystem.org
Systematized Nomenclature of Dentistry (SNODENT)	SNODENT is a systematized nomenclature of dentistry containing dental diagnoses, signs, symptoms, and complaints.	American Dental Association	www.ada.org
Systematized Nomenclature of Medicine—Clinical Terms (SNOMED CT)	SNOMED CT is a comprehensive clinical terminology and infrastructure that enables a consistent way of capturing, sharing, and aggregating health data across specialties and sites of care.	International Health Terminology Standards Development Organisation	www.ihtsdo.org/snomed-ct/
Universal Medical Device Nomenclature System (UMDNS)	UMDNS is a standard international nomenclature and coding system used to facilitate identifying, processing, filing, storing, retrieving, transferring, and communicating data about medical devices.	ECRI Institute (formerly the Emergency Care Research Institute)	www.ecri.org/Products/Pages/UMDNS.aspx
Health, Research, and Comparative Data			
Unified Medical Language System (UMLS)	A program initiated by the National Library of Medicine to build an intelligent, automated system that can understand biomedical concepts, words, and expressions and their interrelationships.	National Library of Medicine	www.nlm.nih.gov/research/umls/
MedlinePlus	MedlinePlus brings together authoritative information from the National Library of Medicine, National Institutes of Health, and other government agencies and health-related organizations. MEDLINE searches are included. MedlinePlus also provides drug information, a medical encyclopedia, interactive patient tutorials, and timely health news.	US National Library of Medicine and National Institutes of Health	www.nlm.nih.gov/medlineplus/
Agency for Healthcare Research and Quality (AHRQ)	AHRQ supports research and provides information on the quality of healthcare, patient safety issues, and healthcare costs.	Department of Health and Human Services	www.ahrq.gov
Medicare Provider Analysis and Review (MEDPAR)	The MEDPAR database is used for administrative purposes to collect information on Medicare claims and consists of data such as diagnosis related groups (DRGs), ICD-9-CM codes, Medicare coverage information, and patient demographics.	Centers for Medicare and Medicaid Services	www.cms.hhs.gov/MedicareFeeforSvcPartsAB/03_MEDPAR.asp#TopOfPage
American Hospital Directory (AHD)	The AHD provides an inpatient and outpatient Medicare claims database for more than 6,000 hospitals.	American Hospital Directory	www.ahd.com
Statistics			
National Committee on Vital Healthcare and Statistics (NCVHS)	NCVHS serves as a national advisory board to the public on health data, statistics, and information systems.	Department of Health and Human Services	www.ncvhs.hhs.gov

(*Continued on next page*)

Recommended Resources	Description	Sponsoring Organization	Web Site
Health Insurance Portability and Accountability Act (HIPAA) Administrative Simplification (*continued*)			
National Center for Health Statistics (NCHS)	NCHS is a public health statistics agency charged with collecting statistical information critical for improving public health in the United States.	Centers for Disease Control and Prevention	www.cdc.gov/nchs
Centers for Disease Control and Prevention (CDC)	CDC includes federal agencies that oversee health promotion and disease control and prevention activities in the United States.	Centers for Disease Control and Prevention	www.cdc.gov
National Vital Statistics System (NVSS)	NVSS provides statistical information compiled at the state level. Statistics include births, deaths, and fetal deaths.	Centers for Disease Control and Prevention	www.cdc.gov/nchs/nvss.htm
Clinical Resources			
National Institutes of Health (NIH)	NIH is the nation's medical research organization, consisting of 18 separate health institutes, the National Center for Complementary and Alternative Medicine, and the National Library of Medicine.	Department of Health and Human Services	www.nih.gov
National Library of Medicine (NLM)	NLM is the national online library for biomedicine and health science information.	National Institutes of Health	www.nlm.nih.gov
The Visible Human Project	NLM's development of anatomically detailed and three-dimensional representations of normal human bodies.	National Institutes of Health	www.nlm.nih.gov/research/visible/visible_human.html
Virtual Hospital	Virtual Hospital is a digital health sciences library for healthcare providers and patients. It contains thousands of textbooks and booklets.	University of Iowa Health Care	www.vh.org
Compliance Resources			
Department of Health and Human Services (HHS) Office of Inspector General (OIG)	OIG protects the integrity of HHS programs, as well as the health and welfare of the beneficiaries of those programs.	Department of Health and Human Services	www.oig.hhs.gov
Fiscal Year OIG Work Plan	The focused CMS Work Plan assists OIG with the prevention of healthcare fraud, waste, and abuse.	Department of Health and Human Services	www.oig.hhs.gov/publications/workplan.asp
Fraud Prevention and Detection	Resources including compliance programs, corporate integrity agreements, and exclusion programs.	Department of Health and Human Services	www.oig.hhs.gov/fraud.asp
Health Care Compliance Association	The Health Care Compliance Association is a professional association providing its members with compliance news, information, and a variety of related services.	Health Care Compliance Association	www.hcca-info.org
Medicare Reimbursement Resources			
Federal Register	The daily publication of the US Government Printing Office for proposed rules and notices of federal agencies and organizations, as well as executive orders and other presidential documents.	US Government	www.gpoaccess.gov/fr

Recommended Resources	Description	Sponsoring Organization	Web Site
Health Insurance Portability and Accountability Act (HIPAA) Administrative Simplification (*continued*)			
Conditions of Participation (CoPs) and Conditions for Coverage (CfCs)	CMS develops CoPs and CfCs that healthcare organizations must meet to participate in the Medicare and Medicaid programs.	Centers for Medicare and Medicaid Services	www.cms.hhs.gov/ CFCsAndCoPs/
Documentation Guidelines Evaluation and Management Services	Documentation guidelines developed to supplement the CPT evaluation and management service code definitions used for physician reporting.	Centers for Medicare and Medicaid Services	http://www.cms.hhs.gov/ MLNProducts/downloads/ eval_mgmt_serv_guide.pdf
Electronic Code of Federal Regulations (e-CFR)	E-CFR is a sample model of a currently updated version of the Code of Federal Regulations (CFR). The CFR is the official compilation of federal rules and requirements.	National Archives and Records Administration's Office of the Federal Register and the Government Printing Office	http://ecfr.gpoaccess.gov/ cgi/t/text/text-idx?c= ecfr&tpl=%2Findex.tpl
Medicare Administrative Contractor (MAC)	Medicare is replacing fiscal intermediaries (FIs) and carriers with new contract entities, MACs. The full vision includes functional contractors such as quality improvement organizations and Recovery Audit Contractors working with the MACs. By 2010, the MACs will be the central point in the fee-for-service program.	Centers for Medicare and Medicaid Services	www.cms.hhs.gov/ MedicareContractingReform/
Internet-Only Manuals (IOMs)	IOMs provide technical and professional information about the Medicare and Medicaid programs.	Centers for Medicare and Medicaid Services	www.cms.hhs.gov/manuals
Medicare Learning Network (MLN)	The MLN site provides access to a variety of education products to assist providers and beneficiaries and their advocates in understanding the Medicare program.	Centers for Medicare and Medicaid Services	www.cms.hhs.gov/ MLNGenInfo/
MLN Matters	MLN Matters includes informational articles designed to help providers understand new or changed Medicare policy.	Centers for Medicare and Medicaid Services	www.cms.hhs.gov/ MLNMattersArticles/
Medicare Providers	This provider-specific home page is a one-stop resource focused on the informational needs and interests of Medicare providers, including physicians and other practitioners.	Centers for Medicare and Medicaid Services	www.cms.hhs.gov/center/ provider.asp
Electronic Billing and EDI Transactions	This link provides information on the CMS-1500, CMS-1450, and electronic data interchange support.	Centers for Medicare and Medicaid Services	www.cms.hhs.gov/ ElectronicBillingEDITrans/
Medicare Preventive Services	Coding and reporting guidance for preventive services covered under the Medicare program.	Centers for Medicare and Medicaid Services	www.cms.hhs.gov/ PrevntionGenInfo/
Health Information	This site provides Medicare beneficiaries with information about Medicare benefits, publications, and valuable Web sites.	Department of Health and Human Services	www.medicare.gov/Health/ Overview.asp
Quality Improvement Organizations (QIOs)	QIOs contract with CMS to ensure that Medicare beneficiaries receive high-quality healthcare that is medically necessary and appropriate and meets professionally recognized standards of care.	Centers for Medicare and Medicaid Services	www.cms.hhs.gov/ QualityImprovementOrgs/

(Continued on next page)

Recommended Resources	Description	Sponsoring Organization	Web Site
Health Insurance Portability and Accountability Act (HIPAA) Administrative Simplification (*continued*)			
Recovery Audit Contractor (RAC)	The goal of the RAC program is to identify improper payments made on claims of healthcare services provided to Medicare beneficiaries.	Centers for Medicare and Medicaid Services	www.cms.hhs.gov/RAC/ 01_Overview.asp#TopOfPage
CMS Quarterly Provider Update	The update communicates current provider information on regulations, policies, and revisions made to the manual instructions.	Centers for Medicare and Medicaid Services	www.cms.hhs.gov/ QuarterlyProviderUpdates/ EmailUpdates/list.asp
Governmental Data Sets			
Data Elements for Emergency Department Systems (DEEDS)	Developed to create uniform specifications for data entered in emergency department patient records.	National Center for Injury Prevention and Control	www.cdc.gov/ncipc/pub-res/ deedspage.htm
Minimum Data Sets 2.0 and 3.0	A patient-centered assessment instrument that Medicare- and Medicaid-certified nursing facilities must use to conduct a comprehensive, accurate, standardized, reproducible assessment of each resident's functional capacity.	Centers for Medicare and Medicaid Services	www.cms.hhs.gov/ NursingHomeQualityInits/ 01_overview.asp
Inpatient Rehabilitation Facility Patient Assessment Instrument (IRF-PAI)	The IRF-PAI is used to gather data to determine payment for Medicare Part A fee-for-service patients admitted to an inpatient rehabilitation unit or hospital.	Centers for Medicare and Medicaid Services	www.cms.hhs.gov/ InpatientRehabFacPPS/ 04_IRFPAI.asp#TopOfPage
Outcome and Assessment Information Set (OASIS)	A standard core assessment data tool developed to measure the outcomes of adult patients receiving home health services under the Medicare and Medicaid programs.	Centers for Medicare and Medicaid Services	www.cms.hhs.gov/OASIS/ 01_Overview.asp
Nongovernmental Data Sets			
Healthcare Effectiveness Data and Information Set (HEDIS)	HEDIS is a tool used by many health plans to measure performance by measuring important dimensions of care and service.	National Committee for Quality Assurance	www.ncqa.org/tabid/59/ Default.aspx
ORYX	ORYX integrates outcomes and other performance measurement data into the accreditation process. Joint Commission–accredited hospitals collect data on standardized—or core—performance measures.	The Joint Commission	www.jointcommission.org/ AccreditationPrograms/ Hospitals/ORYX/facts_oryx. htm
AHIMA Member Resources			
Communities of Practice (CoP)	The CoP is an online member interaction tool providing up-to-date industry news links to helpful resources, and, most importantly, solutions and ideas from peers.	AHIMA	http://cop.ahima.org/
AHIMA Body of Knowledge	The AHIMA Body of Knowledge offers AHIMA-owned content and links to other materials that encompass the theory and practice of health information management.	AHIMA	http://library.ahima.org/xpedio/ groups/public/documents/ web_assets/bok_home.hcsp
AHIMA Resources: ICD-10-CM/PCS	The AHIMA ICD-10 home page includes information for preparing to convert from ICD-9-CM to ICD-10-CM and ICD-10-PCS.	AHIMA	www.ahima.org/icd10/

Recommended Resources	Description	Sponsoring Organization	Web Site
Health Insurance Portability and Accountability Act (HIPAA) Administrative Simplification (*continued*)			
AHIMA Resources: Coding	The AHIMA coding home page includes information on coding events, coding education, coding roundtables, and more.	AHIMA	www.ahima.org/coding
AHIMA Practice Briefs and Toolkits	This Web site includes links to AHIMA practice briefs and other resources such as the RAC tool kit and sample job descriptions.	AHIMA	www.ahima.org/infocenter/ practice_tools.asp
Standards of Ethical Coding	The standard of professional ethics for health information coding professionals.	AHIMA	www.ahima.org/infocenter/ guidelines/standards.asp
"Managing an Effective Query Process"	This practice brief provides information on managing the query process to improve physician documentation and coding professionals' understanding of unique clinical situations.	AHIMA	http://library.ahima.org/xpedio/ groups/public/documents/ ahima/bok1_040394.hcsp

Prepared by

Judy A. Bielby, MBA, RHIA, CPHQ, CCS

Prepared by (original)

AHIMA Coding Practice Team
Kathy Giannangelo, RHIA, CCS
Susan Hull, MPH, RHIA, CCS
Karen Kostick, RHIT, CCS, CCS-P
Rita Scichilone, MHSA, RHIA, CCS, CCS-P
Mary Stanfill, RHIA, CCS, CCS-P
Sarah Wills-Dubose, MA, MEd, RHIA
Ann Zeisset, RHIT, CCS, CCS-P

American Health Information Management Association. "Internet Resources for Accurate Coding and Reimbursement Practices (Updated)." *Journal of AHIMA* (Updated March 2010).

Abbreviations

AFDC: *Aid to Families with Dependent Children.* One of the Centers for Medicare and Medicaid Services Medicaid eligibility categories.

AHA: *American Hospital Association.* A national association that supports member institutions. For health information, the AHA is the clearinghouse for ICD-9-CM coding issues. AHA is one of the four Cooperating Parties on policy development for the use of ICD-9-CM.

AHIMA: *American Health Information Management Association.* A professional organization for health information management professionals. AHIMA provides seminars and publications supporting the use of ICD-9-CM. It is one of the four Cooperating Parties that approve official coding policy.

AHRQ: *Agency for Healthcare Research and Quality.* The branch of the United States Public Health Service that supports general health research and distributes research findings and treatment guidelines with the goal of improving the quality, appropriateness, and effectiveness of healthcare services.

AMA: *American Medical Association.* An association for physicians that promotes the science and art of medicine. AMA maintains and publishes the Current Procedural Terminology (CPT) coding system.

AP-DRGs: *All-patient diagnosis-related groups.* A case-mix system developed by 3M and used in a number of state reimbursement systems to classify non-Medicare discharges for reimbursement purposes.

APR-DRGs: *All-patient refined diagnosis-related groups.* A case-mix system developed by 3M that includes four distinct subclasses (minor, moderate, major, and extreme) based on the severity of the patient's illness.

BBA: *Balanced Budget Act of 1997.* Public Law 105-33 enacted by Congress on August 5, 1997, that mandated a number of additions, deletions, and revisions to the original Medicare and Medicaid legislation; the legislation that added penalties for healthcare fraud and abuse to the Medicare and Medicaid programs.

BBRA: *Balanced Budget Refinement Act of 1999.* The amended version of the Balanced Budget Act of 1997 that authorizes implementation of a per-discharge prospective payment system for care provided to Medicare beneficiaries by inpatient rehabilitation facilities.

CC: *Complication/comorbidity.* A *complication* is a condition arising after the beginning of hospital observation and treatment that modifies the course of the patient's illness or the medical care required. A *comorbidity* is a preexisting condition that will, because of its presence with a specific principal diagnosis, cause an increase in the patient's length of stay by at least 1 day in 75 percent of cases. Complications and comorbidities generally require coding as additional diagnoses and may affect DRG assignment.

CDS: *Clinical documentation specialist.* A coding professional or nurse who works on the patient floors or alongside the physicians in the clinic setting.

CHAMPUS: *Civilian Health and Medical Program—Uniformed Services.* A federal program providing supplementary civilian-sector hospital and medical services beyond that which is available in military treatment facilities to military dependents, retirees and their dependents, and certain others. Now known as TRICARE.

CHAMPVA: *Civilian Health and Medical Program—Veterans Affairs.* The federal healthcare benefits program for dependents of veterans rated by the Department of Veterans Affairs (VA) as having a total and permanent disability, for survivors of veterans who died from VA-rated service-connected conditions or who were rated permanently and totally disabled at the time of death from a VA-rated service-connected condition, and for survivors of persons who died in the line of duty.

CMI: *Case-mix index.* The average relative weight of all cases treated at a given facility or by a given physician, which reflects the resource intensity or clinical severity of a specific group in relation to the other groups in the classification system; calculated by dividing the sum of the weights of diagnosis-related groups for patients discharged during a given period divided by the total number of patients discharged.

CMS: *Centers for Medicare and Medicaid Services.* Formerly known as HCFA, this government agency is responsible for administration of the Medicare and Medicaid programs. CMS is one of the four Cooperating Parties that approve official coding policy.

COBRA: *Consolidated Omnibus Budget Reconciliation Act of 1975.* The federal law requiring every hospital that participates in Medicare and has an emergency department to treat any patient in an emergency condition or active labor, whether or not the patient is covered by Medicare and regardless of the patient's ability to pay; COBRA also requires employers to provide continuation benefits to specified workers and families who have been terminated but previously had healthcare insurance benefits.

CPG: *Compliance program guidance.* The information provided by the OIG to help healthcare organizations develop internal controls that promote adherence to applicable federal and state guidelines.

DME: *Durable medical equipment.* Medical equipment designed for long-term use in the home, including eyeglasses, hearing aids, surgical appliances and supplies, orthotics and prostheses, and bulk and cylinder oxygen.

DMERC: *Durable medical equipment regional carrier.* A fiscal intermediary designated to process claims for durable medical equipment.

DRA: *Deficit Reduction Act of 2005.* Legislation that provides states the flexibility to reform their Medicaid programs.

DRG: *Diagnosis-related group.* DRGs represent a classification system that categorizes patients who are medically related with respect to their diagnoses and treatments and are statistically similar in their lengths of stay. See MS-DRG.

FI: *Fiscal intermediary.* An organization that contracts with the Centers for Medicare and Medicaid Services to serve as the financial agent between providers and the federal government in the local administration of Medicare Part A claims. This has been transitioned to a Medicare Administrative Contractor (MAC), which pays both Part A and Part B claims. See MAC.

FPL: *Federal poverty level.* The income qualification threshold established by the federal government for certain government entitlement programs.

HAC: *Hospital-acquired condition.* Conditions that are high-cost, high-volume, or both; are assigned to a higher-paying Medicare severity adjusted diagnosis-related group (MS-DRG) when present as a secondary diagnosis (that is, conditions under the MS-DRG system that are complications/comorbidities or major complications/comorbidities); and could reasonably have been prevented through the application of evidence-based guidelines.

HHS: *Department of Health and Human Services.* A government executive branch department that oversees CMS's administration of the Medicare and Medicaid programs and the work of many other government agencies related to healthcare.

HIMS: *Health information management services.* One of several names for the health record department. This name is meant to provide a better description of the function of the department, which is the management of health information.

HIPAA: *Health Insurance Portability and Accountability Act of 1996.* The federal legislation enacted to provide continuity of health coverage, control fraud and abuse in healthcare, reduce healthcare costs, and guarantee the security and privacy of health information. The act limits exclusion for preexisting medical conditions, prohibits discrimination against employees and dependents based on health status, guarantees availability of health insurance to small employers, and guarantees renewability of insurance to all employees regardless of size of organization.

HMO: *Health maintenance organization.* Entity that combines the provision of healthcare insurance and the delivery of healthcare services, characterized by: (1) an organized healthcare delivery system to a geographic area, (2) a set of basic and supplemental health maintenance and treatment services, (3) voluntarily enrolled members, and (4) predetermined fixed, periodic prepayments for members' coverage.

HPMP: *Hospital Payment Monitoring Program.* A program designed to measure, monitor, and reduce the incidence of improper fee-for-service inpatient payments. Replaced the Payment Error Prevention Program (PEPP).

ICD-9-CM: *International Classification of Diseases, 9th Revision, Clinical Modification for Use in the United States.* A diagnostic and procedural classification system published by the National Center for Health Statistics and Centers for Medicare and Medicaid Services in cooperation with the World Health Organization.

ICD-10: *International Classification of Diseases, 10th Revision.* The most recent update of the ICD diagnostic and procedural classification system, currently in use in some parts of the world. Clinical modification (ICD-10-CM) is being developed for implementation in the United States.

ICD-10-PCS: *International Classification of Diseases, 10th Revision, Procedural Classification System.* Procedural classification system being developed in conjunction with ICD-10.

IPA: *Individual practice association, independent physician association, independent practice association,* or *independent provider association.* A form of health maintenance organization (HMO) that consists of a group of physicians who form together as a legal corporation to provide care for the HMO patients.

IPF: *Inpatient psychiatric facility.* An inpatient facility or unit of an existing hospital that specializes in inpatient treatment for psychiatric disorders.

IRF: *Inpatient rehabilitation facility.* An inpatient facility or unit that specializes in post-acute care services for rehabilitation purposes.

IRVEN: *Inpatient Rehabilitation Validation and Entry.* A computerized data-entry system used by inpatient rehabilitation facilities.

LCD: *Local coverage determination.* Coverage rules, at a fiscal intermediary or carrier level, that provide information on what diagnoses justify the medical necessity of a test.

LMRPs: *Local medical review policies.* Documents that define Medicare coverage of outpatient services via lists of diagnoses defined as medically reasonable and necessary for the services provided. These are being transitioned to local coverage determinations.

LOS: *Length of stay.* The total number of patient days for an inpatient episode, calculated by subtracting the date of admission from the date of discharge.

MA: *Medicare Advantage (Medicare Part C).* A preferred provider organization (PPO)-type of coverage for Medicare beneficiaries that offers options such as regional PPOs and specialized health plans for certain diagnoses.

MAC: *Medicare Administrative Contractor.* The Medicare Prescription Drug, Improvement and Modernization Act of 2003 (MMA) allowed the Centers for Medicare and Medicaid Services (CMS) to make significant changes to Medicare's administrative structure. CMS is integrating administration of Medicare Parts A (Fiscal Intermediaries/FI) and B (Carriers) for the fee-for-service benefit into Medicare Administrative Contractors (MACs).

MA-PD: *Medicare Advantage-Prescription Drug.* The Medicare plan that includes medication coverage.

MCC: *Major complication/comorbidity.* A *complication* is a condition arising after the beginning of hospital observation and treatment that modifies the course of the patient's illness or the medical care required. A *comorbidity* is a preexisting condition that will, because of its presence with a specific principal diagnosis, cause an increase in the patient's length of stay by at least 1 day in 75 percent of cases. Medicare has designated certain conditions as MCCs (major complications/comorbidities) that when present as a secondary diagnosis have a greater impact on length of stay and/or resources used to care for the patient and may affect MS-DRG assignment.

MDC: *Major diagnostic category.* A part of the diagnosis-related group system that divides all possible principal diagnoses into 25 mutually exclusive areas. MDCs were formed to ensure that Medicare severity adjusted diagnosis-related groups (MS-DRGs) would be clinically coherent.

MDHs: *Medicare-dependent rural hospitals.* Facilities that are paid based on a formula of diagnosis-related group rate or on their costs for specific time periods, whichever is higher.

MMA: *Medicare Prescription Drug, Improvement, and Modernization Act (MMA) of 2003.* Major changes to the Medicare program, including creation of Medicare Part D drug benefit (2006), creation of Health Savings Accounts, and increased payments to Medicare health maintenance organizations.

MS-DRG: *Medicare Severity Adjusted Diagnosis-Related Group.* MS-DRGs were the significant update by Medicare in 2008 to better account for patients' severity of illness. They represent a classification system that categorizes patients who are medically related with respect to their diagnoses and treatments and are statistically similar in their lengths of stay.

MSP: *Medicare secondary payer.* One of the edits in the outpatient and inpatient code editors that reviews claims to determine if the claim should be paid by another form of insurance, such as workers' compensation or private insurance in the event of a traffic accident.

NCD: *National coverage determination.* The equivalent of a local coverage determination at the national level.

NCHS: *National Center for Health Statistics.* A government agency that works with the Centers for Medicare and Medicaid Services to revise ICD-9-CM codes and approve official coding policy. NCHS is one of the four Cooperating Parties that approve official coding policy.

NCQA: *National Committee for Quality Assurance.* A private not-for-profit accreditation organization whose mission is to evaluate and report on the quality of managed care organizations in the United States.

NCVHS: *National Committee on Vital and Health Statistics.* A public policy advisory board that recommends policy to the National Center for Health Statistics and other health-related federal programs.

OBRA: *Omnibus Budget Reconciliation Act of 1986.* A federal law that requires outpatient visits, either medical or surgical, to be reported using ICD-9-CM and HCPCS for outpatient services billing.

OIG: *Office of the Inspector General.* The office through which the federal government established compliance plans for the healthcare industry.

P4P: *Pay for performance.* A movement toward reimbursing physicians proportionate to the quality of care. Electronic health records (EHRs) can improve quality of care by having functions such as automatic pop-up reminders during electronic charting. Reminders can be programmed into EHR systems to address such issues as contraindications and drug interactions triggered by the data entered. Another aspect of P4P is related to outcomes documented during subsequent patient visits.

PDP: *Prescription drug plan.* Patients who chose to remain in the traditional Medicare coverage plans will have the option of joining a PDP to obtain drug benefits for an additional charge.

PHO: *Physician–hospital organization.* An individual practice association where physicians and hospital(s) join together to provide contracted services. In a PHO, both the hospital and the physician practices share in the risk associated with prepayment of services.

PIP-DCG: *Principal inpatient diagnostic cost group.* A model designed to calculate each beneficiary's relative risk in terms of overall Medicare expenditures.

POA: *Present on admission.* The UB-04 form has an additional field for all diagnoses codes to indicate whether the condition was present on admission. Instructions for accurately reporting conditions as POA are included in the ICD-9-CM Official Coding Guidelines.

PPS: *Prospective payment system.* A government reimbursement plan implemented in 1983 to control the cost of inpatient hospital services to Medicare recipients. Payments were set at a flat rate rather than on a fee-for-service or per-day basis.

QIO: *Quality improvement organization.* The Centers for Medicare and Medicaid Services contracts with private medical review organizations to ensure that the government pays only for medically necessary, appropriate, and high-quality healthcare services. QIOs conduct diagnosis-related group validations to compare the hospital's coding of the case on the claim with the attending physician's documentation in the health record.

RIC: *Rehabilitation impairment category.* A group reflective of the primary need for rehabilitation care.

SCHs: *Sole community hospitals.* Small facilities that are paid based on a formula of diagnosis-related group rate or on their costs for specific time periods, whichever is higher.

SCHIP: *State Children's Health Insurance Program.* The children's healthcare program implemented as part of the Balanced Budget Act of 1997; sometimes referred to as the Children's Health Insurance Program, or CHIP.

SOW: *Scope of work.* The quality improvement organization's (QIO's) contract with the Centers for Medicare and Medicaid Services that specifies the goals and topics for review.

SSI: *Supplemental Security Income.* One of the Centers for Medicare and Medicaid Services Medicaid eligibility categories.

TEFRA: *Tax Equity and Fiscal Responsibility Act of 1982.* The federal legislation that modified Medicare's retrospective reimbursement system for inpatient hospital stays by requiring implementation of diagnosis-related groups and the acute care prospective payment system.

UB-04: *Uniform Bill-2004.* Updated in 2004, this single uniform bill consolidated the numerous forms that hospitals were using to submit bills to third-party payers. The health information management department supplies the clinical data that are placed on the form and ensures their accuracy.

UCDS: *Uniform Clinical Data Set.* A standard set of data about each hospitalization. The UCDS was developed to form the foundation for a new review methodology. The goal is to move from retrospective case-by-case review to a system based on computerized analysis of large databases, which will identify patterns of use and outcome.

UHDDS: *Uniform Hospital Discharge Data Set.* A minimum common core of data on individual hospital discharges in the Medicare and Medicaid programs. Its purpose is to provide uniformity and comparability in hospital discharge data.

UR: *Utilization review.* The process of determining whether the medical care provided to a specific patient is necessary according to preestablished objective screening criteria at time frames specified in the organization's utilization management plan.

VBP: *Value-based purchasing.* Links payment more directly to the quality of care provided. The Centers for Medicare and Medicaid Services has launched VBP initiatives in hospitals, physician offices, nursing homes, home health services, and dialysis facilities.

Annotated Bibliography

3M/Health Information Systems. 2009. *Diagnosis Related Groups Definitions Manual.* **Current Version. Salt Lake City: 3M/Health Information Systems.** The official documentation for the Medicare grouper in use for the current fiscal year of the prospective payment system.

American Health Information Management Association. 2010. *Clinical Coding Workout with Answers,* **2010 ed. Chicago: AHIMA.** *Clinical Coding Workout* challenges coding students and professionals to develop expert skills required for coding accuracy and reimbursement.

American Health Information Management Association. 1990 to present. Coding notes and clinical notes, *Journal of AHIMA.* A monthly column in the *Journal of AHIMA* that features coding advice, the latest peer review organization information, and clinical disease discussions.

American Hospital Association. 1984 to present. *Coding Clinic for ICD-9-CM.* **Chicago: AHA.** Published quarterly by AHA, *Coding Clinic* responds to questions from coders across the country and contains official coding policy, including the official guidelines for ICD-9-CM coding practices. Its content is cleared by the Cooperating Parties prior to publication.

Barta, A., DeVault, K., and Zeisset, A. 2011. *ICD-10-CM Coder Training Manual.* **Chicago: AHIMA.** Experienced ICD-9-CM coders trained by AHIMA-certified ICD-10-CM trainers can use this manual to build their knowledge of ICD-10-CM. In addition to a textual adaptation of AHIMA's "ICD-10-CM Overview: Deciphering the Code," a distance education course that is a prerequisite to AHIMA's ICD-10 Academies, the manual contains references to and explanations of ICD-10-CM coding guidelines and conventions. It provides ICD-10-CM coding exercises at the beginning, intermediate, and advanced level. These exercises emphasize all aspects of the coding classification system to allow students to apply their knowledge of coding principles and definitions. Answers are also provided.

Beers, M.H. 2006. *Merck Manual of Diagnosis and Therapy,* **18th ed. Edited by Porter, R.S., and T.V. Jones. Whitehouse Station, NJ: Merck.** A compendium by body system of common diseases and health conditions. Each disease is presented with typical signs, laboratory tests usually performed to affirm the diagnosis, and potential treatment options.

Bowman, S. 2008. *Health Information Management Compliance: Preventing Fraud and Abuse,* **4th ed. Chicago: AHIMA.** This resource for effective compliance programs in all healthcare settings delivers the latest compliance research and trends in an easy-to-understand format. It includes sample auditing and monitoring tools, guidelines for documentation within existing systems, structures for designing a compliance program, and information on how to prepare for an audit.

Code Write. **Chicago: AHIMA.** The monthly newsletter of the Coding Community of Practice (CoP). Available on the Coding CoP at www.ahima.org/. *Code Write* features articles about issues relevant to the community of professional clinical coders.

Department of Health and Human Services. 2010. *International Classification of Diseases, Ninth Revision, Clinical Modification for Use in the United States.* **Washington, DC: US Government Printing Office.** Everyone who codes manually should have an updated codebook. If an encoder is used, at least one manual should be available for reference. Changes are effective every October 1.

Dorland. 2007. *Dorland's Illustrated Medical Dictionary,* **31st ed. Philadelphia: Saunders.** A traditional medical dictionary used by most transcriptionists. It contains anatomic and disease-oriented illustrations. The book is usually updated annually. Purchase of the new edition of this book every other year or every 2 years is generally acceptable.

Fischbach, F. 2008. *A Manual of Laboratory Diagnostic Tests,* **8th ed. Philadelphia: Lippincott Williams & Wilkins.** A laboratory manual that presents laboratory tests, normal ranges, abnormal ranges, and what the abnormal value indicates. Any manual providing this information would be adequate.

Gahart, B.L. and A. Nazareno. 2009. *2010 Intravenous Medications: A Handbook for Nurses and Allied Health Professionals,* **26th ed. St. Louis: Mosby.** A reference and review guide to indications, potential adverse effects, dosages, and implications for use of drugs administered intravenously.

Garrett, G.S. 2009. *Present on Admission,* **2nd ed. Chicago: AHIMA.** Key issues and concerns arising from these regulations are addressed, especially the new requirement to implement the hospital-acquired condition payment provision on all Medicare claims. This publication explains the details and ramifications of the POA indicator, helping you become your organization's resident POA expert.

Hazelwood, A.C. and C.A. Venable. 2009. *ICD-10-CM and ICD-10-PCS Preview,* **2nd ed. Chicago: AHIMA.** This newly revised, practical introduction will help you to prepare your facility for ICD-10 implementation, as required by the notice of proposed rule making issued by the Centers for Medicare and Medicaid Services, effective October 1, 2011. *The ICD-10-CM and ICD-10-PCS Preview,* 2nd ed. is the perfect guide for professional coders, managers, information systems personnel, clinicians, health insurers, and other users of coded clinical data who need to come up to speed on ICD-10.

Hyde, L.A. and C. Carol Spencer. 2008. *Analyzing the Financial Impact of MS-DRGs.* **Chicago: AHIMA.** Featuring all the crosswalk tables needed to guide the process, *Analyzing the Financial Impact of MS-DRGs* offers a step-by-step approach to conducting a facility-specific analysis. A complication and comorbidity (CC) impact analysis is included, listing the top 30 CCs most commonly reported as the single CC on claims. Coding and documentation improvement opportunities are also identified.

Kennedy, J.S. 2008. *Severity DRGs and Reimbursement: An MS-DRG Primer.* **Chicago: AHIMA.** Responds to healthcare professionals' needs since they are increasingly responsible for knowing the clinical basis behind ICD-9-CM, the logic of any applicable DRG methodology, and the capture and application of this knowledge in every patient's data set. This new resource offers a detailed complication and comorbidity (CC) analysis of all changes in this important ruling.

Lefert, C. and I. Blevins. 2008. *ICD-9-CM Diagnostic Coding for Long-Term Care and Home Care.* **Chicago: AHIMA.** Long-term care and home care staff will benefit from the reinforcement of concepts and skills needed for correct code assignment required for reimbursement and data collection purposes found in *ICD-9-CM Diagnostic Coding for Long-Term Care and Home Care.*

McPhee, S.J., M.A. Papadakis, and L.M. Tierney. 2009. *Current Medical Diagnosis and Treatment 2010,* **49th ed. New York: McGraw-Hill Professional Publishing.** An annual publication that presents most medical illnesses by body system with a straightforward discussion outlining symptoms, differential diagnoses, and typical treatment protocols. Purchasing this text every other year or every 2 years is generally adequate.

Schraffenberger, L.A. 2011. *Basic ICD-9-CM Coding,* **2011 ed. Chicago: AHIMA.** This annual publication offers basic coding instruction, including *Coding Clinic* guidelines. The most current edition should be kept available to coders.

Schraffenberger, L.A. and L. Kuehn. 2011. *Effective Management of Coding Services,* **4th ed. Chicago: AHIMA.** For three editions, *Effective Management of Coding Services* has helped train new and future coding managers and provided a valuable resource for those already in practice. Led by trusted industry leaders at the helm, this essential textbook and reference returns with expanded coverage of the wide variety of tasks, topics, and knowledge necessary to manage the coding function in today's increasingly complex environment.

Scott, K.S. 2008. *Medical Coding for Non-coders: Understanding Coding and Reimbursement in Today's Healthcare Industry.* **Chicago: AHIMA.** This book delivers an introduction to medical coding for noncoding healthcare professionals. An overview of coding and reimbursement systems provides a full understanding of code sets, billing, and fraudulent coding.

Springhouse. 2008. *Springhouse Nurse's Drug Guide,* **10th ed. Ambler, PA: Lippincott Williams & Wilkins.** A reference guide to medication, similar to *Physicians' Desk Reference.*

Sullivan, T.E., G.C. McNeill, and K.E. Wall. 2010. *Implementing ICD-10-CM/PCS for Hospitals.* **Chicago: AHIMA.** This book provides sample tools for implementing ICD-10-CM/PCS within the large hospital facility environment. This toolkit provides a guide to the most comprehensive approach necessary to complete the preparation for ICD-10-CM/PCS. The tools provided in this book can be modified to fit individual, smaller organizations. Using these tools will provide continuity during the project.

Thomson Healthcare. 2009. *Physicians' Desk Reference,* **64th ed. Montvale, NJ: Thomson Healthcare.** The traditional reference manual for pharmacies. It identifies most drugs, their indications, contraindications, dosages, and such. Any current manual that supplies similar information is required.

Way, L. and G.M. Doherty. 2009. *Current Surgical Diagnosis and Treatment,* **13th ed. Norwalk, CT: Appleton and Lange.** An annual publication that presents most surgical illnesses by body system with a straightforward discussion outlining symptoms, surgical options, and typical complications. Purchasing this text every other year or every 2 years is generally adequate.

Wilson, D.D. 2009. *Benchmarking to Improve Coding Accuracy and Productivity.* **Chicago: AHIMA.** Healthcare professionals now have their first comprehensive resource to benchmark and improve coding accuracy and productivity and affect reimbursements. Designed for those accountable for coding compliance and financial performance, as well as for HIM and coding educators, this book offers insight into all areas of the coding function.

World Health Organization and National Center for Health Statistics. 2010. *International Classification of Diseases, Tenth Revision, Clinical Modification for Use in the United States.* **Washington, DC: US Government Printing Office.** The implementation date for ICD-10-CM and ICD-10-PCS in the United States is October 1, 2013. Coding professionals should begin to prepare for the transition to ICD-10-CM and ICD-10-PCS well before the implementation date.

Index